T0188985

Upper Endoscopy for GI Fellows

Douglas G. Adler, MD, FACG, AGAF, FASGE
Editor

Upper Endoscopy for GI Fellows

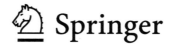
Springer

Editor
Douglas G. Adler, MD, FACG, AGAF,
 FASGE
Gastroenterology and Hepatology,
 Huntsman Cancer Center
University of Utah School of Medicine
Salt Lake City, UT
USA

Videos can also be accessed at
https://link.springer.com/book/10.1007/978-3-319-49041-0

ISBN 978-3-319-84074-1   ISBN 978-3-319-49041-0   (eBook)
DOI 10.1007/978-3-319-49041-0

Printed on acid-free paper

This Springer imprint is published by Springer Nature
The registered company is Springer International Publishing AG
The registered company address is: Gewerbestrasse 11, 6330 Cham, Switzerland

For J and for B

Preface

For most practicing endoscopists, an esophagogastroduodenoscopy (EGD) is the first endoscopic procedure they ever perform. I distinctly remember the very first EGD I ever did as a first-year GI fellow, and the tremendous excitement and anticipation I felt walking into the procedure room for the first time. I was unused to the constricting feel of my gown, gloves, and mask, but was excited to be wearing them. "I'm here," I thought, "I made it." I had already familiarized myself with the endoscope handle and the operation of the control heads and buttons, and was ready to go. After a few minutes of verbal instruction from my attending physician, I was handed the endoscope, the patient was sedated, and we were off. The examination passed uneventfully (for both the patient and myself!) and I remember thinking afterward, "that was so easy!"

Indeed, upper endoscopy (as EGD is sometimes referred to) is deceptively simple. The anatomy is often straightforward and simple to navigate with an upper endoscope, and the foregut is very forgiving to novice endoscopists. It is hard to get lost or disoriented, and simple maneuvers can help you achieve important endoscopic and clinical goals. Like most GI fellows, I soon discovered that there was more to performing an excellent upper endoscopy than simply advancing the endoscope to the duodenum, and that not all examinations were as easy as my first. Variations in anatomy range from simple to highly complex, and mucosal abnormalities could either be overtly pathologic or maddeningly subtle and hard to detect. It quickly became apparent that I needed to learn to recognize and be able to navigate a whole host of postsurgical reconstructions, some of which are commonly encountered and other less so. Some bleeding sources were readily apparent, other defied even the most detailed and careful examination. Some causes of upper abdominal pain were found quickly and easily, others not so much. Despite the steep learning curve and the long hours and late nights involved, this was an exciting journey.

As with most things endoscopic, the more you learn the more you realize you do not know. The depth and breadth of pathology and endoscopic interventions that can be encountered and performed during the course of an upper endoscopy are almost too numerous to count. As months became years, I always found that there was something new to discover in an upper endoscopy; some new illness to identify and some new maneuver to perform. In addition, as my endoscopic skills grew, the range of diagnostic and therapeutic maneuvers I became comfortable performing also grew. Even to this day, 17 years after my first EGD as a GI fellow, I am still adding new diagnostic and therapeutic interventions to my armamentarium. I suspect this trend will continue for as long as I am in practice and new tools and techniques continue to be developed.

I created this book as a handy resource for beginning endoscopists, but my goal is not to produce a book *just* for beginners. My goal was to produce a volume that would be useful all the way through ones training, covering the fundamentals of upper endoscopy (such as how to perform an upper endoscopy and how to treat upper GI bleeding) as well as more complex and involved interventions including the management of Barrett's esophagus, foregut strictures (both benign and malignant), submucosal lesions, complications (how to avoid them, and how to manage them when they happen), and other advanced topics. Each chapter includes many high-quality endoscopic images to highlight key concepts. In addition, each chapter is supplemented with an endoscopic video to give the reader a video library of cases to learn from as well.

Everybody has to start somewhere, and that somewhere is usually an EGD! I hope you find this book to be a valuable tool as you start your endoscopic career.

Salt Lake City, UT, USA   Douglas G. Adler, MD, FACG, AGAF, FASGE

Contents

About the Editor

Douglas G. Adler, MD, FACG, AGAF, FASGE received his medical degree from Cornell University Medical College in New York, NY. He completed his residency in internal medicine at Beth Israel Deaconess Medical Center/Harvard Medical School, Boston, MA. Dr. Adler completed both a general gastrointestinal fellowship and a therapeutic endoscopy/ERCP fellowship at Mayo Clinic in Rochester, MN. He then returned to the Beth Israel Deaconess Medical Center for a fellowship in endoscopic ultrasound. Dr. Adler is currently a tenured Professor of Medicine and Director of Therapeutic Endoscopy at the University of Utah School of Medicine in Salt Lake City, UT. Dr. Adler is also the GI Fellowship Program Director at the University of Utah School of Medicine. Working primarily at the University of Utah School of Medicine's Huntsman Cancer Institute, Dr. Adler focuses his clinical, educational, and research efforts on the diagnosis and management of patients with gastrointestinal cancers and complex gastrointestinal disease, with an emphasis on therapeutic endoscopy. He is the author of more than 300 scientific publications, articles, and book chapters. This is Dr. Adler's sixth textbook on gastroenterology.

Contributors

Douglas G. Adler Gastroenterology and Hepatology, Huntsman Cancer Center, University of Utah School of Medicine, Salt Lake City, UT, USA

Dino Beduya Division of Gastroenterology and Hepatology, University of New Mexico School of Medicine, Albuquerque, USA

Kathryn R. Byrne Division of Gastroenterology, University of Utah, Salt Lake City, UT, USA

David L. Diehl Department of Gastroenterology and Nutrition, Geisinger Medical Center, Danville, PA, USA

John C. Fang Department of Gastroenterology, University of Utah, Salt Lake City, UT, USA

Douglas S. Fishman Section of Gastroenterology, Hepatology and Nutrition, Texas Children's Hospital, Baylor College of Medicine, Houston, TX, USA

Jon D. Gabrielsen Department of General Surgery, Geisinger Medical Center, Danville, PA, USA

Juan Reyes Genere Section of Internal Medicine, Department of Medicine, University of Chicago Medical Center, Chicago, IL, USA

Jeremy Kaplan Division of Gastroenterology and Hepatology, Thomas Jefferson University, Philadelphia, PA, USA

Vivek Kaul Division of Gastroenterology and Hepatology, Center for Advanced Therapeutic Endoscopy, University of Rochester Medical Center & Strong Memorial Hospital, Rochester, NY, USA

C. Andrew Kistler Division of Gastroenterology and Hepatology, Thomas Jefferson University, Philadelphia, PA, USA

Shivangi T. Kothari Division of Gastroenterology and Hepatology, Center for Advanced Therapeutic Endoscopy, University of Rochester Medical Center & Strong Memorial Hospital, Rochester, NY, USA

Linda S. Lee Division of Gastroenterology, Hepatology and Endoscopy, Brigham and Women's Hospital, Harvard Medical School, Boston, MA, USA

Aaron Martin Division of Gastroenterology and Hepatology, Thomas Jefferson University, Philadelphia, PA, USA

Keisha R. Mitchell Section of Gastroenterology, Hepatology and Nutrition, Texas Children's Hospital, Baylor College of Medicine, Houston, TX, USA

Thiruvengadam Muniraj Huntsman Cancer Center, University of Utah School of Medicine, Salt Lake City, UT, USA; Section of Digestive Diseases, Yale University School of Medicine, New Haven, CT, USA

Gulshan Parasher Division of Gastroenterology and Hepatology, University of New Mexico School of Medicine, Albuquerque, USA

Waqar A. Qureshi Section of Gastroenterology and Hepatology, Department of Medicine, Baylor College of Medicine, Houston, TX, USA

Stephen R. Rotman Division of Gastroenterology, Brigham and Women's Hospital, Boston, MA, USA

John R. Saltzman Division of Gastroenterology, Brigham and Women's Hospital, Boston, MA, USA; Harvard Medical School, Brigham and Women's Hospital, Boston, MA, USA

Imran Sheikh Department of Gastroenterology, Fox Chase Cancer Center, Philadelphia, PA, USA

Ali A. Siddiqui Division of Gastroenterology and Hepatology, Thomas Jefferson University, Philadelphia, PA, USA; Department of Gastroenterology, Thomas Jefferson University Hospital, Philadelphia, PA, USA

Uzma D. Siddiqui Center for Endoscopic Research and Therapeutics (CERT), Endoscopic Ultrasound (EUS) and Advanced Endoscopy Training, University of Chicago Medical Center, Chicago, IL, USA

Jianhua Andy Tau Section of Gastroenterology and Hepatology, Department of Medicine, Baylor College of Medicine, Houston, TX, USA

Jeffrey Tokar Department of Gastroenterology, Fox Chase Cancer Center, Philadelphia, PA, USA

Joseph Yoo Division of Gastroenterology and Hepatology, Thomas Jefferson University, Philadelphia, PA, USA

How to Perform a High-Yield Esophagogastroduodenoscopy

Thiruvengadam Muniraj and Douglas G. Adler

Introduction

Esophagogastroduodenoscopy (EGD) provides excellent visualization of the mucosal surfaces of the esophagus, stomach, and proximal duodenum. Performing a high-quality EGD not only includes competence in the procedure with minimal patient discomfort, ensuring the appropriate identification of normal and abnormal findings, and performing therapeutic techniques, but also an understanding of the indications, risks, benefits, and limitations of the procedure. Acquiring the skills to perform upper endoscopy safely, effectively, and comfortably requires a solid understanding on what to look for during the endoscopy. In the past years, quality metrics in health care has been given more importance and various societies have come up with specific quality metric guidelines. This chapter will review how to perform a high-yield upper endoscopic examination. The authors recognize that there are wide variations in practice, but hope to demonstrate examples of good practice in many of the most commonly encountered clinical situations.

Pre-Procedure Management

A good knowledge of pertinent clinical history, indications, contraindications, pertinent past health history (which includes GI surgical history), patient exam findings, issues of informed consent, complications expected, patient education, antibiotic prophylaxis, and anticoagulation management is required prior to starting the endoscopic procedure.

Electronic supplementary material
Supplementary material is available in the online version of this chapter at 10.1007/978-3-319-49041-0_1. Videos can also be accessed at https://link.springer.com/chapter/10.1007/978-3-319-49041-0_1.

T. Muniraj · D.G. Adler (✉)
Huntsman Cancer Center, University of Utah School of Medicine, 30N 1900E 4R118, Salt Lake City, UT 84132, USA
e-mail: douglas.adler@hsc.utah.edu

Patient should be informed of and agree to the procedure and the administration of sedation/anesthesia, after discussion of its benefits, risks, and limitations and possible alternatives.

Sedation and Anesthesia

The level of sedation used for an EGD ranges from no sedation, minimal or moderate sedation, and up to deep and general anesthesia. In general, most upper endoscopic procedures are performed with the patient under moderate sedation, a practice that was formerly referred to as "conscious sedation," with complex procedures or high-risk patients often being examined under general anesthesia. With moderate sedation, the patient, while maintaining respiratory and cardiovascular function, is able to make purposeful responses to verbal or tactile stimulation. While deeper sedation and general anesthesia is administered by anesthesiologists or nurse anesthetists, moderate sedation is generally administered by the endoscopist with the assistance of a RN. Therefore, good knowledge of pharmacologic profiles of sedative agents and skills necessary to resuscitate a deeply sedated patient is warranted to perform endoscopy effectively and safely.

According to American Society of Anesthesiologist (ASA) guidelines, the patient should be fasting at least 2 h after consuming clear liquids and at least 6 h after consuming solids and non-clear liquids prior to the procedure [1].

When there are issues with administering sedation, selected patients may be able to undergo un-sedated endoscopic procedures using smaller caliber endoscopes (less than 6 mm, transnasal) and may tolerate well [2, 3].

Topical Pharyngeal Sprays

Topical pharyngeal sprays with lidocaine, tetracaine, and benzocaine are often used for during upper endoscopy, particularly during moderate sedation or un-sedated procedures. While there are studies showing better patient tolerance with use of these sprays, the risk of aspiration is small but real. Also, methemoglobinemia and anaphylactic reactions are rare but serious complications of topical anesthetic sprays.

Indications

An EGD should be performed only if there is a clear indication, which implies a change in management is probable based on results of endoscopy, and/or after an empirical trial of therapy for a suspected digestive disorder has been unsuccessful, and/or as the initial method of evaluation as an alternative to radiographic studies and/or when a primary therapeutic procedure is contemplated [4] (see Table 1.1). However, specific alarm symptoms should prompt an EGD without other evaluation (see Table 1.2). EGD is generally contraindicated when a perforated viscus is known or suspected, unless the indication for the EGD itself is to *close* the perforation [4]. EGD is generally not indicated for evaluating symptoms considered to be functional in origin (though EGD may sometimes be needed to rule out an organic disease), and in patients with metastatic cancer when the results will not change the management.

Table 1.1 Common indications for EGD [4]

1. Upper abdominal symptoms that persist despite an appropriate trial of therapy
2. Upper abdominal symptoms associated with other symptoms or signs suggesting structural disease (e.g., anorexia and weight loss) or new-onset symptoms in patients older than 50 years of age
3. Dysphagia or odynophagia
4 Esophageal reflux symptoms that persist or recur despite appropriate therapy
5. Persistent vomiting of unknown cause
6 Other diseases in which the presence of upper GI pathology might modify other planned management. Examples include patients who have a history of ulcer or GI bleeding who are scheduled for organ transplantation, long-term anticoagulation, or nonsteroidal anti-inflammatory drug therapy for arthritis and those with cancer of the head and neck
7. Familial adenomatous polyposis syndromes
8. For confirmation and specific histologic diagnosis of radiologically demonstrated lesions: • Suspected neoplastic lesion   • Gastric or esophageal ulcer   • Upper tract stricture or obstruction
9. GI bleeding: • In patients with active or recent bleeding   • For presumed chronic blood loss and for iron deficiency anemia when the clinical situation suggests an upper GI source or when colonoscopy does not provide an explanation
10. When sampling of tissue or fluid is indicated
11. Selected patients with suspected portal hypertension to document or treat esophageal varices
12. To assess acute injury after caustic ingestion
13. To assess diarrhea in patients suspected of having small-bowel disease (e.g., celiac disease)
14. Treatment of bleeding lesions such as ulcers, tumors, vascular abnormalities (e.g., electrocoagulation, heater probe, laser photocoagulation, or injection therapy)
15. Removal of foreign bodies
16. Removal of selected lesions
17. Placement of feeding or drainage tubes (e.g., peroral, percutaneous endoscopic gastrostomy, percutaneous endoscopic jejunostomy)
18. Dilation and stenting of stenotic lesions (e.g., with transendoscopic balloon dilators or dilation systems using guidewires)
19. Management of achalasia (e.g., botulinum toxin, balloon dilation)
20. Palliative treatment of stenosing neoplasms (e.g., laser, multipolar electrocoagulation, stent placement)
21. Endoscopic therapy of intestinal metaplasia
22. Intraoperative evaluation of anatomic reconstructions typical of modern foregut surgery (e.g., evaluation of anastomotic leak and patency, fundoplication formation, pouch configuration during bariatric surgery)
23. Management of operative complications (e.g., dilation of anastomotic strictures, stenting of anastomotic disruption, fistula, or leak in selected circumstances)

Table 1.2 Alarm symptoms prompting EGD

Unintentional weight loss
Dysphagia
Odynophagia
Hematemesis/Melena
Refractory acid reflux

Table 1.3 Identification of landmarks

Vocal cords/hypopharynx
Top of gastric folds
Z line
Greater and lesser curvature of stomach
Pyloric orifice
Duodenal bulb
Second part of duodenum
Post-surgical anatomy

Procedural Technique

It should be stressed that the technique advocated herein is not the only or ideal manner in which to perform an upper endoscopy, and individual techniques vary (Video 1.1).

The upper endoscope instrument controls consist of insertion section with optical system which is 9.2 mm in diameter, air/water buttons, a control head for left/right (small wheel) deflection, a control head for up/down deflection (big wheel), biopsy channel port (two ports in large therapeutic endoscopes), Narrow Band Imaging (NBI) or similar electronic enhancement button, and video/picture controls which can include zoom or near focus, depending on the instrument. Using the thumb, index, and middle fingers, most buttons and knobs can be controlled simultaneously with ease. Beginners should learn on how to set up the endoscopy cart, adjusting the light settings and connecting accessories such as heating probe or APC to an electrosurgical generator as needed.

Prior to starting endoscopy, the patient should be positioned in the left lateral decubitus position with the head of the bed elevated and a bite block should be inserted to allow the scope to pass through when the patient is sedated. The bite block protects the patient's teeth from the endoscope and protects the endoscope from the patient's teeth. Endoscopists should be familiar with intubating the esophagus in supine patients as this if often essential to the performance of upper endoscopy in ICU patients. Most EGD exams involve the identification of specific landmarks to ensure the completeness of the procedure (see Table 1.3).

Esophageal Intubation

The most challenging part of upper endoscopy for beginners is often the intubation of the esophagus. The intubation of esophagus should be done under direct visualization. The endoscope should, in general, not be advanced blindly or with undue force. In patients undergoing conscious sedation or in minimally sedated patients, sometimes it is useful to ask the patient to swallow when the scope enters the posterior pharynx to help relax the upper esophageal sphincter. Some endoscopists use the left index or middle finger to direct the scope into the posterior pharynx. Flexing the neck at this time may be useful to facilitate the endoscope passage to the posterior pharyngeal area.

Direct Visualization of Hypopharynx, Upper Esophageal Sphincter

The landmarks to guide entry into the upper esophageal orifice are present in and can be directly identified in the hypopharynx. In practice, this consists of visualizing the vocal cords and piriform sinuses and locating the upper esophageal sphincter (UES) just posterior to these. The UES is usually located 15–18 cm from the incisors, at the level of thyroid cartilage.

Despite adequate visualization of landmarks, occasionally it may difficult to intubate the UES, especially if the patient is inadequately sedated, or having issues with prominent cervical spine or neck mobility or has had prior head and neck surgery for oncologic issues.

Zenker's Diverticulum

During endoscopy, the presence of a Zenker's diverticulum often creates difficulty in UES intubation due to either compression of the normal esophageal lumen and/or obscuring the lumen from view. In addition, some patients have a prominent cricopharyngeal bar. It is prudent to consider and think about a possibility of a Zenker's diverticulum in elderly patients to reduce the risk of the procedure.

Examination of Esophagus

Under direct vision, the lumen of the esophagus is carefully visualized. This is done by insertion of the endoscope in the esophagus, along with air insufflation and direct observation. The scope can be gently torqued clockwise and anticlockwise manner to examine all the sides of the esophagus. Use of the tip deflection knobs is usually not necessary in the esophagus, except when performing some interventions such as taking biopsies. The aortic pulsation is normally located approximately at 20–25 cm from the upper incisors.

Identifying the Gastroesophageal Junction (GEJ)/ Squamo-Columnar Junction/Z Line

In adults, the GEJ is typically located approximately 35-40 cm from the upper incisors. This is an important mark to remember. The location of the top of the gastric folds can be noted, and the distance from the GEJ to the upper incisors can be noted. The squamo-columnar junction is represented by the clear demarcation of the pale pearl colored esophageal mucosa to salmon pink gastric mucosa and called as "Z line." If salmon-colored pink mucosa extends cephalad from top of gastric folds, this suggests Barrett's esophagus.

Hiatal Hernia

Normally, the diaphragmatic hiatus squeezes the esophagus at or just below the GE junction. The position of the hiatus can be visualized by the contraction waist seen the lower esophagus, which is more easily observed when the patient sniffs or during deep breathing. A hiatal hernia is diagnosed if the Z line is more than 2 cm above the hiatus. Hiatal hernia also typically examined and confirmed during retroflexion in the stomach (see Fig. 1.1).

Examination of the Stomach

After esophageal evaluation, the endoscope is then passed into the lumen of the stomach itself. When patient is in left lateral position, this maneuver is usually easily accomplished. Intubation into the stomach is confirmed by identification of the characteristic rugal folds.

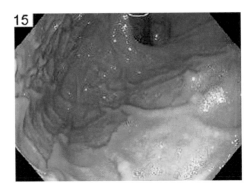

Fig. 1.1 Retroflexion in stomach

Identifying Lesser/Greater Curvature/Anterior/Posterior

Once the endoscope passes the GE junction, it usually enters the stomach along the lesser curvature, and the light shines on the greater curvature demonstrating the longitudinal rugal folds. The gastric wall to the left usually represents the anterior gastric wall, while the rightward stomach represents the posterior gastric wall.

Suction, Irrigation, and Air Insufflation

As a general rule, a good first thing to do after entering the stomach is to suction and remove any residual fluid in the fundus to reduce the risk of aspiration. Sometimes there may be retained food, blood, or mucus impairing mucosal visualization. A thorough water irrigation, with alternating suction helps to improve mucosal evaluation. Simethicone drops mixed in the water used for irrigation augment visibility by clearing gas bubbles or these can be washed away with a power flush, if available. Although air insufflation is necessary to distend the stomach for better visualization, too much air insufflation should be avoided as it may cause retching, vomiting, and even mucosal trauma from acute distension.

Examination of the Pylorus and Incisura

After suctioning, and optimally distending the stomach, the endoscope should be directed to the pylorus. The pylorus and the peri-pyloric area are examined carefully for any mucosal irregularities that would warrant biopsy or treatment. After slightly withdrawing from the pylorus, the tip is deflected upwards to examine the incisura angularis.

Examination of Gastric Body and Antrum

With an adequately distended stomach, the antrum and the body can then be carefully examined along both the lesser and greater curvatures, and along their anterior and posterior walls. The endoscope should be withdrawn almost up to the GE junction for a complete "long view" examination.

Retroflexion in the Stomach

After optimal distension of stomach with air, retroflexion is performed in order to view areas such as the fundus, cardia, and GE junction that otherwise would have limited tangential visualization during initial entry into the stomach. Also, selective examination of the incisura angularis is frequently performed again in the retroflexed view. In retroflexion, the endoscope is rotated and using counterclockwise and clockwise rotation the entire GE junction, lesser curve, and gastric cardia can be examined effectively (see Fig. 1.1).

Pyloric Intubation

As in esophageal intubation, pyloric intubation should be performed under direct visualization without blind advancement. The pyloric channel is visualized easily by identifying the radiating gastric folds which converge to the pyloric orifice (see Fig. 1.2).

Intubation of the pylorus may be difficult at times, due to spasms (commonly) or the presence of pyloric stenosis (rarely). Sometimes an ulcer in the pyloric channel may make pyloric intubation difficult or can produce bleeding, which is usually limited. By using gentle air insufflation, the pylorus may be visualized and the scope tip is gently placed into the pyloric orifice and with slight pressure the endoscope usually easily passes through the duodenum.

Examination of the Duodenum

Duodenal Bulb

Once the pylorus is intubated, the duodenal bulb is visualized. The bulb is then identified immediately after entering the pyloric orifice, by appreciating the small-bowel-type mucosa. The bulb is often chamber-like and can appear somewhat cavernous even in a normal individual. The duodenal bulb should be carefully examined in anterior, posterior, medial, and lateral walls as lesion in this area can easily be missed. During evaluation of the duodenal bulb, the endoscope may sometimes fall back into the stomach, which is normal.

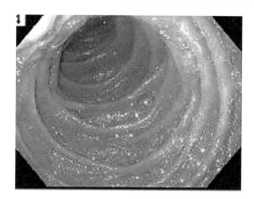

Fig. 1.3 Second part of duodenum

Second Portion of the Duodenum

The most common maneuver to pass around the duodenal sweep into the second portion of the duodenum involves flexing the tip of the endoscope by deflecting the tip upwards (coming back on the large wheel) while rotating the shaft of the endoscope clockwise. Once the scope is passed beyond the bulb, the concentric rings of circular duodenal folds are seen, which are known as the valves of Kerckring (also, valvulae conniventes). The folds projecting into the lumen of the small intestine serve as a landmark for the 2nd portion of the duodenum (see Fig. 1.3). Using torque maneuvers, the duodenal lumen is visualized and the scope is passed at least to the level just beyond the ampulla. Paradoxical motion on scope withdrawal at this level is useful to examine distal 2nd part of duodenum and the beginning of the 3rd duodenum. Limited exam of the ampulla can be performed, but in some patients the ampulla cannot be identified with a forward viewing scope even with careful attempts to do so (see Fig. 1.4). Care should be taken to withdraw very slowly along the duodenal sweep as the endoscope tends to fall out very quickly and lesion at the sweep may be missed.

Repeat Examination of Esophagus

Once the 1st and 2nd portion of the duodenum is examined well, the scope may be withdrawn back into the stomach. After withdrawing from the scope from the stomach, the endoscope should again be slowly withdrawn in the esophagus to carefully not to miss any subtle findings such as a gastric inlet patch (heterotopic gastric mucosa) [5] (see Fig. 1.5). Any lesion noted in the esophagus can be localized in relation to the centimeters from the upper incisors.

Examination of Larynx

Following complete examination of esophagus, the larynx and vocal cords can be examined on withdrawal as well if needed. This may be important especially when patient has symptoms of hoarseness of voice or severe GERD symptoms.

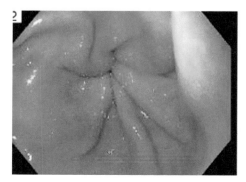

Fig. 1.2 Pyloric orifice with converging folds

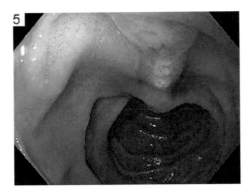

Fig. 1.4 Limited exam of the ampulla

Using a Side-Viewing Endoscope (Duodenoscope)

The lateral wall of the second portion of the duodenum as well as the ampulla can be difficult to examine effectively with regular forward viewing endoscope. Competence with passing the side-viewing endoscope may be helpful in situations when there is bleeding in the medial wall of the duodenum or when biopsy needs to be obtained from the ampulla or in patients with Familial Adenomatous Polyposis (FAP) who need to undergo careful duodenal surveillance for ampullary and non-ampullary adenomas.

Using Double-Channel Endoscopes and Therapeutic Channel Endoscopes

For selective therapeutic procedures, an endoscope with a dual-channel treatment capability may be very useful. The currently available T2 endoscopes have slightly larger outer diameter (12.6 mm), with two channels: one 3.7-mm-diameter channel and another 2.8-mm-diameter channel. This endoscope allows full suction capability with a single instrument loaded or simultaneous use of two endoscopic accessories instruments. There is a single larger channel (T1) endoscope with outer diameter 10 mm available which is often used when placing luminal stents as it has a larger channel (3.7 mm) when compared to regular endoscope (2.8 mm). The T1 endoscope is often referred to as a "therapeutic endoscope" as it is rarely used for diagnostic purposes. Therapeutic endoscopes or double-channel endoscopes are often used in patients with active upper gastrointestinal bleeding, in the performance of endoscopic mucosal resection, the placement of stents, or other interventional settings.

Using Ultra-Thin Endoscopes

In the presence of severe narrowing due to strictures, or performing diagnostic endoscopy in an un-sedated patient,

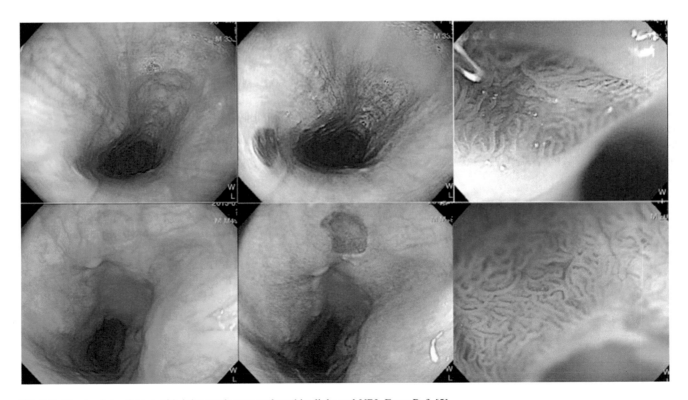

Fig. 1.5 Proximal esophagus with inlet patch seen under white light and NBI. From Ref. [5]

an ultra-slim endoscope may be used. The outer diameter of this scope is typically in the 5-mm range, and the channel port has an inner diameter of 2.2 mm. This endoscope can be passed via the transnasal route as well.

Identifying Abnormal Lesions

A clear understanding of normal anatomy and normal endoscopic findings of the esophagus, stomach, and duodenum is necessary prior to interpretation of abnormal endoscopic findings. Novice endoscopists should consider obtaining and referring to an endoscopic atlas frequency to familiarize themselves with the common appearance of a variety of with endoscopic findings (see Table 1.4). Repetitive exposure to a wide variety of endoscopic findings will help one to appreciate subtle findings and clearly delineate the normal from the abnormal.

Biopsy—*When and Where to Take Biopsy*

Biopsy forceps should be deployed close to the tip of the endoscope so as to maximize mechanical advantage. Sometimes biopsies must be obtained at a significant distance from the tip of the endoscope, but this makes the maneuver much more difficult. After opening the forceps, applying a firm pressure on the target site, grab the tissue and snap the forceps back into the scope.

Esophagus

Esophageal biopsies can sometimes be difficult as the forceps are often parallel to the esophageal wall, as opposed to perpendicular (or nearly so) as in the rest of the GI tract. In the esophagus, biopsies can be facilitated by using the tip of the endoscope to drive the forceps into a position that is more *en face* to the mucosa. If just obtaining random biopsies of the esophagus (i.e., to rule out eosinophilic esophagitis in a patient with dysphagia), another option is to open the biopsy forceps over the target tissue, place it flush over the mucosa, and apply suction to collapse the lumen. This will generally allow sufficient mucosa to go into the biopsy forceps, which is then closed to capture the tissue.

Gastroesophageal Reflux Disease (GERD)

Biopsies directed to irregularities of the esophageal mucosa are rarely warranted in patients with GERD and esophagitis. Biopsies in an esophageal–gastric junction with inflammatory aspects are not recommended.

Table 1.4 Some of the abnormal lesions to be familiarized in EGD

Esophagus
Zenker's diverticulum
Inlet patch
Esophagitis—Peptic, infectious, eosinophilic, pill induced
Schatzki ring
Esophageal stricture
Extrinsic compression of the esophagus
Esophageal tumors
MW tear
Esophageal varices
Hiatal hernia
Cameron lesion
Stomach
Erythema versus gastritis
Gastric cancer
MALToma
Dieulafoy lesion
Ulcers, erosions
GAVE
Gastropathy
Gastric varices
AVM
Submucosal lesions—GIST, Pancreatic rest, lipoma, pseudocyst
Duodenum
Ulcer
Ampullary adenoma or mass
Duodenal polyp(s)
Brenner's glands
Peri-ampullary diverticulum
Celiac villous atrophy

Reflux Esophagitis

Esophagitis from acid reflux is usually apparent in the distal esophagus at or near to the level of the GE junction. If the distal esophagus is normal with areas of esophagitis in the mid- or proximal esophagus, then these are less likely to be acid related. Longitudinal linear mucosal breaks, which if severe can be confluent and extend circumferentially or upwards are the findings in reflux esophagitis, are also rarely biopsied.

Eosinophilic Esophagitis (EoE)

EoE can be suspected in patients with a variety of findings including a narrow-caliber esophagus, a ringed esophagus, mucosal linear furrows, or white plaques. In patients with suspected EoE, two to four biopsies of the proximal esophagus and two to four biopsies of the distal esophagus should be performed. Also, at the time of initial diagnosis, biopsies from gastric antrum and duodenum can be performed as needed to rule out other causes of esophageal eosinophilia and to exclude a more systemic process like eosinophilic gastroenteritis [6]. Some patients with suspected EoE should be treated with a 2-month course of proton pump inhibitor (PPI) prior to endoscopic biopsies to exclude PPI responsive esophageal eosinophilia (PPI-REE), although in practice many endoscopists biopsy the esophagus anytime the mucosa is suspicious for EoE [6].

Infectious Esophagitis

In patients with suspected infectious esophagitis, the site of biopsy varies according to the suspected etiology based on the morphology of the esophageal ulcerations. For suspected cytomegalovirus (CMV) esophagitis, biopsies should be taken from the base (center) of the ulcers. If patients have esophagitis suspected to be due to Herpes Simplex Virus (HSV), biopsies should be from the edges of the ulcers. Targeted biopsies and exfoliative cytology should be performed for suspected esophageal candidiasis.

Monilial (Candida) Esophagitis

Patients with white plaques in the esophagus often do not need to have a definitive biopsy obtained if the appearance is strongly suggestive of fungal infection. Typically, these patients are treated empirically with an oral antifungal, i.e., fluconazole. If a definitive sample is desired, either a biopsy or a brush cytology specimen is usually adequate to confirm the diagnosis (see Fig. 1.6).

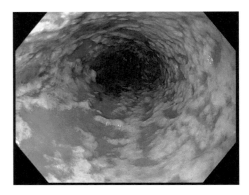

Fig. 1.6 Candida esophagitis

Barrett's Esophagus (BE)

BE should be considered when there is extension of salmon-colored mucosa into the tubular esophagus extending ≥ 1 cm proximal to the gastroesophageal junction (GEJ) with biopsy confirmation of intestinal metaplasia. Endoscopic biopsy should not be performed in the presence of a normal Z line or a Z line with only <1 cm of variability [7]. In patients with suspected BE, some have recommended at least 8 random biopsies should be obtained to maximize the yield of IM on histology. In patients with short (1–2 cm) segments of suspected BE in whom 8 biopsies may be unobtainable, at least 4 biopsies per cm of circumferential BE, and one biopsy per cm in tongues of BE, should be obtained [7]. The current GI society guideline recommend that endoscopic surveillance should employ four-quadrant biopsies at 2-cm intervals in patients without dysplasia and 1-cm intervals in patients with prior dysplasia, which is slightly more than the previously followed per Seattle protocol [8, 9] (see Fig. 1.7).

Stomach

Any concerning or suspicious gastric mucosal areas should typically be biopsied facilitate a diagnosis, be it for gastritis, malignancy, or other processes. Certain conditions like gastric antral vascular ectasia (GAVE), portal hypertensive gastropathy, angioectasias, and pancreatic rests are often diagnosed by the typical endoscopic appearance, and in these cases biopsies are rarely indicated [10] (see Fig. 1.8).

Dyspepsia

In patients undergoing EGD for dyspepsia as the sole indication, routine biopsies of normal-appearing esophageal mucosa or GE junction mucosa are generally discouraged. Conversely, biopsies of normal-appearing gastric mucosa for the detection of *Helicobacter pylori* (HP) infection, if the HP infection status is unknown, are recommended [11, 12].

Helicobacter Pylori

When obtaining biopsies from the gastric body and antrum for the detection of HP infection, the 5-biopsy Sydney System has been suggested for taking specimens from the lesser and greater curve of the antrum within 2–3 cm of the pylorus, from the lesser curvature of the corpus (4 cm proximal to the angularis), from the middle portion of the

Fig. 1.7 Barrett's esophagus **a** under white light **b** under NBI. Reprinted from Ref. [9], with permission from Elsevier

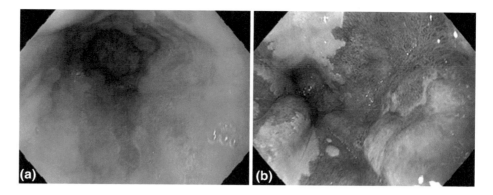

Gastric Ulcers

The main role of endoscopy in an uncomplicated gastric ulcer is to confirm the diagnosis and to rule out malignancy [14]. However, given the low incidence of gastric cancer in the USA, there are no clear data to support routine biopsies on all gastric ulcers. If the ulcer is suggestive of malignancy due to associated mass, raised edges, irregular borders, or other signs of malignancy biopsy should be performed. However, as malignant ulcers may initially have a benign appearance, some endoscopists perform biopsies in all gastric ulcers. Such biopsies should be taken from base and the edge of the ulcer [14].

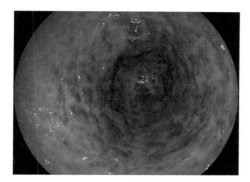

Fig. 1.8 Endoscopic appearance of gastric antral vascular ectasia (GAVE)

Duodenum

In the absence of other signs or symptoms associated with an increased risk of celiac disease, routine biopsies of the normal-appearing duodenal mucosa to detect celiac disease are not recommended [11]. However, in immuno-compromised patients undergoing EGD for dyspepsia as the sole indication, routine biopsies of the normal-appearing duodenum for the detection of GVHD in post-allogeneic tissue transplantation patients and for opportunistic infections are recommended [11, 12]. Duodenal ulcers are extremely unlikely to be malignant, and therefore routine biopsy of these ulcers is not recommended. Patients with duodenal ulcers often undergo gastric biopsies to rule out HP infection, even in the absence of obvious gastritis.

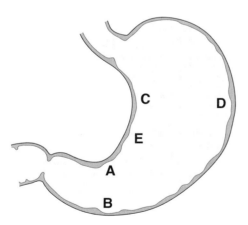

Fig. 1.9 Locations of gastric biopsy per updated Sydney 5-biopsy system **a** lesser curvature of the antrum **b** greater curvature of the antrum **c** lesser curvature of the body **d** greater curvature. Reprinted from Ref. [11], with permission from Elsevier

Celiac Disease

If suspicion for celiac disease is high, duodenal biopsies should be obtained even if the serology is negative. At least 4 biopsies from distal duodenum and 2 biopsies from the duodenal bulb should be obtained [15].

greater curvature of the corpus (8 cm from the cardia), and one from the incisura angularis [11, 13] (see Fig. 1.9) [11]. In practice, many endoscopists do not take this many biopsies and simply sample the body and the antrum.

Quality Indicators in EGD

The American Society for Gastrointestinal Endoscopy (ASGE), the American College of Gastroenterology (ACG), and the American Gastroenterological Association (AGA) have always promoted the importance of performing a high-quality endoscopy. A high-quality endoscopy is a complete examination in which patients receive an rightly indicated procedure, correct diagnoses are recognized or excluded, any therapy provided is appropriate, and all steps that minimize risk have been taken [16, 17]. Recent guidelines from all the GI societies have proposed specific metrics addressing all the aspects of endoscopy such as following high performance target are complete examination of the esophagus, stomach, and duodenum, including retroflexion in the stomach with photo documentation.

Conclusion

All practicing endoscopists should be able to perform a high-yield upper endoscopy in an efficient manner. Individual techniques vary, but there is remarkable agreement on general best practices in most of the common situations encountered in upper endoscopy. Careful evaluation and biopsy of the esophagus, stomach, and duodenum can help answer clinical questions in a variety of clinical situations.

References

1. Practice guidelines for sedation and analgesia by non-anesthesiologists. Anesthesiology 2002;96:1004–17.
2. Preiss C, Charton JP, Schumacher B, Neuhaus H. A randomized trial of unsedated transnasal small-caliber esophagogastroduodenoscopy (EGD) versus peroral small-caliber EGD versus conventional EGD. Endoscopy. 2003;35:641–6.
3. Horiuchi A, Nakayama Y, Hidaka N, Ichise Y, Kajiyama M, Tanaka N. Prospective comparison between sedated high-definition oral and unsedated ultrathin transnasal esophagogastroduodenoscopy in the same subjects: pilot study. Dig Endosc Off J Jpn Gastroenterol Endosc Soc. 2009;21:24–8.
4. Early DS, Ben-Menachem T, Decker GA, et al. Appropriate use of GI endoscopy. Gastrointest Endosc. 2012;75:1127–31.
5. Chung CS, Lin CK, Liang CC, Hsu WF, Lee TH. Intentional examination of esophagus by narrow-band imaging endoscopy increases detection rate of cervical inlet patch. Dis Esophagus Off J Int Soc Dis Esophagus/ISDE. 2015;28:666–72.
6. Dellon ES, Gonsalves N, Hirano I, Furuta GT, Liacouras CA, Katzka DA. ACG clinical guideline: Evidenced based approach to the diagnosis and management of esophageal eosinophilia and eosinophilic esophagitis (EoE). Am J Gastroenterol. 2013;108:679–92 quiz 93.
7. Shaheen NJ, Falk GW, Iyer PG, Gerson LB. ACG clinical guideline: diagnosis and management of barrett's esophagus. Am J Gastroenterol. 2016;111:30–50.
8. Levine DS, Blount PL, Rudolph RE, Reid BJ. Safety of a systematic endoscopic biopsy protocol in patients with Barrett's esophagus. Am J Gastroenterol. 2000;95:1152–7.
9. Cameron GR, Jayasekera CS, Williams R, Macrae FA, Desmond PV, Taylor AC. Detection and staging of esophageal cancers within Barrett's esophagus is improved by assessment in specialized Barrett's units. Gastrointest Endosc. 2014;80:971–83 e1.
10. Prachayakul V, Aswakul P, Leelakusolvong S. Massive gastric antral vascular ectasia successfully treated by endoscopic band ligation as the initial therapy. World J Gastrointest Endosc. 2013;5:135–7.
11. Yang YX, Brill J, Krishnan P, Leontiadis G. American gastroenterological association institute guideline on the role of upper gastrointestinal biopsy to evaluate dyspepsia in the adult patient in the absence of visible mucosal lesions. Gastroenterology. 2015;149:1082–7.
12. American gastroenterological association institute guideline on the role of upper gastrointestinal biopsy to evaluate dyspepsia in the adult patient in the absence of visible mucosal lesions: clinical decision support tool. Gastroenterology. 2015;149:1119.
13. Dixon MF, Genta RM, Yardley JH, Correa P. Classification and grading of gastritis. The updated Sydney system. international workshop on the histopathology of gastritis, Houston 1994. Am J Surg Pathol. 1996;20:1161–81.
14. Banerjee S, Cash BD, Dominitz JA, et al. The role of endoscopy in the management of patients with peptic ulcer disease. Gastrointest Endosc. 2010;71:663–8.
15. Rubio-Tapia A, Hill ID, Kelly CP, Calderwood AH, Murray JA. ACG clinical guidelines: diagnosis and management of celiac disease. Am J Gastroenterol. 2013;108:656–76 quiz 77.
16. Rizk MK, Sawhney MS, Cohen J, et al. Quality indicators common to all GI endoscopic procedures. Gastrointest Endosc. 2015;81:3–16.
17. Park WG, Shaheen NJ, Cohen J, et al. Quality indicators for EGD. Gastrointest Endosc. 2015;81:17–30.

Nonvariceal Upper Gastrointestinal Bleeding

Stephen R. Rotman and John R. Saltzman

Introduction

Upper gastrointestinal bleeding (UGIB) is defined as bleeding in the gastrointestinal tract originating between the mouth and the ligament of Treitz. Nonvariceal UGIB is responsible for over 300,000 hospitalizations per year in the USA and is the primary reason for urgent endoscopy. The mortality rate for UGI bleeding is significant, although in recent years, it has been declining with the use of effective medical and endoscopic therapies [1]. Gastroenterologists will typically manage UGIB cases from presentation through evaluation, treatment, and follow-up care on a routine basis on inpatient services. The technical approach to the endoscopic treatment of UGIB is a set of skills that must be learned for treating bleeding effectively in clinical practice. There are multiple guidelines that detail the recommended approach to the management of patients with UGIB [2–7]. In this chapter, the evaluation and management of patients with suspected or established nonvariceal UGIB are discussed, with a focus on the various endoscopic techniques and tools.

Initial Management

Initial therapy for patients with acute UGIB includes resuscitation with immediate placement of at least two large-bore ($\geq$18-gauge) peripheral intravenous catheters [8, 9]. Establishment of large-bore vascular access is critical for the delivery of appropriate volumes and types of fluid, or in some cases, blood product, for resuscitation and hemodynamic stabilization of the patient. By comparison, an 18-gauge intravenous catheter allows for a maximum fluid flow rate of 105 mL/min, whereas a 20-gauge intravenous catheter allows for a maximum fluid flow rate of 60 mL/min. In patients with compromised ability to protect their airway, altered mental status, or ongoing and severe hematemesis, elective endotracheal intubation should be considered. Intubation is recommended in cases of active vomiting or significant hematemesis because of the increased risk of clinically significant aspiration during endoscopy.

A restrictive strategy to the administration of blood transfusions has been shown to benefit most patients with acute UGIB [10]. This includes refraining from packed red blood cell transfusions when the hemoglobin is $\geq$7 g per deciliter in cases of acute UGIB without ongoing active bleeding or active coronary disease. Prior management strategies included initial nasogastric tube placement and lavage to evaluate for an upper GI source of bleeding. However, the use of nasogastric tubes is no longer recommend because of their low negative predictive value, as well as a lack of benefit in patient outcomes in clinical studies [3, 11].

Medical Therapies

Many medications have been used as part of the management of patients with acute UGIB. These include antacids, histamine-2-receptor antagonists, proton pump inhibitors

Electronic supplementary material
Supplementary material is available in the online version of this chapter at 10.1007/978-3-319-49041-0_2. Videos can also be accessed at https://link.springer.com/chapter/10.1007/978-3-319-49041-0_2.

S.R. Rotman · J.R. Saltzman
Division of Gastroenterology, Brigham and Women's Hospital, Boston, MA 02115, USA
e-mail: stephen.rotman@gmail.com

J.R. Saltzman (✉)
Harvard Medical School, Brigham and Women's Hospital, Boston, MA 02115, USA
e-mail: jsaltzman@bwh.harvard.edu

(PPIs), and octreotide. Antacids and histamine-2-receptor antagonists can increase intragastric pH but have been superseded by PPIs.

The use of PPIs in the initial management of patients with suspected UGIB is now widely adopted as part of the treatment of acute UGIB since a landmark study in 1997 showed improved outcomes with the use of PPI versus placebo [12]. PPI use allows patients to achieve a gastric pH of >6.0 and decreases rates of further ulcer bleeding, allowing for more rapid patient stabilization and facilitation of other medical and endoscopic therapies [13]. Early PPI use also aides in initial ulcer healing [14]. A recent meta-analysis has shown that twice-daily IV PPI bolus is noninferior to an IV PPI bolus dose followed by a continuous infusion [15]. Thus, either a PPI twice-daily bolus or IV infusion may be given to patients with acute UGIB. There is also data that suggest that oral PPI therapy is similarly effective to IV PPI therapy in the setting of bleeding [16]. In patients on IV PPI therapy, once the bleeding has been stabilized or stopped, patients may be safely transitioned to an oral PPI. In patients receiving endoscopic therapy for high-risk lesions, the switch to an oral PPI typically occurs after 72 h without the evidence of rebleeding.

Many patients with UGIB will present while on therapeutic antithrombotic agents. It has been shown that therapeutic endoscopy is effective and can be safely performed in patients with an INR of ≤2.5 [17]. Vitamin K or fresh frozen plasma can be administered as part of resuscitation prior to endoscopy in cases of ongoing active bleeding. When patients present on other antithrombotic agents including aspirin, thienopyridines, or novel oral anticoagulants, the endoscopist must consider the indication for therapy and consequences, including potential for adverse events if the antithrombotic agent is stopped in the setting of UGIB. In the setting of acute bleeding, these agents are typically withheld, but should be restarted after the bleeding is controlled if the indication is secondary prevention [18, 19]. It has been recommended that aspirin and warfarin are restarted within one to three days or four to seven days, respectively, following control or bleeding [3]. Decisions on antithrombotic management should be carried out in collaboration with the prescribing physicians, considering the risks of bleeding if these medications are continued and the risks of thrombotic events if these medications are withheld.

Risk Stratification

Risk stratification in acute UGIB can be accomplished by the use of validated risk scores. These can be used to separate low-risk patients (who can often be discharged after endoscopy) from high-risk patients who will benefit from more

resources, including intensive care unit (ICU) level of care and urgent endoscopy [2, 3]. Several UGIB risk stratification scores exist including the Rockall score, the Glasgow-Blatchford score, (GBS), and the AIMS65 score [20–22].

The GBS and AIMS65 scores use only the clinical information available at the time of initial presentation to the emergency department. The AIMS65 score includes five factors: serum albumin <3.0 g/dL, INR >1.5, altered mental status, systolic blood pressure <90 mm Hg, and age ≥65 years. In the AIM65 score, each factor is assigned a score of 1 and high-risk patients have an AIMS score >1. Patients with a GBS score of 0–2 and an AIMS65 score of 0 can be considered for outpatient management, while patients with a GBS >10 or an AIMS65 >2 should be considered for ICU management and an urgent endoscopy following adequate volume resuscitation [23, 24].

Endoscopic Management

In the management of UGIB, in addition to the stabilization of the patient, volume resuscitation, medical therapy, and endoscopy should be performed. Endoscopic therapy can often completely stop active bleeding and prevent rebleeding. Upper endoscopy is more than 90% sensitive in identification of a bleeding site, with sensitivity inversely related to the time elapsed between patient presentation and the timing of the endoscopic procedure. After hemodynamic resuscitation and stabilization, multiple guidelines recommend that all patients with acute UGIB should undergo upper endoscopy within 24 h of the patient's initial presentation. Urgent endoscopy (less than 12 h after presentation) has not been shown to be superior to early endoscopy (within 24 h of presentation). However, urgent endoscopy may be beneficial for patients with suspected ongoing active bleeding or for patients with high-risk prognostic scores following hemodynamic stabilization. All lesions should be photographed prior to and after endoscopic intervention to provide proper documentation of the initial lesion and its response to endoscopic treatment.

The goals of endoscopy are to identify and treat lesions that are actively bleeding or contain high-risk stigmata of recent bleeding (Table 2.1). High-risk stigmata of recent hemorrhage (SRH) include actively bleeding lesions (spurting or oozing) (Fig. 2.1), nonbleeding visible blood vessels within an ulcer, and adherent blood clots covering a lesion (Fig. 2.2). These stigmata are important to recognize because they are the lesions with the greatest risk of having a rebleeding event. High-risk SRH should generally be treated when identified by endoscopy. The management of adherent clots is most controversial as the bleeding risk depends on the bleeding stigmata underneath the clot. A commonly

Table 2.1 Stigmata of recent hemorrhage in descending order from highest risk to lowest risk for further bleeding

	Further bleeding (average) (%)	Prevalence (%)
Spurting bleeding	80	9
Nonbleeding visible vessel	44	10
Adherent clot	20	12
Active oozing	10	6
Flat pigmented spot	10	8
Clean-based ulcer	5	55

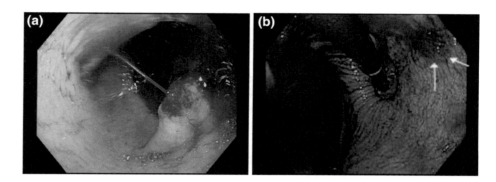

Fig. 2.1 a Actively spurting bleeding. **b** Active oozing blood from an ulcer

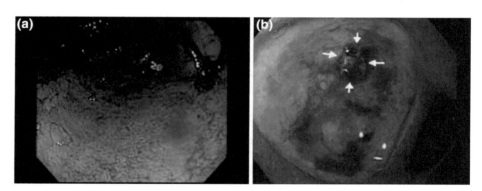

Fig. 2.2 a Adherent clot on gastric ulcer. **b** Duodenal ulcer with a visible vessel surrounded by *arrows*

employed endoscopic technique to evaluate lesions underneath visible clots is to inject dilute epinephrine at the base of the clot and then to cold guillotine the clot off the lesion using a snare without using shearing force. The underlying area is then vigorously irrigated. If a bleeding or a nonbleeding visible vessel is uncovered, further endoscopic therapy is indicated [25].

Measures to Improve Visibility

Direct Irrigation

Irrigation during endoscopy is important not only to identify the bleeding site, but also to prepare the target tissue for intervention. Irrigation of suspected bleeding lesions is done with water or saline directed onto the lesion until adequate visualization is achieved. Most current endoscopes include ports and accessories to deliver a forward-directed water jet through the tip of the endoscope, allowing for easy and copious directed delivery of irrigating fluid. When significant air bubbles are present, addition of simethicone to the irrigating fluid in the water bottle can aide in visualization. Irrigation of an ulcer should not be deferred out of fear for provoking bleeding. Irrigation can help to identify the precise location of the SRH and can provide the operator information needed to determine which endoscopic tool or approach is optimal.

If a large volume of blood or clot is present, a standard endoscope may not provide enough suction capacity to clear the area. In these cases, a large channel or dual-channel therapeutic endoscope can be used to facilitate more effective suctioning of fluid and/or clots. A large capacity external suction device can also be attached to the biopsy port of an endoscope for patients with large amounts of intraluminal contents requiring aspiration bypassing the suction inside of the endoscope housing connected to the endoscope processor and allowing for more effective suctioning.

Pharmacologic Methods

Several pharmacologic agents have been used in UGIB to help clear the stomach contents in an effort to facilitate improved visualization during endoscopy. Intravenous erythromycin used prior to endoscopy can help with gastric visualization. Erythromycin is a motilin-like prokinetic agent, promoting gastric contractions and subsequent gastric emptying. Erythromycin at 250 mg bolus or 3 mg/kg infusion administered over 30 min (intravenously) is effective clinically and should be administered 30–120 min prior to the anticipated endoscopy. Metoclopramide 10 mg IV has also been used as a prokinetic agent to promote clearance of gastric debris and blood from the stomach prior to endoscopy, although there is less available data concerning its efficacy. These prokinetic agents improve gastric visualization and potentially reduce the need for repeat endoscopy [26].

Endoscopic Therapeutic Methods

Once a source of bleeding has been identified, there are many instruments and techniques in the endoscopist's armamentarium to provide treatment and to prevent rebleeding (Table 2.2). Rebleeding is a major source of morbidity and mortality. Endoscopic techniques for bleeding control include injection therapies, contact and noncontact thermal devices, mechanical devices such as endoscopic clips and band ligation, radiofrequency ablation, and the use of a combination of techniques. Other novel tools include hemostatic sprays, but these are not currently approved by the FDA.

Table 2.2 Commonly used modalities for endoscopic therapy

Injection therapy
– Epinephrine (1:10,000)
– Sclerosant agents (alcohol, ethanolamine, and polidocanol)
– Tissue adhesives (cyanoacrylate glue and thrombin/fibrin)
Thermal therapy
– Contact: heater probe, bipolar probe, and monopolar probe
– Noncontact: APC
Mechanical therapy
– Hemoclips
– Over-the-scope clips
– Endoscopic band ligation
Combination therapy
– Injection + thermal therapy
– Injection + mechanical therapy

Injection Therapies

Injection therapy is primarily performed with dilute epinephrine, although saline alone may be used if epinephrine is not available [27]. Injection therapies induce hemostasis by producing a tamponade effect on the area and epinephrine causes vasoconstriction reducing local blood flow, although this effect is less than the primary fluid tamponade. Epinephrine is generally diluted to 1:10,000. This may be done by adding 1 mL of 1:1000 epinephrine into a syringe containing 9 mL of saline. The concentration can be further reduced in patients with serious cardiac comorbidities to 1:100,000, especially when used near the gastroesophageal junction where its use may cause more systemic cardiac effects. Patients with contraindications to epinephrine can receive saline alone as the injectate. Saline alone can be used as an injectant to produce tamponade if epinephrine is not available.

The general technique of injection is to introduce a standard endoscopic injection catheter through the working channel of the endoscope until the tip is visible. Then, the injection needle is advanced and locked in position. Different injection needles with different diameters allow for variability in the amount of force needed to introduce the needle into the submucosa. It is recommended to inject into multiple locations surrounding the bleeding lesion with a four-quadrant technique, although some lesions with active bleeding may achieve hemostasis after only one injection. If the needle is not inserted deep enough to reach the submucosal space, injected fluid will leak into the lumen when the syringe is depressed. If this happens, one can readjust the needle by pulling the injection catheter out of the mucosa and then reinserting at the same or a different location in an effort to reach the submucosa with the needle tip. Of note, some pressure is required to introduce the injection needle tip into the submucosa. Alternatively, the injection can be started with the tip of the needle in the lumen and the probe advanced during injection to find the submucosal space.

Injection can be used to help control bleeding of various etiologies, including from vessels within ulcers, vascular malformations, and Dieulafoy's lesions, as well as when a discrete lesion is not visualized due to active bleeding. In the stomach, 8–10 mL total injection can be used in multiple injections of about 2 mL each, although there is no absolute number or volume of injections. Higher doses are more likely to cause cardiovascular side effects, and this should be kept in mind, especially when epinephrine is used near the gastroesophageal junction.

Soon following the injection, the area around the lesion will develop pallor and the hemostatic effects are seen when any active bleeding slows or stops. Use of injection monotherapy is not recommended because it is less effective than other monotherapies or combination therapies and is less durable as it is associated with higher rates of rebleeding. Rather, injection therapy is often used as a prelude to a second treatment (thermal or mechanical therapy) once bleeding has abated and visualization has been improved.

Injection therapy can be used to treat a myriad of bleeding lesions because of the short-lived effect of vasoconstriction and temporary cessation of bleeding. In situations where there is overwhelming bleeding obscuring visualization despite irrigation, injection of epinephrine can help slow bleeding and ultimately identify and thus allow treatment of the source. Injection therapy is most helpful to slow or stop bleeding; thermal and/or mechanical therapy can subsequently be applied to achieve complete and durable hemostasis.

Other injection agents include sclerosants (although these are usually used in the treatment of bleeding varices if band ligation has failed or is not available). These agents can be used for nonvariceal bleeding sources as well. Sclerosants include ethanol, polidocanol, and ethanolamine. These agents induce local inflammation and fibrosis of a bleeding vessel. Other agents that can be injected include cyanoacrylate and fibrin glues. Cyanoacrylate glue is a liquid material that transforms (polymerizes) into a solid after injection. This can be particularly useful in bleeding gastric varices, whereby the glue becomes an artificial thrombus in the varix reducing blood flow by occluding the vessel. Fibrin glue has also been used endoscopically as a form of injection therapy. Fibrinogen and factor XIII are mixed with thrombin and calcium. In this manner, the clotting cascade is activated and clotting is promoted. Cyanoacrylate and fibrin glue may be of limited availability.

Thermal Therapies

Contact thermal therapies used for the control of UGIB include heater and bipolar probes, as well as monopolar therapies [27]. The technique for the use of heater and bipolar therapies involves controlling bleeding by simultaneously compressing and cauterizing a bleeding vessel, known as coaptive coagulation. Heater and bipolar therapies do not require a grounding pad applied to the patient as the electrical circuit is completed within the device itself. Once in widespread use, heater probes rarely are utilized in current practice and bipolar electrocautery devices are now commonly employed to treat GI bleeding. Heater probes are quite effective and, if available, are still an excellent choice for treating upper GI bleeds.

While the bipolar probe can be used multi-directionally, with either a perpendicular or tangential approach, a heater probe can be used perpendicularly only. The larger 10 French probes can deliver thermal energy over a larger area

than the smaller 7 French probes and are felt to be more effective, although the 10 French probes require a therapeutic endoscope with a large channel size.

The technique of applying endoscopic cautery using either a bipolar or heater probe is similar for both devices. First, the probe is advanced out of the tip of the endoscope and into the lumen for a short distance, so that the tip is visualized endoscopically (Video 2.1). If the probe is too far out of the scope, it can be difficult to control and the operator will lose mechanical advantage. The endoscope should be positioned as close to the lesion as possible for the control of therapy to maximize visualization and efficiency of endoscopic maneuvers. The probe should make direct contact with the bleeding vessel and be held in place with direct pressure to ensure continued contact. Moderate-to-firm pressure is usually used in the stomach due to its relatively thick wall, and mild-to-moderate pressure is typically used in the rest of the gastrointestinal tract, such as in the small bowel or esophagus where the walls are thinner. One suggested technique uses four to six pulses of energy for approximately 10 s each, although many variations exist. No gold standard on the number and duration of therapy exists as these depend on the specifics of the lesion being treated and on its location. The endpoint for therapy is the cessation of bleeding and visible cauterization of the target lesion, which often appears flattened following successful therapy application.

Energy levels recommended are 10–15 W in the duodenum and 15–20 W in the stomach. After each round of therapy, the target lesion can be inspected for ongoing bleeding, adverse events, and the need for additional therapy. If the probe is stuck to the vessel, removal of the probe can sometimes trigger rebleeding. Some devices allow water irrigation directly through the probe to minimize the risk of the probe adhering to the coagulum and can be irrigated after each application of cautery.

Monopolar therapy can also treat bleeding vessels and has been extensively used to treat endoscopically induced bleeding, such as bleeding occurring during endoscopic submucosal dissection (ESD). However, there is much less clinical data available on the use of monopolar cautery for the control of acute UGIB. One monopolar probe is a rotatable probe with flat jaws (Coagrasper, Olympus Corporation, Center Valley, PA), used to capture and compress tissue while delivering thermal energy. The technique involved with this device is different from the coaptive coagulation technique used for the heater and bipolar probes. By using monopolar forceps, the bleeding lesion is grasped and "tented" toward the scope. Cautery is used at higher power settings, such as 50 W, for shorter durations of 1–2 s [28]. Monopolar cautery requires the use of a grounding pad, similar to that used for polypectomy. This pad should not be placed over any implanted metal, such as a joint replacement.

Argon plasma coagulation (APC) is a noncontact, superficial method of thermal therapy that induces destruction of bleeding lesions or aberrant vessels and vascular malformations. APC uses argon gas that is electrically conducted creating a high-energy plasma. It is unlike heater, bipolar, or monopolar probe therapies, as it does not touch or compress the tissue targeted for therapy. APC uses monopolar energy, and a grounding pad must be placed on the patient prior to use. The probes for APC are available in a variety of configurations, including with those tips that are end-firing and circumferential. Cautery will seek the closest mucosal surface to the probe, regardless of probe type. APC has, in general, a lesser degree of tissue penetration than other hemostatic methods.

APC technique involves passing the probe carefully through the endoscope as the probe can easily kink and advancing the probe close to the target tissue. The probe needs to be only a few millimeters away from the target but should *not* make contact with the mucosa. Contact of the probe may cause dissection of charged argon gas through the wall and result in perforation. Pulses of argon gas and ionization charge are controlled by a foot pedal. The lesion may be "sprayed" or "painted" with the goal being adequate treatment of the tissue, with a white charring of the superficial layer of the mucosa (Fig. 2.3).

APC can be used in the treatment of bleeding from vascular malformations, radiation-induced rectal bleeding, or gastric antral vascular ectasia (GAVE). In a lesion that

spreads, such as GAVE, APC is effective in treating a large involved area. The tissue is sprayed as the APC probe or endoscope is moved along a lesion and large amount of mucosa can therefore be quickly treated. Repeated treatments are often required for cases of GAVE, with typically three to four treatment sessions required depending on the extent of GAVE. The tip of the APC probe will collect charred material if there is contact with the tissue. The probe should then be removed from the endoscope removing the charred material with gauze, following which the probe may be reintroduced through the endoscope for resuming treatment.

During treatment with APC, there will be a buildup of visible gas in the lumen. This buildup of gas is expected, and the argon gas should be intermittently suctioned completely during the course of therapy, requiring removal of the probe unless a double-channel therapeutic scope is used. APC may also be used to treat upper GI tumor bleeding (Video 2.1), although there is a risk of rebleeding and little available data on its effectiveness (Fig. 2.4).

Radiofrequency Ablation

Radiofrequency ablation (RFA) is another treatment modality that delivers superficial cautery and can be used in the treatment of GAVE and vascular malformations. There are several types of probes available, including a rotatable

Fig. 2.3 a. Arteriovenous malformation with classic spider appearance. **b** Tissue destruction (AVM) after APC therapy. Charring of the tissue is seen

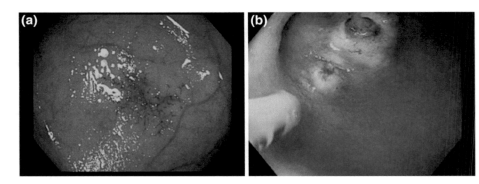

Fig. 2.4 a Bleeding esophageal tumor. **b** Bleeding esophageal tumor after the treatment with APC therapy

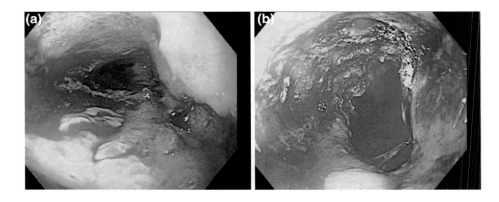

RFA probe that can be deployed through the scope, as well as a 60 or 90° probe that attaches externally to the scope tip. The probe needs to make direct and solid contact with the target area in order to provide effective cautery. The through-the-scope probe can be rotated in order to accomplish adequate positioning and tissue contact. Using a pedal connected to the generator, RFA is delivered with a set energy and time pulse. Each area of the lesion should be treated with two successive pulses, with a typical energy per pulse of 12 J/cm^2.

Mechanical Hemostasis Using Clips

Endoscopic through-the-scope clips are commonly used to treat bleeding lesions [29, 30]. They can be used on actively bleeding lesions as well as on lesions with stigmata of recent bleeding, such as visible vessels within ulcers, vascular malformations, and Dieulafoy's lesions (Fig. 2.5). Most available clips can be rotated, opened, and closed repeatedly as needed prior to the deployment. Ideal lesions for clips include those that are accessible, vessels less than 2 mm in diameter and ulcers that are pliable (not firm or indurated). Difficult locations for clip application include high on the lesser curvature of the stomach and the posterior wall of the duodenum. Clips can also be applied successfully for closure of Mallory–Weiss tears (Fig. 2.6).

The technique of through-the-scope clip application starts with the passage of the clip catheter. The clip should be closed and then passed through the working channel of the endoscope. Once visible endoscopically, the clip can be opened and rotated to the desired position by the assistant working with the endoscopist. Clip rotation is beneficial for ideal hemoclip placement, especially in challenging locations. The goal of the therapy is to target the lesion with the clip as well as any feeding vessel. If targeting a visible vessel in an ulcer base, the clip should ideally span across the vessel. The delivery catheter is then extended such that the clip is engaged with the targeted tissue. As with thermal

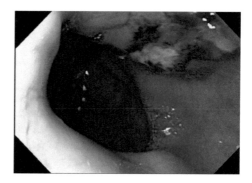

Fig. 2.6 Mallory–Weiss tear with oozing

therapies, the scope should be as close to the target lesion as possible for best mechanical advantage in order to effectively deploy the hemoclip. Suction helps enable the hemoclip to sit flush against the target tissue. If the endoscopist is satisfied with the position, the clip can be closed. If the clip placement or position is not appropriate, it can be opened again and its position can be changed. Once in the desired position, the clip can then be deployed, thereby separating it from the catheter (Video 2.1). After firing and deployment, it is sometimes necessary to gently move the delivery catheter slightly forward and backward to fully separate the delivery system from the clip.

When a target lesion is on a wall that is difficult to approach and not amenable to perpendicular clip placement, clips can still be used. In these situations, the clip is extended only slightly out of the endoscope. The alignment of the clip should be made to be flushed with the mucosa. The clip can then be manipulated to rest onto the lesion tangentially (as if it is being laid flat). Then, the clip can be closed and deployed. Multiple clips can be placed in one area, and once the visible vessel has been clipped, placing a clip on each side of the vessel may ablate the blood flow from a feeding vessel. It some situations, it may be difficult to place a hemoclip directly on a vessel. When this occurs, clips should be placed on each side of the lesion to ligate the feeding vessel.

Clips typically stay in place for several weeks following which they slough off, although they may remain in place much longer, especially if attached to underlying muscularis propria. Patients receiving clips must be made aware that some clips may not be MRI compatible and a plain radiograph can confirm whether they are present. Most current clips are approved by the FDA as conditionally MRI compatible, safe up to a 3 T magnet MRI. Clips can also be utilized in combination with injection therapy. The use of clips may follow injection with dilute epinephrine, especially if the target lesion is initially difficult to visualize due to active bleeding or when treating large arteries, such as Dieulafoy's lesions, the left gastric artery, or the gastro-duodenal artery. Injection therapy can be used after the

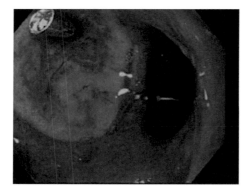

Fig. 2.5 Duodenal ulcer shown in Fig. 2.2b after hemoclip placement

application of clips when there is residual oozing following successful placement of the clips.

Over-the-Scope Clips

A recent addition to mechanical hemostasis is the over-the-scope clip (OTSC). These are larger clips, more similar to a clamp, that is fitted to the end of the endoscope. These OTSCs can be used to treat larger lesions, such as large vessels within bleeding ulcers (i.e., Dieulafoy's lesions, the left gastric artery, or the gastroduodenal artery), or to treat cases of recurrent or refractory bleeding (Fig. 2.7) [31]. The OTSC is attached to the end of the scope similar to a banding device. There is a release thread that is pulled through the scope, similar to a banding device, and attached to a wheel that is in turn attached to the channel port of the endoscope. The target lesion is drawn using full suction into a cap at the end of the endoscope, and the wheel is turned deploying the over-the-scope clip. These clips are large enough that they may cover an entire bleeding ulcer. When placing these clips, they should be applied directly over the lesion in a straight-on approach.

Band Ligation

Endoscopic band ligation is a technique most often used in the treatment of esophageal or gastroesophageal varices. However, band ligation has also been used to treat Dieulafoy's (Fig. 2.8) and Cameron (Fig. 2.9) lesions.

Spray Therapies

Several new topical hemostatic powders have become available as endoscopic treatment modalities for UGIB [32]; however, these are not currently FDA approved. TC-325 is an inorganic powder that sprayed onto a bleeding site. The

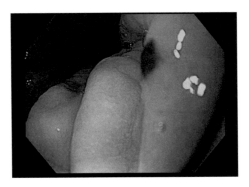

Fig. 2.8 Dieulafoy's lesion

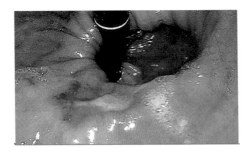

Fig. 2.9 Cameron lesion

endoscopic technique is to advance the spray catheter through the scope, which is placed near the targeted bleeding lesion. The endoscopist then presses a trigger releasing CO_2 and applying TC-325 under pressure to the bleeding site. The compound adheres to the lesion causing a mechanical tamponade, activating platelets and coagulation factors, as well as desiccating the tissue. TC-325 has been shown to be useful in the treatment of bleeding ulcers, Dieulafoy's lesions, malignancy, and post-sphincterotomy bleeding [33, 34]. However, the lesion must be actively bleeding at the time of therapy in order for the therapy to be effective. In addition, lesions with a significant risk of further bleeding should be treated with an additional modality, such as hemoclips, to decrease rebleeding risk.

Adjuncts to Therapy

Cap

Clear caps attached to the tip of the endoscope can be used to help manage difficult locations of UGIB treatment [35]. Caps can aid in visualization by allowing for compression of tissue with the cap, such that SRH can be seen behind folds or in difficult intestinal turns. The use of the cap can thus bring a lesion into better view and facilitating endoscopic therapy. The cap can also be used to help remove large blood clots, which is facilitated by suction into the rimmed cap [36].

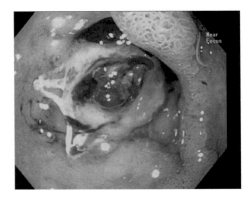

Fig. 2.7 Over-the-scope clip applied to a duodenal ulcer

Doppler Probe

A Doppler probe can be passed through the endoscope's working channel and used to interrogate a bleeding lesion. The probe should be placed in contact with the target lesion with mild pressure and is used in the low or medium depth settings with an auditory signal. The lesion can be interrogated starting at the vessel or center and extending radially in four-quadrants to fully assess the lesion. The Doppler probe can be used before therapy to determine whether there is blood flow in the case of indeterminate lesions (Video 2.1). Following therapy of a bleeding lesion, the Doppler probe can also confirm cessation of blood flow or determine whether there is residual blood flow. It has been shown that lesions with cessation of blood flow following treatment are much less likely to rebleed than those with continued blood flow. It appears that Doppler criteria are better at predicting successful endoscopic treatment than traditional visual criteria, such as flattening of the treated vessel following cautery. Doppler probes have not disseminated widely into clinical use at this time, although this could change going forward.

Recurrent Bleeding

Recurrent bleeding occurs in 10–20% of patients who undergo endoscopic therapy for UGIB. Patients with rebleeding after initial control represent a subset of patients with more severe bleeding associated with a higher mortality. A repeat endoscopy with another attempt at endoscopic therapy should typically be performed in patients with recurrent UGIB [37]. Select patients with severe bleeding, such as with ongoing hemodynamic compromise or bleeding from large arteries or in difficult endoscopic locations, may directly proceed with interventional radiology/angiography or surgery. However, the majority of patients with rebleeding deserve another endoscopic attempt due to the efficacy of endoscopic therapy and reduced complication rate compared to other interventions.

At the time of an endoscopy for rebleeding, the choice of endoscopic therapy depends on the exact findings. The same therapy as initially given can be applied a second time, or a different therapy can be applied. If a thermal therapy was initially used, hemoclips may be preferable so that the tissue is not further damaged, to decrease the risk of perforation. If hemoclips were initially used, additional hemoclips can be applied or the patient may be treated with thermal therapy without concern for conducting electric current if the metallic clip is inadvertently contacted. An OTSC can also be deployed to control recurrent upper GI bleeding.

Conclusions

Acute upper GI bleeding remains a major source of morbidity and mortality. It is also responsible for a large number of hospitalizations and significant healthcare expenditure in the USA. While the majority of patients with acute upper GI bleeding will spontaneously stop bleeding, patients with ongoing or severe bleeding or high-risk stigmata of recent hemorrhage require endoscopic therapy. There are a multitude of tools that can be used to endoscopically identify, treat, and prevent bleeding. It is important for endoscopists to be familiar with all available resources in order to optimally manage patients with acute upper GI bleeding.

References

1. Abougergi MS, Travis AC, Saltzman JR. The in-hospital mortality rate for upper GI hemorrhage has decreased over 2 decades in the United States: a nationwide analysis. Gastrointest Endosc. 2015;81 (4):882–8.
2. Barkun AN, Bardou M, Kuipers EJ, et al. International Consensus Upper Gastrointestinal Bleeding Conference Group. International consensus recommendations on the management of patients with nonvariceal upper gastrointestinal bleeding. Ann Intern Med. 2010;152(2):101–13.
3. Laine L, Jensen DM. Management of patients with ulcer bleeding. Am J Gastroenterol. 2012;107:345–60.
4. Dworzynski K, Pollit V, Kelset A, et al. Management of acute upper gastrointestinal bleeding: summary of NICE guidance. BMJ. 2012;344:e3412.
5. Gralnek IM, Dumonceau JM, Kuipers EJ, et al. Diagnosis and management of nonvariceal upper gastrointestinal hemorrhage: European Society of Gastrointestinal Endoscopy (ESGE) Guideline. Endoscopy. 2015;47(10):a1–46.
6. Sung JJ, Chan FK, Chen M, et al. Asia-Pacific Working Group consensus on non-variceal upper gastrointestinal bleeding. Gut. 2011;60:1170–7.
7. Hwang JH, Fisher DA, Ben-Menachem T, et al. Standards of practice Committee of the American Society for Gastrointestinal Endoscopy. The role of endoscopy in the management of acute non-variceal upper GI bleeding. Gastrointest Endosc. 2012;75:1132–8.
8. Simon TG, Travis AC, Saltzman JR. Initial assessment and resuscitation in nonvariceal upper gastrointestinal bleeding. Gastrointest Endosc Clin N Am. 2015;25(3):429–42.
9. Kumar NL, Travis AC, Saltzman JR. Initial management and timing of endoscopy in nonvariceal upper GI bleeding. Gastrointest Endosc. 2016;84(1):10–7.
10. Villanueva C, Colomo A, Bosch A, et al. Transfusion strategies for acute upper gastrointestinal bleeding. N Engl J Med. 2013;368 (1):11–21.
11. Huang ES, Karsan S, Kanwal F, et al. Impact of nasogastric lavage on outcomes in acute GI bleeding. Gastrointest Endosc. 2011;74:971–80.
12. Khuroo MS, Yatoo GN, Javid G, et al. A comparison of omeprazole and placebo for bleeding peptic ulcer. N Engl J Med. 1997;336:1054–8.

13. Lau JY, Sung JJ, Lee KK, et al. Effect of intravenous omeprazole on recurrent bleeding after endoscopic treatment of bleeding peptic ulcers. N Engl J Med. 2000;343:310–6.

14. Lau JY, Leung WK, Wu JC, et al. Omeprazole before endoscopy in patients with gastrointestinal bleeding. N Engl J Med. 2007;356:1631–40.

15. Sachar H, Vaidya K, Laine L. Intermittent vs Continuous proton pump inhibitor therapy for high-risk bleeding ulcers. A systematic review and meta-analysis. JAMA Intern Med. 2014;174(11):1755–62.

16. Sung JJ, Suen BY, Wu JC, et al. Effects of intravenous and oral esomeprazole in the prevention of recurrent bleeding from peptic ulcers after endoscopic therapy. Am J Gastroenterol. 2014;109 (7):1005–10.

17. Wolf AT, Wasan SK, Saltzman JR. Impact of anticoagulation on rebleeding following endoscopic therapy for nonvariceal upper gastrointestinal hemorrhage. Am J Gastroenterol. 2007;102 (2):290–6.

18. Sung JJ, Lau JY, Ching JY, et al. Continuation of low-dose aspirin therapy in peptic ulcer bleeding: a randomized trial. Ann Intern Med. 2010;152(1):1–9.

19. Witt DM, Delate T, Garcia DA, et al. Risk of thromboembolism, recurrent hemorrhage, and death after warfarin therapy interruption for gastrointestinal tract bleeding. Arch Intern Med. 2012;172 (19):1484–91.

20. Blatchford O, Murray WR, Blatchford M. A risk score to predict need for treatment for upper-gastrointestinal haemorrhage. Lancet. 2000;356:1318.

21. Saltzman JR, Tabak YP, Hyett BH, Sun X, Travis AC, Johannes RS. A simple risk score accurately predicts in-hospital mortality, length of stay, and cost in acute upper GI bleeding. Gastrointest Endosc. 2011;74:1215–24.

22. Hyett BH, Abougergi MS, Charpentier JP, Kumar NL, Brozovic S, Claggett BL, et al. The AIMS65 score compared with the Glasgow-Blatchford score in predicting outcomes in upper GI bleeding. Gastrointest Endosc. 2013;77:551–7.

23. Mustafa Z, Cameron A, Clark E, Stanley AJ. Outpatient management of low-risk patients with upper gastrointestinal bleeding: can we safely extend the Glasgow Blatchford Score in clinical practice? Eur J Gastroenterol Hepatol. 2015;27(5):512–5.

24. Abougergi MS, Charpentier JP, Bethea E, et al. A Prospective, multicenter study of the AIMS65 score compared with the Glasgow-Blatchford score in predicting upper gastrointestinal hemorrhage outcomes. J Clin Gastroenterol. 2016;50(6):464–9.

25. Jensen DM, Kovacs TO, Jutabha R, et al. Randomized trial of medical or endoscopic therapy to prevent recurrent ulcer hemorrhage in patients with adherent clots. Gastroenterology. 2002;123:407–13.

26. Barkun AN, Bardou M, Martel M, Gralnek IM, Sung JJ. Prokinetics in acute upper GI bleeding: a meta-analysis. Gastrointest Endosc. 2010;72:1138–45.

27. Bucci C, Rotondano G, Marmo R. Injection and cautery methods for nonvariceal bleeding control. Gastrointest Endosc Clin N Am. 2015;25(3):509–22.

28. Saltzman JR, Thiesen A, Liu JJ. Determination of optimal monopolar coagulation settings for upper GI bleeding in a pig model. Gastrointest Endosc. 2010;72:796–801.

29. Saltzman JR, Strate LL, Di Sena V, et al. Prospective trial of endoscopic clips versus combination therapy in upper GI bleeding (PROTECCT–UGI bleeding). Am J Gastroenterol. 2005;100 (7):1503–8.

30. Brock AS, Rockey DC. Mechanical hemostasis techniques in nonvariceal upper gastrointestinal bleeding. Gastrointest Endosc Clin N Am. 2015;25(3):523–33.

31. Manta R, Galloro G, Mangiavillano B, et al. Over-the-scope clip (OTSC) represents an effective endoscopic treatment for acute GI bleeding after failure of conventional techniques. Surg Endosc. 2013;27:3162–4.

32. Barkun AN, Moosavi S, Martel M. Topical hemostatic agents: a systematic review with particular emphasis on endoscopic application in GI bleeding. Gastrointest Endosc. 2013;77(5):692–700.

33. Chen YI, Barkun AN. Hemostatic powders in gastrointestinal bleeding: a systematic review. Gastrointest Endosc Clin N Am. 2015;25(3):535–52.

34. Yau AHL, Ou G, et al. Safety and efficacy of Hemospray® in upper gastrointestinal bleeding. Can J Gastroenterol Hepatol. 2014;28(2):72–6.

35. Rajala MW, Ginsberg GG. Tips and tricks on how to optimally manage patients with upper gastrointestinal bleeding. Gastrointest Endosc Clin N Am. 2015;25(3):607–17.

36. Moreels TG, et al. Distal cap to facilitate removal of blood clots during endoscopic hemostasis for upper gastrointestinal bleeding. Endoscopy. 06/2009; 41 Suppl 2:E152.

37. Lau JY, Sung JJ, Lam YH, Chan AC, et al. Endoscopic retreatment compared with surgery in patients with recurrent bleeding after initial endoscopic control of bleeding ulcers. N Engl J Med. 1999;340(10):751–6.

Variceal Upper GI Bleeding

3

Jianhua Andy Tau and Waqar A. Qureshi

Abstract

Variceal hemorrhage is one the most harrowing situations encountered by GI fellows in training. It will be encountered frequently and emergently. Management of acute variceal hemorrhage demands sound endoscopic technique, prompt resuscitation, and medical therapy with antibiotics and somatostatin analogues. Despite advances in techniques and algorithms, the mortality rate and re-bleeding rate associated with variceal hemorrhage remain high. The Child-Pugh class, size of the varix, and endoscopic presence of high-risk stigmata determine the choice between non-selective beta blocker (NSBB) and endoscopic variceal ligation in the primary prevention of esophageal hemorrhage, while secondary prevention requires both. Proper dosing and tolerance of NSBB is challenging but can preclude further endoscopic surveillance. Gastric varices are defined by their location. They are less common, but more challenging. Glue injection and TIPS are currently the prominent tools used in both acute hemorrhage and secondary prevention, while primary prevention is typically avoided.

Esophageal Varices

Gastroesophageal variceal hemorrhage is one of the most common fatal complications of cirrhosis. Advancements in medical therapies along with guidelines from multiple societies have reduced mortality due to variceal hemorrhage from 40 to 15% over the past two decades [1, 2].

The development of gastroesophageal varices (GOV) correlates with the severity of cirrhosis (Child-Pugh Class),

Electronic supplementary material

Supplementary material is available in the online version of this chapter at 10.1007/978-3-319-49041-0_3. Videos can also be accessed at https://link.springer.com/chapter/10.1007/978-3-319-49041-0_3.

J.A. Tau · W.A. Qureshi (✉)
Department of Medicine, Section of Gastroenterology and Hepatology, Baylor College of Medicine, 7200 Cambridge Street, Ste 10C, Houston, TX 77030, USA
e-mail: waqmd@yahoo.com; wqureshi@bcm.edu

J.A. Tau
e-mail: tau@bcm.edu

and even more directly, the hepatic venous pressure gradient (HPVG), a proxy for the portal pressure. The HPVG is the difference between the wedged hepatic venous pressure and the free hepatic venous pressure. Forty percent of Child A patients will have varices; the incidence doubles to 80% in Child C patients [3]. Likewise, patients with HVPG < 10 mm Hg have virtually no risk of developing variceal hemorrhage, while HPVG > 20 mm Hg predicts higher rates of bleeding, re-bleeding, and mortality [4–6]. Among cirrhotic patients who do not have varices, 7–8% will develop them per year. Among cirrhotic patients who have varices, 5–15% will bleed for the first time per year [7]. Among cirrhotic patients who have bled from varices, 60% will bleed again per year [8, 9] (Fig. 3.1).

Endoscopy plays a critical role in every aspect of the management of patients with varices and variceal hemorrhage including hemostasis of acute hemorrhage, screening, and primary and secondary prophylaxis. While many modalities are under investigation, there are currently no reliable methods of predicting which cirrhotic patients will have esophageal varices without endoscopy [10]. As such, all patients

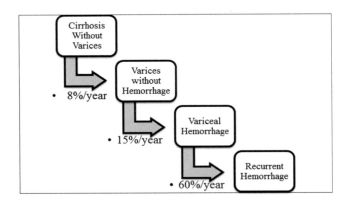

Fig. 3.1 Natural history of portal hypertension: annual risks of varices and variceal

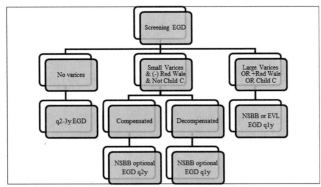

Fig. 3.3 Primary prophylaxis algorithm

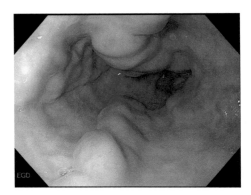

Fig. 3.2 Large (grade 3) esophageal varices

newly diagnosed with cirrhosis should undergo screening endoscopy to assess for varices (Fig. 3.2). The screening endoscopy will determine who to treat, with what to treat, and the how long until the next surveillance endoscopy.

Options for prophylaxis against recurrent bleeding from esophageal varices include non-selective beta blockers and/or endoscopic esophageal variceal ligation (EVL). Non-selective beta blockers (propranolol and nadolol) reduce portal pressures via beta-1 adrenergic blockage of cardiac output and beta-2 adrenergic blockage of splanchnic vasoconstriction. The combination reduces portal pressures. The dose of NSBBs is adjusted to a target heart rate of 50–55 or a decrease in 25% of baseline heart rate. Esophageal variceal ligation is a local therapy at the level of the varices themselves and has no effect whatsoever on portal pressures. As such, NSBBs are in theory useful for the prevention of the two other forms of decompensation from portal hypertension (ascites, hepatic encephalopathy), while EVL prevents only variceal bleeding.

Primary Prophylaxis (Fig. 3.3)

If no esophageal varices are detected on initial screening endoscopy, the suggested surveillance interval is 2–3 years, depending on whether the offending etiology of cirrhosis is resolved or not. If, for example, the offending etiology is alcohol or HCV, and the patient is abstinent or cured, respectively, then an interval of 3 years is acceptable. Non-selective beta blockers are not recommended as a large multicenter randomized controlled trial showed no differences between placebo and non-selective beta blockers in preventing the development of varices [11]. The goal for these patients is to prevent decompensation by treating the root cause of cirrhosis and any other offending processes—including obesity, alcohol, and viral hepatitis. Recent studies suggest statins may also be of benefit in cirrhosis by decreasing fibrogenesis, improving liver microcirculation, and decreasing portal pressure in cirrhosis [12]. If at any time these patients develop decompensated cirrhosis—ascites, hepatic encephalopathy, or variceal bleeding—they should undergo EGD at that time, and EGD should be repeatedly annually. Simply speaking, once a cirrhotic patient develops ascites, variceal hemorrhage, or hepatic encephalopathy, they should undergo annual variceal screening on a lifelong basis or until they undergo liver transplantation.

If esophageal varices are detected on screening EGD, three specific parameters should be noted and documented, as they determine risk of hemorrhage (high versus low) and thus the choice of prophylaxis:

(1) Size (small, <5 mm; large, >5 mm)
(2) Red wale marks or other high-risk stigmata (cherry red spot, white nipple sign)
(3) Child-Pugh Class.

Table 3.1 Pros and cons of NSBB versus EVL

		NSBB	EVL
Pros		1. Low cost	1. Done at screening EGD
		2. No repeat EGD risk (never again)	2. Fewer contraindications
		3. Reduces portal HTN (ascites/HE)	3. Fewer side effects
			4. No titration
Cons		1. 15% intolerance	1. Post-EVL ulcer bleeding
		2. 15% contraindication	2. Repeat EGD risk
		3. Under dosing (HR > 55)	3. Cost of endoscopy
		4. Indefinite therapy	4. Does not reduce portal HTN (ascites/HE)

High-risk patients are defined as patients with:

- Medium/large varices (>5 mm) regardless of red wale or Child Class
  or
- Small varices (<5 mm) with red wale signs/stigmata
  or
- Small varices (<5 mm) in a Child C patient.

Low-risk patients are defined as patients with:

- Small varices (<5 mm) without red wale signs/stigmata in a Child A patient.

Primary prophylaxis in high-risk patients can administered be via either non-selective beta blockers (NSBB) or (not and) endoscopic variceal ligation (EVL). The decision should be a function of resources, expertise, patient preference, and risks. (Table 3.1).

The pros of NSBB are low cost and none of the risks of endoscopy. Most significantly, once NSBB is initiated appropriately, *no repeat endoscopy is required*. The cons include a relative or absolute contraindication rate of over 15% (bradycardia, hypotension, peripheral vascular disease, asthma, insulin-dependent diabetes, refractory ascites, SBP), while another 15% of patients simply stop due to intolerance from side effects (most commonly dizziness, fatigue, weakness, sexual side effects, or dyspnea). NSBB should likely be avoided in patients with refractory ascites or spontaneous bacterial peritonitis as studies have shown increased mortality in these subsets of patients [13, 14]. In addition, treatment is life long, as discontinuation results in return of bleeding risk. Propranolol has a higher side effect rate (17%) than nadolol (10%) [15]. The other risk is inadequate dose titration to reach a resting heart rate 50–55 or decrease in baseline heart rate by 25%.

The benefit of EVL is that it can be done at the time of screening EGD, and there is a lower adverse event rates than NSBB (4% versus 13%). However, the adverse events are more serious, specifically bleeding from ligation-induced ulcers, which have in rare cases been fatal. In addition, once started, repeat EVL must be done within 2–4 weeks until varices are obliterated, then another EGD in 1–3 months to

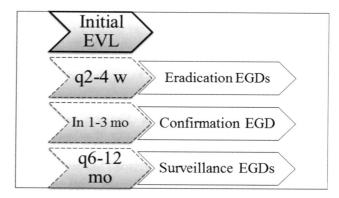

Fig. 3.4 EVL follow up

ensure obliteration, and finally, every 6–12 months to check for recurrence (Fig. 3.4). In general, it is reasonable to start patients without contraindications on NSBB, and if they cannot tolerate them, switch to the EVL option. Among the subpopulation of patients who have small varices with red wales or Child C Class (Group 2 and 3 above), EVL may be technically more difficult given the smaller variceal size so NSBB is preferred over EVL. Among the subpopulation of patients with medium/large varices without red wale signs or Child C Class, NSBB are preferred over EVL, as well.

Primary prophylaxis in low-risk patients is considered optional with non-selective beta blocker to reduce the progression to large varices. There is no long-term evidence to back this recommendation currently. There is no role for EVL. For these patients, upper endoscopy every 1–2 years is recommended. If patients have no signs of decompensation, EGD every 2 years is reasonable. If patients have decompensated cirrhosis, surveillance EGD every year is indicated. As with high-risk patients, if any signs of decompensation develop, they are to have endoscopy at the time of decompensation and repeat endoscopy every year.

Acute Esophageal Variceal Hemorrhage

The patient with active variceal hemorrhage should be admitted to the intensive care unit for immediate circulatory resuscitation, intubation in patients with hematemesis or severe encephalopathy or difficulties protecting their airway, and close hemodynamic monitoring. Endoscopy should be done as soon as possible (usually taken to mean <12 h). Crystalloid or albumin infusions should be used to achieve and maintain hemodynamic stability and tissue perfusion. Red blood cell transfusion should aim for a Hgb 7–8 g/dL. Liberal transfusion strategies targeting Hb 9–11 g/dL have been shown in a randomized controlled trial to be associated with increased mortality likely due to increased portal pressures [16]. There are no specific guidelines concerning transfusion targets for INR or platelets in these patients, but their use as adjunctive therapy to achieve hemostasis is reasonable. There is, in general, no coagulopathy or thrombocytopenia so severe as to preclude endoscopic attempts at hemostasis.

Beyond adequate resuscitation, there is perhaps no medical therapy more beneficial than antibiotics in the bleeding cirrhotic patient. Antibiotic prophylaxis decreases sepsis, recurrence of bleeding, and death [17]. The number needed to treat (NNT) is 4 to prevent sepsis and 22 to prevent death [18]. The most commonly used agents are third-generation cephalosporins (Ceftriaxone 1 g IV every 24 h), given high rates of quinolone resistance in the USA and among this patient population who are often on SBP prophylaxis with quinolones.

Along with antibiotics, intravenous vasoactive medications (Terlipressin, Somatostatin, Octreotide) should be started prior to endoscopy. Octreotide is the only available formulation in the USA. It has been shown to control acute hemorrhage and decrease transfusion requirements, but its effect on mortality is less convincing. [19]. Vasoactive medications should be continued for up to 5 days, because this is the peak period of recurrent hemorrhage, though they can be stopped 24 h after the last evidence of hemorrhage. Upon discontinuation of vasoactive medications, the patient should transition seamlessly to NSBBs or TIPS before discharge if appropriate in selected patients. Pre-procedure intravenous erythromycin may help clear the stomach of blood and clots.

There are two endoscopic therapies for esophageal varices—esophageal variceal ligation (EVL) and endoscopic sclerotherapy (EST).

Endoscopic Sclerotherapy (EST)

EST involves injecting a sclerosing agent into the variceal lumen or immediately adjacent to the varix. EST controls acute variceal bleeding in 70% of patients [20]. There are wide range of sclerosants including sodium tetradecyl sulfate, sodium morrhuate, ethanol, polidocanol, and ethanolamine oleate.

Injections begin distally near the cardia, starting below any bleeding site and working upward in a spiral manner. The sclerosant is injected in 1–3 mL volumes at a time per varix via a needle tip catheter through the working channel of the endoscope. The sclerosant induces thrombosis immediately upon entering the vessel, while adjacent injection creates a tamponade effect via edema and inflammation of adjacent tissue. Overtime, these areas develop fibrosis and obliterate the varix. If bleeding occurs immediately upon retraction of the needle, tamponade can be achieved by simply advancing the endoscope into the stomach and using the body of the endoscope to tamponade.

EST is advantageous for its low cost and no need for second oral intubation like EVL. However, it is less effective and, most importantly, has a much higher complication rate than EVL, specifically more early re-bleeding and esophageal strictures. Other adverse events of EST include fever, retrosternal discomfort/pain, dysphagia, esophageal perforation, mediastinitis, pleural effusion, bronchoesophageal fistula, acute respiratory distress syndrome, and infection. Bacteremia is not uncommon following EST. Endoscopic sclerotherapy is reserved for situations in which EVL is not technically feasible or has failed, and is no longer recommended for secondary prophylaxis of variceal hemorrhage.

Esophageal Variceal Ligation (EVL)

Esophageal variceal ligation (banding) is the endoscopic therapy of choice for controlling esophageal variceal hemorrhage (see Video 3.1 and Figs. 3.5 and 3.6). EVL is superior to endoscopic sclerotherapy in regards to recurrent bleeding, local adverse events including ulceration and stricture formation, time to variceal obliteration, and survival [21]. The band ligator consists a friction-fitting transparent cylindrical cap preloaded with elastic bands, which attaches

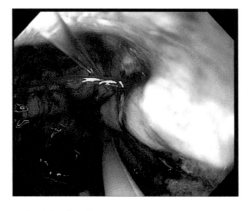

Fig. 3.5 Active bleeding from an esophageal varix

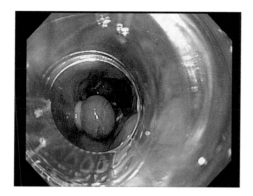

Fig. 3.6 View of a varix post-banding

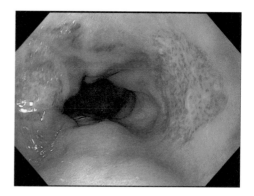

Fig. 3.7 Post-banding ulcers seen two weeks after banding

over the endoscope tip; a spool that fits onto the biopsy port via a Velcro strap; and a trip wire connecting the two, which is passed up through the endoscopic channel.

The procedure involves two intubations. First, a thorough diagnostic upper GI evaluation is done to identify all sources of bleeding and specifically to identify the size, number of esophageal varices, and any high-risk stigmata (wales, white nipple, etc.). The endoscope is withdrawn, and the band ligator is attached onto the endoscope. After re-intubation, banding begins distally from the GE junction upwards, often in a spiral pattern. Starting distally allows for complete visualization and avoids the potential risk of dislodging a band during advancement of the endoscope past a previously captured varix. Once the bulging varix is visualized, the tip is pointed toward it and continuous suction is applied, prolapsing the varix into the cap. Once the screen "reds out," the spool is twisted and the trip wire releases one of the loaded bands over the varix. Active bleeding or high risk stigmata for bleeding (white nipple/fibrin cap or red wale signs) are the ideal targets for banding. During variceal-band ligation, transient bleeding can occur because of rupture of the varix, but this is usually self limited. The procedure is repeated for each column of varices, moving upwards in a spiral fashion until all columns of varices are flattened, which is ideally achieved before reaching the mid-esophagus. Patient can be placed on liquid diet after the procedure for the first 12–24 h, and then advanced as tolerated. Placement of a naso-gastric tube is typically avoided lest the bands are dislodged, though there is no evidence to our knowledge to support this.

After 3–5 days, ligated sites inevitably slough and produce consistent shallow ulcerations from 3 to 7 days after application (Figs. 3.7 and 3.8). Early re-bleeding occurs in about 10–20% of patients and the majority occurs within the first 5 days. The bleeding is typically due to post-EVL induced ulcers in the setting of high portal pressure, which appears to occur more commonly in patients undergoing EVL after an episode of acute bleeding, with reports as high as 14% [22]. Ligation-induced ulcers heal at a mean of

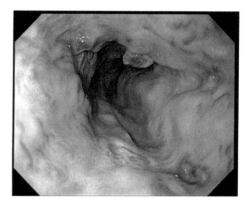

Fig. 3.8 In this photograph, a post-banding ulcer is seen at 6 o'clock while numerous red areas called "wale signs" are seen

14 days compared with 21 days for those resulting from sclerotherapy [23]. Proton pump inhibitors may decrease post-EVL ulcer size but have not been demonstrated to significantly reduce bleeding risk [24].

Endoscopy should be repeated every 2–4 weeks until varices have been eradicated, which typically requires 2–4 sessions [25]. Then a follow-up EGD should be performed in 1–3 months after obliteration and then every 6–12 months thereafter [26].

Salvage Therapy

For patients in whom all the above attempts at hemostasis have failed or who re-bleed (10–20%), balloon tamponade and covered self-expanding metals stents (SEMS) can be temporizing measures until TIPS can be placed (<24 h). Balloon tamponade is effective in temporarily achieving hemostasis in over 80% of cases but carries an alarming 20% mortality rate from aspiration, asphyxiation due to upward migration into the airway, or esophageal perforation. In addition, bleeding recurs after deflation of the balloon the majority of the time [27]. Intubation for airway protection and sedation is a must when using balloon tamponade. Self-expanding metal stents are feasible, effective, and likely safer, but require technical experience and risk migration [28–30]. Patients with early re-bleeding after initial EVL should typically have another endoscopic attempt at hemostasis. TIPS is the final salvage pathway for all patients with refractory esophageal hemorrhage regardless of history of hepatic encephalopathy [31]. Success rates are variable and highly based on local expertise.

Secondary Prophylaxis

Once a patient has had an episode of variceal hemorrhage, they have a 60% of re-bleeding annually without prophylaxis. When they do re-bleed, they die one third of the time [32, 33]. Besides those who have contraindications to NSBBs or are post-TIPS, all patients who survive variceal hemorrhage should in theory receive the combination of NSBBs and (not or) EVL. NSBB should be started *prior* to leaving the hospital, and as early as 24 h from the last evidence of bleeding. The immediate addition of NSBB after EVL and 5 days of Octreotide decreases re-bleeding significantly (38–14%) [34].

If TIPS is used to control the acute hemorrhage, no further prophylaxis is indicated as portal pressures should have normalized, though re-evaluation of TIPS via dedicated doppler ultrasound every 6 months to ensure patency is indicated. In general, TIPS should not be used as a first-line therapy. Even though bleeding is reduced with TIPS compared to medical therapy, there is significant increase in costs and rates of hepatic encephalopathy, less improvement in Child-Pugh class, and identical survival rates [35]. TIPS should be reserved for those who fail both NSBB and EVL or potentially two subpopulations who have shown mortality benefit with TIPS as secondary prophylaxis: Child C (Score < 14) and Child B patients with active hemorrhage at time of endoscopy [36, 37].

Finally, addition of a long acting nitrate (isosorbide mononitrate) to NSBBs is not recommended because the combination has more side effects (headache, dizziness) without superiority with respect to bleeding or mortality [38].

Gastric Varices

Gastric varices (GV) are rare relative to esophageal varices, and thus, available data to guide our medical decisions concerning GV is not as robust as it is for esophageal varices. GV are classified according to their location within the stomach (Sarin Classification), as either GOV or isolated

gastric varices (IGV). GOV are divided into GOV1, which are esophageal varices that extend below the gastroesophageal junction along the lesser curve of the stomach, and GOV2, which are those that extend beyond the gastroesophageal junction into the fundus of the stomach. IGV are divided into IGV1, which are those located in the fundus (aka fundal varices), and IGV2, which are isolated ectopic varices located anywhere else in the stomach. GOV1 account for 75%, GOV2 21%, IGV1 less than 2%, and IGV2 4% of all GVs [39].

Primary Prophylaxis

The incidence of bleeding among cardiofundal varices is 16, 36, and 44% at 1, 3, and 5 years, respectively [40]. However, primary prophylaxis for GV is not recommended at this time due to lack of data. The most common practice when GV are detected for the first time is to "look but don't touch."

Acute Gastric Variceal Hemorrhage

Patients with acute gastric variceal bleeding receive the same medical therapy as described above for esophageal varices, specifically ICU admission, resuscitation with restrictive transfusion strategy, antibiotics, and vasoactive medications. However, in terms of endoscopic therapy, GOV1 specifically differ from all other GV. A bleeding GOV1, which is an extension of an esophageal varix, is treated as esophageal varix with EVL, while all other gastric varices (IGV1, IGV2, GOV2) are treated with tissue adhesives (cyanoacrylate or fibrin glue) and not EVL. There is scant data on therapy for IGV2, but in general, most experts treat them like IGV1. The main complications from cyanoacrylate injections include re-bleeding from glue cast extruding early (4.4%), sepsis (1.3%), and embolic phenomenon (0.7–3%) [41]. Embolic complications can be fatal in some cases. The complication-related mortality is 0.5%.

At our institution, cyanoacrylate is injected with lipiodol in a 1:1 ratio with 1 ml aliquots per varix injection. The lipiodol (poppy-seed oil) is radio-opaque and can be watched under fluoroscopy to make embolization less likely while delaying the polymerization time of the cyanoacrylate. A few months after injection, the cyanoacrylate is naturally extruded into the stomach lumen [42]. Most case series report >90% success rates with the use of tissue adhesives like cyanoacrylate [43] (see Figs. 3.9 and 3.10 to see pre- and post-glue injection of gastric varices and Video 3.2. Figure 3.11 shows an actively bleeding gastric varix). Cyanoacrylate may be injected under EUS guidance and some used coils with glue.

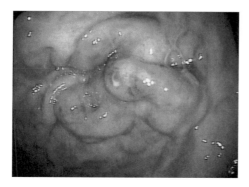

Fig. 3.9 This photograph shows gastric varices pre-glue injection with stigmata of recent bleeding

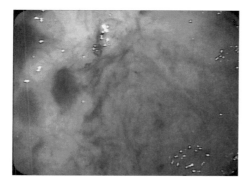

Fig. 3.10 This photograph shows the gastric varices post-glue injection. The gastric varices frequently collapse once glue is injected and blood can no longer flow through the varices

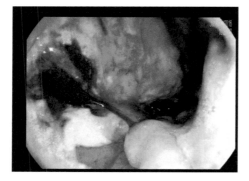

Fig. 3.11 A bleeding gastric varix is seen in a stomach with food. This patient had endotracheal intubation so that banding could be performed safely

Salvage Therapy

If refractory or re-bleeding occurs, balloon tamponade can be used as a bridge to TIPS, which is the salvage treatment of choice in patients bleeding from cardiofundal varices, GOV2, and IGV1. The larger Linton–Nachlas tube is preferred over the Sengstaken–Blakemore tube because of the

Table 3.2 Endoscopic pearls for EVL, endoscopic sclerotherapy, cyanoacrylate injection

EVL	Endoscopic sclerotherapy	Cyanoacrylate injection
1. Procedure of choice in esophageal varices 2. Avoid use in gastric varices, except GOV1 3. Avoid use in rectal varices	1. Use only when EVL not possible 2. Higher incidence of post procedure pain 3. Causes transient dysphagia, chest pain	1. Effective for bleeding gastric varices 2. Can be used in duodenal and rectal varices 3. Not cleared for use by the FDA in the US

large volume (600 mL) of its single gastric balloon, allowing an appropriate compression of the fundal varices [44]. Contrary to what is suggested in esophageal variceal bleeding, a second-attempt endoscopic therapy is usually not considered and patients usually undergo TIPS with early re-bleeding [45].

Secondary Prophylaxis

Re-bleeding rates in most large series range from 10 to 20% [43]. After successful hemostasis, secondary prophylaxis with repeat sessions performed every 2–4 weeks is indicated until obliteration is achieved. Usually, this takes 2–4 sessions. Cyanoacrylate injections may be superior to NSBB alone in preventing re-bleeding [46]. While addition of NSBB to serial cyanoacrylate injections for GV does not seem to add any additional protection from re-bleeding [47], given that many patients have concomitant EV and GV, NSBBs are still recommended and used as an adjunct to endoscopic therapy for secondary prophylaxis. TIPS is a very effective therapy to prevent GV re-bleeding, but TIPS-treated patients have more hepatic encephalopathy and long-term morbidity requiring hospitalization [48–50]. Thus, it remains controversial whether TIPS should be universally applied for secondary prophylaxis or reserved as a salvage therapy only.

Conclusion

Varices and, more importantly, variceal bleeding remain common and deadly. In conjunction with prompt resuscitation, antibiotics, and somatostatin analogues, a variety of endoscopic techniques are available treat acute hemorrhage (Table 3.2). Endoscopic therapies remain the first-line treatment for esophageal variceal bleeding, which is the most commonly encountered source of bleeding in patients with portal hypertension. The severity of liver disease, size of the varices, and presence of high-risk stigmata dictate prevention strategies with either non-specific beta blockers, EVL, or both. GV are less commonly treated by endoscopy, but endoscopic options exist in these patients.

References

1. Graham DY, Smith JL. The course of patients after variceal hemorrhage. Gastroenterology. 1981;80(4):800–9.
2. Carbonell N, Pauwels A, Serfaty L, et al. Improved survival after variceal bleeding in patients with cirrhosis over the past two decades. Hepatology. 2004;40:652–9.
3. Pagliaro L, D'Amico G, Pasta L, Politi F, Vizzini G, Traina M, et al. Portal hypertension in cirrhosis: Natural history. In: Bosch J, Groszmann RJ, editors. Portal Hypertension. Pathophysiology and treatment. Oxford, UK: Blackwell Scientific; 1994. p. 72–92.
4. Groszmann RJ, Bosch J, Grace N, Conn HO, Garcia-Tsao G, Navasa M, et al. Hemodynamic events in a prospective randomized trial of propranolol vs placebo in the prevention of the first variceal hemorrhage. Gastroenterology. 1990;99:1401–7.
5. Moitinho E, Escorsell A, Bandi JC, Salmeron JM, Garcia-Pagan JC, Rodes J, et al. Prognostic value of early measurements of portal pressure in acute variceal bleeding. Gastroenterology. 1999;117:626–31.
6. Monescillo A, Martinez-Lagares F, Ruiz del Arbol L, Sierra A, Guevara C, Jimenez E, et al. Influence of portal hypertension and its early decompression by TIPS placement on the outcome of variceal bleeding. Hepatology. 2004;40:793–801.
7. Merli M, Nicolini G, Angeloni S, Rinaldi V, De Santis A, Merkel C, et al. Incidence and natural history of small esophageal varices in cirrhotic patients. J Hepatol. 2003;38:266–72.
8. Bosch J, Garcia-Pagan JC. Prevention of variceal rebleeding. Lancet. 2003;361:952–4.
9. D'Amico G, Pagliaro L, Bosch J. Pharmacological treatment of portal hypertension: an evidence-based approach. Semin Liver Dis. 1999;19:475–505.
10. Riggio O, Angeloni S, Nicolini G, et al. Endoscopic screening for esophageal varices in cirrhotic patients. Hepatology. 2002;35:501–2.
11. Groszmann RJ, Garcia-Tsao G, Bosch J, et al. for the Portal hypertension collaborative group. Beta-blockers to prevent gastroesophageal varices in patients with cirrhosis. N Engl J Med 2005;353:2254–61.
12. Abraldes JG, Albillos A, Banares R, et al. Simvastatin lowers portal pressure in patients with cirrhosis and portal hypertension: a randomized controlled trial. Gastroenterology. 2009;136:1651–8.
13. Serste T, Melot C, Francoz C, et al. Deleterious effects of beta blockers on survival in patients with cirrhosis and refractory ascites. Hepatology. 2010;52:1017–22.
14. Mandorfer M, et al. Nonselective β blockers increase risk for hepatorenal syndrome and death in patients with cirrhosis and spontaneous bacterial peritonitis. Gastroenterology. 146(7):1680–90.
15. Bolognesi M, Balducci G, Garcia-Tsao G, Gatta A, Gines P, Merli M, et al. Complications in the medical treatment of portal hypertension. Portal hypertension III. Proceedings of the third Baveno international consensus workshop on definitions, methodology and therapeutic strategies. Oxford, UK: Blackwell Science; 2001. p. 180–203.
16. Villanueva C, Colomo A, Bosch A, et al. Transfusion strategies for acute upper gastrointestinal bleeding. N Engl J Med. 2013;368:11–21.
17. Bernard B, Grange JD, Khac EN, et al. Antibiotic prophylaxis for the prevention of bacterial infections in cirrhotic patients with gastrointestinal bleeding: a meta-analysis. Hepatology. 1999;29:1655–61.
18. Chavez-Tapia NC, Barrientos-Gutierrez T, Tellez-Avila FI, Soares-Weiser K, Uribe M. Antibiotic prophylaxis for cirrhotic patients with upper gastrointestinal bleeding. Cochrane Database Syst Rev. 2010;(9):CD002907. Review. PubMed PMID: 20824832.
19. Wells M, Chande N, Adams P, et al. Meta-analysis: vasoactive medications for the management of acute variceal bleeds. Aliment Pharmacol Ther. 2012;35:1267–78.
20. Higashi H, Kitano S, Hashizume M, Yamaga H, Sugimachi K. A prospective randomized trial of schedules for sclerosing esophageal varices. 1 versus 2 week intervals. Hepatogastroenterology 1989;36:337–40.
21. Laine L, Cook D. Endoscopic ligation compared with sclerotherapy for treatment of esophageal variceal bleeding. A meta-analysis. Ann Intern Med. 1995;123:280–7.
22. Petrasch F, Grothaus J, Mossner J, et al. Differences in bleeding behavior after endoscopic band ligation: a retrospective analysis. BMC Gastroenterol. 2010;10:5.
23. Young MF, Sanowski RA, Rasche R. Comparison and characterization of ulcerations induced by endoscopic ligation of esophageal varices versus endoscopic sclerotherapy. Gastrointest Endosc. 1993;39:119–22.
24. Shaheen NJ, Stuart E, Schmitz SM, et al. Pantoprazole reduces the size of postbanding ulcers after variceal band ligation: a randomized, controlled trial. Hepatology. 2005;41:588–94.
25. Saeed ZA, Stiegmann GV, Ramirez FC, et al. Endoscopic variceal ligation is superior to combined ligation and sclerotherapy for esophageal varices: a multicenter prospective randomized trial. Hepatology. 1997;25:71–4.
26. Garcia-Tsao G, Bosch J. Varices and variceal hemorrhage in cirrhosis: a new view of an old problem. Clin Gastroenterol Hepatol. 2015;13:2109–17.
27. Avgerinos A, Armonis A. Balloon tamponade technique and efficacy in variceal haemorrhage. Scand J Gastroenterol Suppl. 1994;207:11–6.
28. Dechene A, El Fouly AH, Bechmann LP, Jochum C, Saner FH, Gerken G, et al. Acute management of refractory variceal bleeding in liver cirrhosis by self-expanding metal stents. Digestion. 2012;85(3):185–91.
29. Holster IL, Kuipers EJ, van Buuren HR, Spaander MC, Tjwa ET. Self-expandable metal stents as definitive treatment for esophageal variceal bleeding. Endoscopy. 2013;45(6):485–8.
30. Hsu YC, Chung CS, Tseng CH, Lin TL, Liou JM, Wu MS, et al. Delayed endoscopy as a risk factor for in-hospital mortality in cirrhotic patients with acute variceal hemorrhage. J Gastroenterol Hepatol. 2009;24(7):1294–9.
31. McCormick PA, Dick R, Panagou EB, et al. Emergency transjugular intrahepatic portasystemic stent shunting as salvage treatment for uncontrolled variceal bleeding. Br J Surg. 1994;81:1324–7.
32. D'Amico G, Pagliaro L, Bosch J. Pharmacological treatment of portal hypertension: an evidence-based approach. Semin Liver Dis. 1999;19:475–505.
33. Bosch J, Garcia-Pagan JC. Prevention of variceal rebleeding. Lancet. 2003;361:952–4.
34. de la Pena J, Brullet E, Sanchez-Hernandez E, et al. Variceal ligation plus nadolol compared with ligation for prophylaxis of variceal rebleeding: a multicenter trial. Hepatology. 2005;41:572–8.
35. Escorsell A, Banares R, Garcia-Pagan JC, Gilabert R, Moitinho E, Piqueras B, et al. TIPS versus drug therapy in preventing variceal rebleeding in advanced cirrhosis: a randomized controlled trial. Hepatology. 2002;35:385–92.
36. Garcia-Pagan JC, Caca K, Bureau C, et al. Early use of TIPS in patients with cirrhosis and variceal bleeding. N Engl J Med. 2010;362:2370–9.

37. Garcia-Pagan JC, Di Pascoli M, Caca K, et al. Use of early-TIPS for high-risk variceal bleeding: results of a post-RCT surveillance study. J Hepatol. 2013;58:45–50.
38. Gluud LL, Langholz E, Krag A. Meta-analysis: isosorbidemononitrate alone or with either beta-blockers or endoscopic therapy for the management of oesophageal varices. Aliment Pharmacol Ther. 2010;32:859–71.
39. Sarin SK, Lahoti D, Saxena SP, et al. Prevalence, classification and natural history of gastric varices: a long-term follow-up study in 568 portal hypertension patients. Hepatology. 1992;16:1343–9.
40. Kim T, Shijo H, Kokawa H, et al. Risk factors for hemorrhage from gastric fundal varices. Hepatology. 1997;25:307–12.
41. Cheng LF, Wang ZQ, Li CZ, et al. Low incidence of complications from endoscopic gastric variceal obturation with butyl cyanoacrylate. Clin Gastroenterol Hepatol. 2010;8:760–6.
42. Wang YM, Cheng LF, Li N, et al. Study of glue extrusion after endoscopic N-butyl-2-cyanoacrylate injection on gastric variceal bleeding. World J Gastroenterol. 2009;15:4945–51.
43. Garcia-Pagan JC, et al. Management of Gastric Varices. Clinical Gastroenterology and Hepatology. 2014;12:919–28.
44. Teres J, Cecilia A, Bordas JM, et al. Esophageal tamponade for bleeding varices: controlled trial between the Sengstaken-Blakemore tube and the Linton-Nachlas tube. Gastroenterology. 1978;75:566–9.
45. Chau TN, Patch D, Chan YW, et al. "Salvage" transjugular intrahepatic portosystemic shunts: gastric fundal compared with esophageal variceal bleeding. Gastroenterology. 1998;114:981–7.
46. Mishra SR, Chander SB, Kumar A, et al. Endoscopic cyanoacrylate injection versus beta-blocker for secondary prophylaxis of gastric variceal bleed: a randomised controlled trial. Gut. 2010;59:729–35.
47. Hung HH, Chang CJ, Hou MC, et al. Efficacy of non-selective beta-blockers as adjunct to endoscopic prophylactic treatment for gastric variceal bleeding: a randomized controlled trial. J Hepatol. 2012;56:1025–32.
48. Mahadeva S, Bellamy MC, Kessel D, et al. Cost effectiveness of N-butyl-2-cyanoacrylate (Histoacryl) glue injections versus transjugular intrahepatic portosystemic shunt in the management of acute gastric variceal bleeding. Am J Gastroenterol. 2003;98:2688–93.
49. Lo GH, Liang HL, Chen WC, et al. A prospective, randomized controlled trial of transjugular intrahepatic portosystemic shunt versus cyanoacrylate injection in the prevention of gastric variceal rebleeding. Endoscopy. 2007;39:679–85.
50. Procaccini NJ, Al-Osaimi AM, Northup P, et al. Endoscopic cyanoacrylate versus transjugular intrahepatic portosystemic shunt for gastric variceal bleeding: a single-center US analysis. Gastrointest Endosc. 2009;70:881–7.

Foreign Body Removal

4

Juan Reyes Genere and Uzma D. Siddiqui

Abstract

Foreign bodies in the upper gastrointestinal tract may be the result of intentional ingestion of household objects, unintentional food impaction, or a migrated gastrointestinal device. Managing these foreign bodies hinges on the patient history, physical characteristics of the foreign body, and an assessment of risk for complications. When endoscopic intervention is indicated, determining the timing to intervention and a retrieval strategy are needed. There are many endoscopic retrieval devices and techniques developed to suit the diverse circumstances encountered in gastrointestinal foreign bodies. This chapter discusses the current management and endoscopic retrieval strategies for gastrointestinal foreign bodies.

Introduction

In the USA, there are 100,000 new cases of gastrointestinal foreign bodies reported each year [1]. The majority of these cases (80%) occur in children who unintentionally ingest small objects such as coins, toys, or batteries [1]. Gastrointestinal foreign bodies in adults are less frequent, but their circumstances are diverse. Foreign bodies in adults may be the result of unintentional food impaction, intentional ingestion of household objects, or iatrogenic from gastrointestinal device migration. Managing a gastrointestinal foreign body is a multistep processes that may require endoscopic intervention. Many devices and techniques are available to meet the diverse circumstances of gastrointestinal foreign body retrieval, and they will be discussed in detail in this chapter.

Electronic supplementary material

Supplementary material is available in the online version of this chapter at 10.1007/978-3-319-49041-0_4. Videos can also be accessed at https://link.springer.com/chapter/10.1007/978-3-319-49041-0_4.

J.R. Genere
Department of Medicine, Section of Internal Medicine, University of Chicago Medical Center, 5841 S. Maryland Ave., MC 3051, Chicago, IL 60637, USA
e-mail: juan.reyesgenere@uchospitals.edu

U.D. Siddiqui (✉)
Center for Endoscopic Research and Therapeutics (CERT), Endoscopic Ultrasound (EUS) and Advanced Endoscopy Training, University of Chicago Medical Center, 5700 S. Maryland Avenue, MC 8043, Chicago, IL 60637, USA
e-mail: usiddiqui@bsd.uchicago.edu

Epidemiology

Most gastrointestinal foreign bodies in adults are encountered in the setting of a food bolus or impaction within the esophagus [2, 3]. Food impactions are generally unintentional and occur in patients between 30 and 80 years old, with greater incidence in older patients who are edentulous [3–5]. In up to 52–88% of esophageal food impaction cases, there is underlying esophageal disease [4, 5]. The most common predisposing esophageal condition is a peptic stricture or Schatzki ring (Fig. 4.1) [4–6]. Eosinophilic esophagitis (EoE)-associated food impactions have been increasing over the past 1–2 decades and are seen in up to 30% food impaction cases [7], especially in white males, between 20 and 30 years old [7, 8]. Intentional foreign body ingestions involve swallowing objects such as spoons, razors, and batteries. These types of foreign bodies are strongly associated with children, those with mental illness, intoxicated patients, or for the purpose of secondary gain (i.e., prisoners trying to gain admittance to a medical ward) [3, 9].

Fig. 4.1 Esophageal stricture located distal to an esophageal food impaction that was endoscopically removed

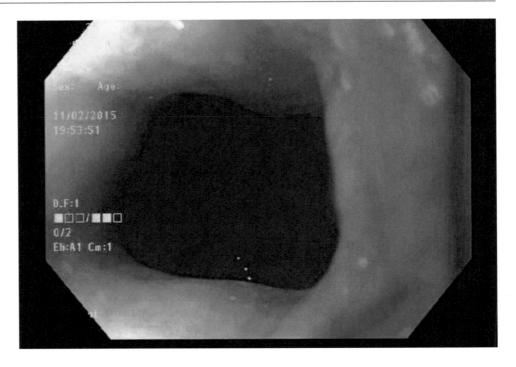

Diagnosis

History and Physical

History is the most important element in diagnosing a gastrointestinal foreign body. Swallowing poorly chewed food, intentionally ingesting a true foreign body, or a history of gastrointestinal device placement can direct diagnostic and therapeutic approach. This is especially important in cases where a foreign body can cause mucosal injury or is unlikely to pass spontaneously [10].

The symptoms of foreign body esophageal impaction include dysphagia 47%, nausea and vomiting 21%, "feeling of food getting stuck" 20%, and chest or epigastric pain 15% [3]. Patients who are present with drooling and inability to manage secretions may have complete esophageal obstruction, which requires emergent endoscopic treatment [10]. Intentionally ingested foreign body may present more often with epigastric pain (55%) or without symptoms at all in 30% of cases [9].

Physical examination should first inspect the oropharynx and assess for hypoxia or respiratory distress, which would suggest a foreign body located in the respiratory tract. Further examination needs to evaluate for complications necessitating surgical intervention, such as acute abdomen, peritonitis, or subcutaneous emphysema of the chest.

Imaging

Plain radiography (X-rays) of the chest, or abdomen, is generally the initial diagnostic test. X-rays can often confirm the presence of a foreign body and characterize the shape, size, and number of objects ingested [11]. Combining posterior-anterior and lateral X-ray views is critical, as this adds another reference point to better localize a foreign body. Foreign bodies diagnosed on a single-view X-ray, on the other hand, may be misleading and delay retrieval (Fig. 4.2). The sensitivity of X-ray is variable (42–90%), with improved sensitivity in the cervical esophagus and intra-abdominal regions [11–13]. The composition of the foreign body must also be considered as radiopaque materials (metal, glass, or stone) can be detected by X-ray, while radiolucent materials (animal bones, food, or plastic) may not [14].

X-ray can also detect signs such as a new pleural effusion, hydrothorax, subcutaneous emphysema, or free air in the abdomen, all of which may indicate a perforation [11]. A prompt surgical consult is indicated if any of these are seen.

CT scans have a much higher sensitivity (97%) than X-ray in detecting foreign bodies [11] and may offer more information in complicated cases. However, even with CT scans, radiolucent materials may still not be visualized [11, 14]. Oral contrast studies are not recommended due to

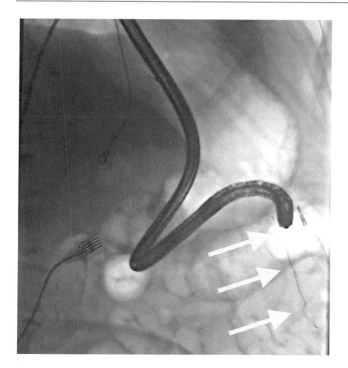

Fig. 4.2 This is a fluoroscopic image taken during an esophagogastroduodenoscopy to evaluate for a migrated esophageal stent (*arrows*). The stent appeared to be located in the proximal small bowel, however, on push enteroscopy (as pictured) no stent was seen. The stent was subsequently found in the descending colon on sigmoidoscopy, and it was successfully removed

associated risk for aspiration in the setting of a high-grade esophageal obstruction. In addition, oral contrast can coat or cover the foreign object which may impair endoscopic removal by obscuring its visibility [10, 15].

Endoscopy

Endoscopy simultaneously confirms the diagnosis and location of a foreign body, as well as providing therapeutic management. Intentionally ingested foreign bodies may require endoscopic intervention up to 76% of the time [10]. Determining the indication and time for endoscopy are the most important aspects of management, and this is a complex, multistep process. In the following sections, the approach to managing foreign bodies will be discussed in detail.

Management

Initial Evaluation

The initial evaluation of a gastrointestinal foreign body should focus on identifying the need for immediate surgical

management. A prompt surgical consult and initiation of antibiotics is necessary for gastrointestinal tract perforation with signs of peritonitis, acute abdomen, pneumomediastinum, or pneumoperitoneum. If there are symptoms of respiratory distress or signs of hypoxia, then airway management with elective intubation may be warranted, as well as consultation with otolaryngology or pulmonary for bronchoscopy. After assessing the need for surgical or pulmonary consultation, the next step is to determine the indication and timing for endoscopic intervention (Fig. 4.3).

Emergent Cases

Emergent endoscopic intervention is required in three types of cases (1) patients presenting with drooling and inability to manage secretions, suggesting complete esophageal obstruction [10]; (2) ingestion of disk batteries, which may cause electrochemical mucosal damage in the esophagus within hours of impaction [10, 16, 17]; (3) sharp objects located in the esophagus, as these are at high risk for mucosal injury [10].

Non-emergent Cases

Time for endoscopic retrieval of a foreign body in non-emergent cases is best before 12–24 h [18, 19]. Waiting to intervene on foreign esophageal impactions longer than this increases complications and reduces the rates of successful endoscopic retrieval [18, 19].

Esophageal foreign bodies are generally an urgent matter [10]. The esophagus is a delicate structure adjacent to vital structures including the pericardium, aorta, and lung pleura. Compromise of the esophageal mucosa integrity can lead to substantial complications from leakage of gastric juices into the mediastinum, to arterial perforation [17]. Special care should be taken in cases of impacted animal bones and objects larger than 3 cm, as these are predictive of esophageal perforation [19]. Blunt objects impacted in the esophagus that are causing symptoms may be the result ongoing ischemic pressure injury and these require expedited removal as well [10]. On the other hand, observation for 12–24 h to monitor for spontaneous passage is appropriate in asymptomatic patients who have ingested blunt objects, such as coins [10].

In the stomach or duodenum, some foreign bodies are still managed urgently [10]. Sharp or pointed objects are associated with the increased risk of perforations up to 35% of the time if left to pass spontaneously [10, 20]. Magnets may lead to mucosal pressure ischemia, perforation, or fistulization if they come into contact with other magnets, or metals, in the gastrointestinal tract [10, 21]. Batteries causing active mucosal injury or objects that may not pass the duodenal sweep (length >6 cm) should also be removed urgently [10].

Fig. 4.3 Algorithm for
managing gastrointestinal foreign
bodies. *. FB that are associated
with mucosal injury or failure of
SP including sharp objects,
damaged batteries, or objects
wider than 2.5 cm. **. FB
indicated for SP are at low risk to
cause mucosal injury or intestinal
obstruction including non-sharp
objects that have passed the
stomach and are <6 cm in length
and <2.5 cm in width. *FB*
Foreign body, *SP* Spontaneous
passage

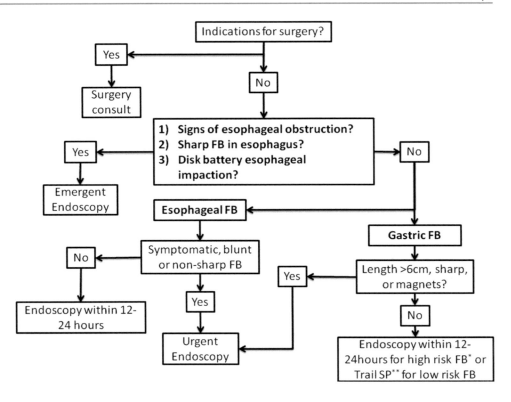

Fig. 4.4 Abdominal X-ray of a
2.2-cm coin located in the
stomach of a 17-month-old male
(*arrow*). This was managed
conservatively with trail of
spontaneous passage and serial
X-rays

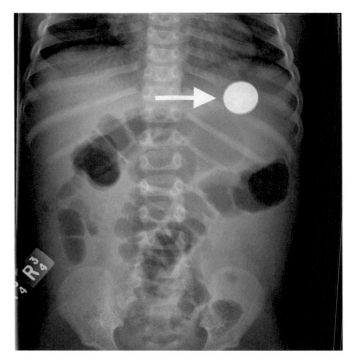

Allowing spontaneous passage is appropriate when a foreign body does not meet criteria for timely removal, has passed the esophagus, and is at low risk to cause obstruction or mucosal injury, as demonstrated in Fig. 4.4 [10, 21, 22]. Monitoring for signs of peritonitis and obtaining periodic X-rays are important to assess the need for retrieval and assure adequate passage over time [10]. The general time intervals indicating that a foreign body has failed to pass and requires retrieval are 3–4 weeks in the stomach and 48 h in the intestines [9, 10]. Exceptions to this apply to batteries (both disk and cylindrical types) in the stomach where failed passage requiring retrieval is at 48 h [10]. Additionally, objects that are wider than 2.5 cm may not pass the pylorus and close monitoring, or non-urgent endoscopic retrieval, should be considered [10].

Medical Therapy

Medical therapies can be used specifically for managing esophageal food impactions, albeit they have a limited role in contemporary practice due to lack of efficacy. Various agents have been used to facilitate the passage of impacted food bolus (including benzodiazepines, calcium channel blockers, anticholinergic, nitrates, and effervescent agents) with the most studied being papain and glucagon [23].

Papain is a proteolytic, trypsin-like enzyme that is diluted in water and administered by mouth to treat meat impactions through its digestive properties [23]. Recently, Morse et al. [24] showed that 87% of protein bolus impaction cases can be successfully treated with oral administration of papain without adverse events [24]. However, papain is not recommended in current guidelines due to historical evidence showing inconclusive efficacy, along with serious adverse events such as aspiration pneumonitis [23, 25].

Glucagon is a polypeptide hormone that can relax the lower esophageal sphincter and, thereby, potentially relieve an impacted esophageal food bolus [26]. Glucagon has been shown to be successful in up to 39.5% of cases, without adverse events [27]. Glucagon alone is not recommended due to its moderate efficacy, but it may be used in combination with endoscopy [10]. The current ASGE guidelines recommend administration of IV glucagon while preparing for endoscopic retrieval to allow a trail of passage prior instrumentation [10].

Endoscopic Retrieval

Upper gastrointestinal foreign bodies can be retrieved successfully with flexible endoscopy >90% of the time [15, 28, 29]. There are many devices available to facilitate foreign body retrieval (Fig. 4.5). Although there have been no studies comparing the efficacy of available devices, the most commonly used are rat-toothed forceps and snare [29]. Endoscopic strategies may be different in each case of foreign body retrieval, depending on the circumstance and object characteristics (Table 4.1).

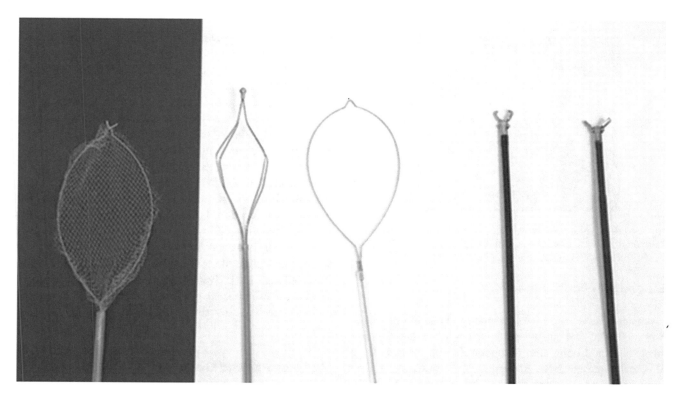

Fig. 4.5 Endoscopic devices pictured from *left* to *right*: Retrieval Roth net, retrieval basket, snare, rat-tooth forceps, and an alligator forceps. From Smith and Wong [55]

Table 4.1 Summary of endoscopic devices and techniques used in foreign body removal by foreign body type

Type of foreign body (FB)	Retrieval device(s)	Technique(s)
Esophageal food impaction	• Rat-tooth forceps • Roth net • Snare	• Pull technique • Combined pull, then push technique
Sharp FB	• Latex hood (first-line) • Overtube (second-line) • Rubber tipped forceps	• Always utilize protective devices to prevent mucosal injury during retrieval
Blunt FB	• Roth net • Retrieval baskets • Rat-tooth forceps	• Overtubes for removing disk batteries
Long FB	• Snare • Retrieval basket	• Remove by the object's long axis • Double snare technique
Phytobezoars	• Forceps and snare • Guidewire • Bezoaratom	• Dissolution with Coca-Cola® • Piecemeal disruption with overtube
Gastric band	• Guidewire • Snare • Mechanical lithotripter	• Endoscopic band cutting, then removal
Self-expanding metal stent (SEMS)	• Snare or forceps • SEMS	Simple cases: • Loop retrieval mechanism Embedded stents: • Distal-to-proximal invagination • Stent-in-stent retrieval

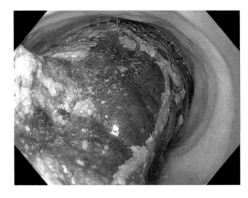

Fig. 4.6 Esophageal food impaction related to an esophageal cancer. This food impaction was removed by piecemeal extraction. An esophageal stent was placed following the extraction

Esophageal Food Impactions

Esophageal food impactions are managed endoscopically by two methods: The push technique describes the advancement of a food bolus into the stomach with an endoscope. This technique has been advocated in the past, and it has a low rate of complications if done with extreme care [5]. The pull technique is the preferred approach, however, given that pushing a food bolus blindly through a potential stricture may result in mucosal injury or perforation. The pull technique involves retrograde extraction of a food bolus. In some cases piecemeal removal is used if a bolus is large or has a soft consistency (Fig. 4.6). Some endoscopists prefer a hybrid "pull-push" technique that employs piecemeal extraction to reduce the size of a food bolus, so it can be safely advanced into the stomach. The most commonly used devices for food impactions are rat-toothed forceps, snares, or nets [3–5]. None of these devices have been shown to be superior to one another.

Other devices and techniques are an option for difficult cases of esophageal food impaction. Endoscope caps used for band ligation, or mucosectomy can be used for suctioning onto a food bolus for extraction [30]. Another method involves guiding an esophageal dilation balloon distal to an impacted food bolus, inflating the balloon slightly to capture the food bolus, and then pulling it out of the esophagus [31]. Even electrocautery has been described to fracture an impacted pill in the esophagus, although this method clearly carries risks to mucosal injury [32].

Sharp or Pointed Objects

Sharp foreign bodies encountered include razor blades, safety pins, glass, broken plastic, or pens (Fig. 4.7a) and special care must be taken during retrieval. Protective devices, such as a latex hood or an overtube, are designed to

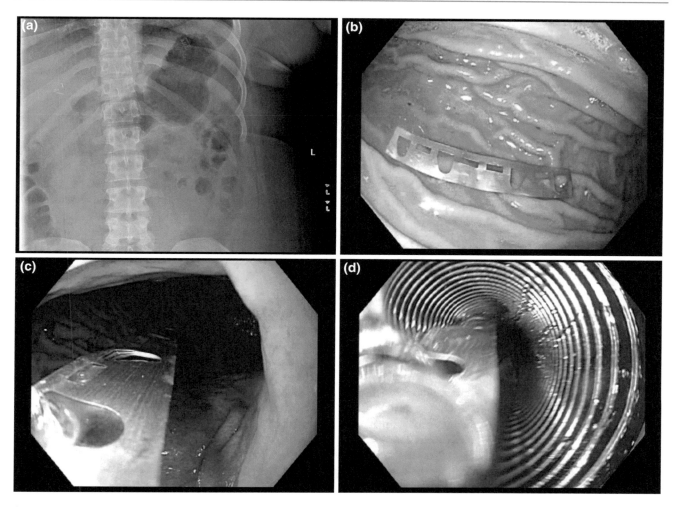

Fig. 4.7 Endoscopic retrieval of an intentionally ingested razorblade: **a**. Abdominal X-ray showing a razorblade in the gastric cardia **b**. Endoscopic image of the razorblade **c**. Grasping the razorblade using endoscopic forceps **d**. Retrieving the razorblade through an overtube

cover the sharp ends of forgein bodies and they are necessary tools for retrieving sharp foreign bodies. (Fig. 4.7b–d). Latex hoods are simple devices that are fitted over the scope end to cover sharp objects [29]. Once the object is secured, the scope is withdrawn and the retracted hood will be pushed forward into a covering position as it passes through the lower esophageal sphincter [29]. Overtubes are used to remove sharp objects when latex hoods are not indicated or cannot be used (Fig. 4.7d). An overtube is essentially a long plastic tube that works as a channel for the endoscope to pass through the oropharynx, esophagus, and into the stomach [33]. The overtube housing protects the mucosa when retrieving a sharp foreign body. It also serves to protect the airway and facilitate repeated reintroduction of the endoscope if needed [29]. Deciding to use an overtube should be judicious, however, as they can cause mucosal injury or other complications including esophageal rupture, ulceration, and bleeding [29, 33, 34].

Blunt Objects

Commonly encountered blunt objects include batteries, coins, or magnets. Disk batteries are best retrieved using a retrieval basket or net and with an overtube to protect the airway during retrieval [10]. Inflating a balloon (as described in Chap. 5.1) has also been described for removing disk batteries impacted in the esophagus. Magnets can be recovered with retrieval nets, and coins can be retrieved with rat-toothed forceps, graspers, or retrieval nets [15].

Large Objects

Objects that are too large to pass through the gastrointestinal tract are also difficult to remove. Large objects may need to be secured with a snare or net, then maneuvered to be removed by its long axis [1, 10]. A two-channel scope allowing two devices to be used simultaneously, such as two snares or graspers, is advantageous when managing long objects that are difficult to maneuver otherwise [1, 15]. For all large objects, it is recommended to use a long overtube that extends beyond the gastroesophageal junction to aid in safe retrieval [10].

Gastric Bezoars

Bezoars are conglomerate masses composed of poorly digested materials and may result in gastrointestinal blockage, ulceration, or other complications [35]. Gastric phytobezoars are the most common type, and these are composed of plant materials [35]. Phytobezoars can be dissolved with Coca-Cola® and treated endoscopically. The mechanism of Coca-Cola® dissolving phytobezoars is not completely understood, but it is believed to involve the combined digestive effects of sodium bicarbonate, carbonic acid, phosphoric acid, and carbonation bubbles [35]. Oral administration of Coca-Cola® alone can dissolve 60% of phytobezoars, and this increases to 94% with addition of endoscopic fragmentation [36]. Forceps and snares care the most typical devices used to piecemeal a phytobezoar, and generally this requires an overtube to allow repeated intubations with the endoscope [15]. Other endoscopic methods for phytobezoar disruption have also been described in combination with dissolving agents. For example, guidewire-mediated fragmentation has been described as a safe fragmentation technique, and this can be used with Coca-Cola® administration [37]. Another method of dissolution involves endoscopically injecting the phytobezoar directly with water or Coca-Cola® [35]. A bezoaratom has been described in a case report as a device that is specifically designed to treat bezoars. The device uses an oval polyfilament snare to secure and break bezoars manually with a crank [35, 38]; however, the device is not currently available in the USA. Endotherapy is generally insufficient for treating non-phytobezoars, and these may require surgical management.

Migrated Device Retrieval

Complications related to upper gastrointestinal therapeutic devices might necessitate endoscopic removal. Adjustable gastric bands for weight loss are typically placed around the gastric cardia to restrict oral intake. These bands can be adjusted by insufflation of air through a port that is surgically placed under the skin. Gastric bands may need to be removed due to erosion and migration into the stomach in 0.6–3% of cases [39]. Surgical removal was previously the only option for eroded gastric bands. However, with advancements in endoscopic devices, they can now be

removed safely using an endoscopic mechanical lithotripter (Fig. 4.8). Dogan et al. [40] showed that endoscopic removal of gastric bands was successful and without complication in 10/13 of cases, using a gastric band cutter device that is similar to a mechanical lithotripter [40]. Our experience using an endoscopic mechanical lithotripter to remove an eroded gastric band is illustrated in the video linked to this chapter (Video 4.1).

Esophageal self-expanding stents can migrate, break, or cause tissue injury, all of which require removal. Esophageal stent removal can be safe [41], but there are associated complications including stricture, ulceration, fistula, perforation, and hemorrhage if they have embedded into the mucosa [15]. Self-expanding stents are generally successfully removed with a retrieval mechanism, such as a loop, that can be pulled with a snare or forceps [15]. Embedded stents are more challenging to remove, and various techniques have been proposed for this situation including distal to proximal invagination (with or without guidewire-assisted peeling), overtube-assisted retrieval, retrieval hooks, and stent-in-stent placement [15, 42]. The stent-in-stent retrieval is the only technique requiring a staged procedure by first placing a fully covered stent within the embedded stent for two weeks to cause necrosis of embedded tissues. This results in the embedded stent to dislodge, so it may be easily removed at a later time [15].

Special Considerations

Prisoners and patients with mental illness present special challenges when managing foreign bodies. These patients often have recurrent intentional foreign body ingestions, which seem to have a lower success rate of endoscopic retrieval [43]. Despite this, surgery is an unfavorable option given post-operative intestinal adhesions may predispose to more complicated encounters in future foreign body ingestions [44]. Thus if initial retrieval attempts fail, then repeat endoscopy or trial of spontaneous passage in this patient group is preferred. A rat-toothed forceps or polypectomy snare may be the best device to remove intentionally ingested foreign bodies, and they have been associated with a high rate of success [9].

Drug packers transport illegal substances by concealing them in the gastrointestinal tract and this behavior may be present with medical complications, such as pain or obstruction. An accurate radiographic diagnosis with location and number of ingested drug packets is important, both from a medical and legal perspective [45]. CT has a greater sensitivity than plain radiography, however, X-ray has a high specificity if drug packets are detected with this imaging modality [45]. Drug packing is generally managed by spontaneous trail of passage, and endoscopic retrieval

Fig. 4.8 Gastric band that eroded into the stomach and was removed endoscopically

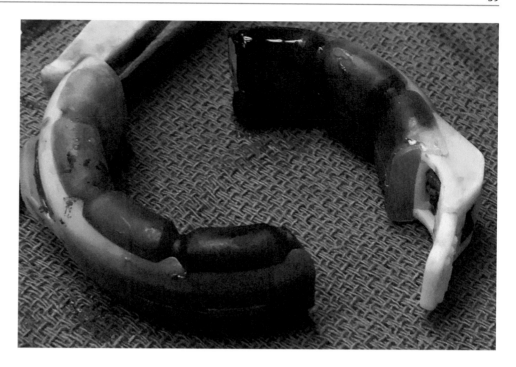

should be avoided as instrumentation may lead to package rupture and patient intoxication [10, 46]. Drug packers presenting with signs of acute drug intoxication, ileus, obstruction, or peritonitis, however, require immediate surgical intervention [47].

Failure to Retrieve Endoscopically

Alternative approaches to management are needed when flexible endoscopy is not successful in retrieving foreign bodies. Flexible endoscopy has a high success rate, but the failure rate can be up to 22% in populations that intentionally ingest objects that are challenging to remove [43]. Proximal esophageal impactions may be difficult to remove with a flexible endoscope and rigid endoscopic retrieval has been shown to be effective in this situation [48]. Rigid endoscopy remains second-line therapy, however, given association with mucosal injury, and post-intervention dysphagia [48]. Surgery may be indicated in 1–5% of cases, which is usually only after endoscopic failure. Factors that predict the need for surgery include ingestion of multiple objects, endoscopic failure, age >70, objects greater than 3 cm, and impaction time >40 h [43, 49].

Complications

Complications related to foreign bodies vary between the circumstances of the foreign body. In patients who have

intentionally ingested a true foreign body, complication rates between 3.6 and 7% have been reported with no associated deaths [9, 50]. The complications range from minor mucosal injuries to perforations requiring surgery. True foreign bodies are most often found in the stomach [9, 43, 50], and this is consistent with the duodenum and stomach being a frequent site of injury [9]. Mucosal perforations develop more often in patients who have had >48 h until intervention or had shorter foreign bodies (<7 cm) that were beyond the pylorus [9].

Unintentional foreign bodies have a greater range of complication rates. Esophageal food impactions are reported to have 0–10% complication rates in the literature [4, 5, 7, 8]. Most of these complications were minor mucosal injuries, although Sengupta et al. [8] reported 3% perforations in a population with prevalent eosinophilic esophagitis. Other types of unintentional foreign body ingestion such as animal bones, dentures, and tooth picks may have a complication rate from 2.8 to 50% [18, 19, 51]. Cases involving animal bone ingestion (especially fish bones) are associated with higher complications, as these are known to be predictive of mucosal injury [19]. Other factors predictive of complications include delayed intervention >12 h, object sharpness, objects >3 cm, location at the upper esophagus, or objects not see on X-ray [8, 18, 50, 51].

Complications associated with gastrointestinal device removal have also been reported. Migrated esophageal stent removal may be associated with complications in 10.6% of cases, and most of these are minor including minor bleeding, mucosal tearing, or pain [41]. Data for complications related to gastric band removal are limited, but Dogan et al. [40] reported no complications in their case series.

Managing complications depends on severity. Minor complications that do not perforate through the gastrointestinal mucosa can usually be managed conservatively with NPO and allowing the area to heal. Esophageal perforation management is dependent on the size of the defect, patient's clinical progression, and their co-morbidities [52, 53]. Small perforations or mucosal tears can be treated with antibiotics and consideration of covered stent placement [52–54]. Patients who develop signs of sepsis, or when conservative measures fail, need surgical repair [53].

Conclusion

Gastrointestinal foreign bodies can be a harmful medical problem and oftentimes challenging to manage. Gastrointestinal foreign bodies may be the result of underlying gastrointestinal disease, psychiatric disorders, secondary gain, or gastrointestinal device malfunction, and each circumstance is uniquely approached. Most cases of foreign bodies will not require endoscopic management, but early endoscopic intervention is advantageous if removal is needed. Flexible endoscopy is the first line tool for removal, and the gastroenterologist should be familiar with the array of devices and techniques used for successful retrieval of foreign bodies.

Acknowledgements Irving Waxman MD, Gautham Reddy MD, Bruce Bissonnette MD, Natalia Lipin MD

References

1. Kay M, Wyllie R. Pediatric foreign bodies and their management. Curr Gastroenterol Rep. 2005;7(3):212–8.
2. Webb WA. Management of foreign bodies of the upper gastrointestinal tract: update. Gastrointest Endosc. 1995;41(1):39–51.
3. Conway WC, Sugawa C, Ono H, Lucas CE. Upper GI foreign body: an adult urban emergency hospital experience. Surg Endosc. 2007;21(3):455–60.
4. Sperry SLW, Crockett SD, Miller CB, Shaheen NJ, Dellon ES. Esophageal foreign-body impactions: epidemiology, time trends, and the impact of the increasing prevalence of eosinophilic esophagitis. Gastrointest Endosc. 2011;74(5):985–91.
5. Longstreth GF, Longstreth KJ, Yao JF. Esophageal food impaction: epidemiology and therapy. A retrospective, observational study. Gastrointest Endosc. 2001;53(2):193–8.
6. Byrne KR, Panagiotakis PH, Hilden K, Thomas KL, Peterson KA, Fang JC. Retrospective analysis of esophageal food impaction: differences in etiology by age and gender. Dig Dis Sci. 2007;52 (3):717–21.
7. Mahesh VN, Holloway RH, Nguyen NQ. Changing epidemiology of food bolus impaction: is eosinophilic esophagitis to blame? J Gastroenterol Hepatol. 2013;28(6):963–6.
8. Sengupta N, Tapper EB, Corban C, Sommers T, Leffler DA, Lembo AJ. The clinical predictors of aetiology and complications among 173 patients presenting to the emergency department with oesophageal food bolus impaction from 2004-2014. Aliment Pharmacol Ther. 2015;42(1):91–8.
9. Palta R, Sahota A, Bemarki A, Salama P, Simpson N, Laine L. Foreign-body ingestion: characteristics and outcomes in a lower socioeconomic population with predominantly intentional ingestion. Gastrointest Endosc. 2009;69(3 Pt 1):426–33.
10. Ikenberry SO, Jue TL, Anderson MA, Appalaneni V, Banerjee S, Ben-Menachem T, et al. Management of ingested foreign bodies and food impactions. Gastrointest Endosc. 2011;73(6):1085–91.
11. Guelfguat M, Kaplinskiy V, Reddy SH, DiPoce J. Clinical guidelines for imaging and reporting ingested foreign bodies. Am J Roentgenol. 2014;203(1):37–53.
12. Pinto A, Muzj C, Gagliardi N, Pinto F, Setola FR, Scaglione M, et al. Role of imaging in the assessment of impacted foreign bodies in the Hypopharynx and Cervical Esophagus. Semin Ultrasound CT MRI. 2012;33(5):463–70.
13. Faggian A, Berritto D, Iacobellis F, Reginelli A, Cappabianca S, Grassi R. Imaging patients with alimentary tract perforation: literature review. Semin Ultrasound CT MRI [Internet]. [cited 2015 Oct 10]; Available from: http://www.sciencedirect.com/science/article/pii/S0887217115000955.
14. Aras MH, Miloglu O, Barutcugil C, Kantarci M, Ozcan E, Harorli A. Comparison of the sensitivity for detecting foreign bodies among conventional plain radiography, computed tomography and ultrasonography. Dentomaxillofacial Radiol. 2010;39 (2):72–8.
15. Chauvin A, Viala J, Marteau P, Hermann P, Dray X. Management and endoscopic techniques for digestive foreign body and food bolus impaction. Dig Liver Dis. 2013;45(7):529–42.
16. Kimball SJ, Park AH, Rollins MD, Grimmer JF, Muntz H. A review of esophageal disc battery ingestions and a protocol for management. Arch Otolaryngol Head Neck Surg. 2010;136 (9):866–71.
17. Loots DP, du Toit-Prinsloo L, Saayman G. Disk battery ingestion: a rare cause of perforation of the brachiocephalic artery. Forensic Sci Med Pathol. 2015;11(4):614–7.
18. Hong KH, Kim YJ, Kim JH, Chun SW, Kim HM, Cho JH. Risk factors for complications associated with upper gastrointestinal foreign bodies. World J Gastroenterol WJG. 2015;21(26):8125–31.
19. Sung SH, Jeon SW, Son HS, Kim SK, Jung MK, Cho CM, et al. Factors predictive of risk for complications in patients with oesophageal foreign bodies. Dig Liver Dis Off J Ital Soc Gastroenterol Ital Assoc Study Liver. 2011;43(8):632–5.
20. Smith MT, Wong RKH. Foreign bodies. Gastrointest Endosc Clin N Am. 2007;17(2):361–82.
21. Lee JH, Lee JS, Kim MJ, Choe YH. Initial location determines spontaneous passage of foreign bodies from the gastrointestinal tract in children. Pediatr Emerg Care. 2011;27(4):284–9.
22. Weiland ST, Schurr MJ. Conservative management of ingested foreign bodies. J Gastrointest Surg. 2002;6(3):496–500.
23. Khayyat YM. Pharmacological management of esophageal food bolus impaction. Emerg Med Int. 2013;2013:924015.
24. Morse CR, Wang H, Donahue DM, Garrity JM, Allan JS. Use of proteolytic enzymes in the treatment of proteinaceous esophageal food impaction. J Emerg Med. 2015.
25. Lee J, Anderson R. Best evidence topic report. Proteolytic enzymes for oesophageal meat impaction. Emerg Med J EMJ. 2005;22(2):122–3.
26. Weant KA, Weant MP. Safety and efficacy of glucagon for the relief of acute esophageal food impaction. Am J Health-Syst Pharm AJHP Off J Am Soc Health-Syst Pharm. 2012;69(7):573–7.

27. Haas J, Leo J, Vakil N. Glucagon Is a safe and inexpensive initial strategy in esophageal food bolus impaction. Dig Dis Sci. 2015.

28. Triadafilopoulos G, Roorda A, Akiyama J. Update on foreign bodies in the esophagus: diagnosis and management. Curr Gastroenterol Rep. 2013;15(4):1–6.

29. Diehl DL, Adler DG, Conway JD, Farraye FA, Kantsevoy SV, Kaul V, Kethu SR, Kwon RS, Mamula P, Rodriguez SA, Tierney WM. Endoscopic retrieval devices. Gastrointest Endosc. 2009;69(6):997–1003.

30. Chiu K-W, Lu L-S, Wu T-C, Chiou S-S. Novel low-cost endoscopic cap for esophageal foreign objects: a case report. Medicine (Baltimore). 2015;94(17):e796.

31. Anand R, Garg S, Dubin E, Dutta S. A novel endoscopic method to relieve food impaction using an inflatable balloon. Case Rep Gastrointest Med. 2015;2015:357253.

32. Syal G, Klair JS, Dang S. An innovative technique for management of esophageal pill impaction. Gastrointest Endosc. 2015;82(2):422–3.

33. Wells CD, Fleischer DE. Overtubes in gastrointestinal endoscopy. Am J Gastroenterol. 2008;103(3):745–52.

34. Dennert B, Ramirez FC, Sanowski RA. A prospective evaluation of the endoscopic spectrum of overtube-related esophageal mucosal injury. Gastrointest Endosc. 1997;45(2):134–7.

35. Iwamuro M, Okada H, Matsueda K, Inaba T, Kusumoto C, Imagawa A, et al. Review of the diagnosis and management of gastrointestinal bezoars. World J Gastrointest Endosc. 2015;7(4):336–45.

36. Ladas SD, Kamberoglou D, Karamanolis G, Vlachogiannakos J, Zouboulis-Vafiadis I. Systematic review: Coca-Cola can effectively dissolve gastric phytobezoars as a first-line treatment. Aliment Pharmacol Ther. 2013;37(2):169–73.

37. Senturk O, Hulagu S, Celebi A, Korkmaz U, Duman AE, Dindar G, et al. A new technique for endoscopic treatment of gastric phytobezoars: fragmentation using guidewire. Acta Gastro-Enterol Belg. 2014;77(4):389–92.

38. Kurt M, Posul E, Yilmaz B, Korkmaz U. Endoscopic removal of gastric bezoars: an easy technique. Gastrointest Endosc. 2014;80(5):895–6.

39. Snow JM, Severson PA. Complications of adjustable gastric banding. Surg Clin North Am. 2011;91(6):1249–64.

40. Dogan ÜB, Akin MS, Yalaki S, Akova A, Yilmaz C. Endoscopic management of gastric band erosions: a 7-year series of 14 patients. Can J Surg J Can Chir. 2014;57(2):106–11.

41. Van Halsema EE, Wong Kee Song LM, Baron TH, Siersema PD, Vleggaar FP, Ginsberg GG, et al. Safety of endoscopic removal of self-expandable stents after treatment of benign esophageal diseases. Gastrointest Endosc. 2013;77(1):18–28.

42. Weigt J, Barsic N, Malfertheiner P. A novel approach to esophageal stent removal in the setting of proximal stenosis and failure of the primary retrieval mechanism. Endoscopy. 2015;47(S 01):E129–30.

43. Dalal PP, Otey AJ, McGonagle EA, Whitmill ML, Levine EJ, McKimmie RL, et al. Intentional foreign object ingestions: need for endoscopy and surgery. J Surg Res. 2013;184(1):145–9.

44. Evans DC. Intentional ingestions of foreign objects among prisoners: a review. World J Gastrointest Endosc. 2015;7(3):162.

45. Reginelli A, Russo A, Uraro F, Maresca D, Martiniello C, D'Andrea A, et al. Imaging of body packing: errors and medico-legal issues. Abdom Imaging. 2015;40(7):2127–42.

46. De Bakker JK, Nanayakkara PWB, Geeraedts LMG, de Lange ESM, Mackintosh MO, Bonjer HJ. Body packers: a plea for conservative treatment. Langenbecks Arch Surg Dtsch Ges Für Chir. 2012;397(1):125–30.

47. Yegane R-A, Bashashati M, Hajinasrollah E, Heidari K, Salehi N-A, Ahmadi M. Surgical approach to body packing. Dis Colon Rectum. 2009;52(1):97–103.

48. Gmeiner D, von Rahden BHA, Meco C, Hutter J, Oberascher G, Stein HJ. Flexible versus rigid endoscopy for treatment of foreign body impaction in the esophagus. Surg Endosc. 2007;21(11):2026–9.

49. Lee H-J, Kim H-S, Jeon J, Park S-H, Lim S-U, Jun C-H, et al. Endoscopic foreign body removal in the upper gastrointestinal tract: risk factors predicting conversion to surgery. Surg Endosc. 2015.

50. Huang BL, Rich HG, Simundson SE, Dhingana MK, Harrington C, Moss SF. Intentional swallowing of foreign bodies is a recurrent and costly problem that rarely causes endoscopy complications. Clin Gastroenterol Hepatol. 2010;8(11):941–6.

51. Lai ATY, Chow TL, Lee DTY, Kwok SPY. Risk factors predicting the development of complications after foreign body ingestion. Br J Surg. 2003;90(12):1531–5.

52. Markar SR, Mackenzie H, Wiggins T, Askari A, Faiz O, Zaninotto G, et al. Management and outcomes of esophageal perforation: a national study of 2564 patients in england. Am J Gastroenterol [Internet]. 2015 Oct 6 [cited 2015 Oct 31]; Available from: http://www.nature.com.proxy.uchicago.edu/ajg/journal/vaop/ncurrent/full/ajg2015304a.html.

53. Nesbitt JC, Sawyers JL. Surgical management of esophageal perforation. Am Surg. 1987;53(4):183–91.

54. Van Heel NCM, Haringsma J, Spaander MCW, Bruno MJ, Kuipers EJ. Short-term esophageal stenting in the management of benign perforations. Am J Gastroenterol. 2010;105(7):1515–20.

55. Smith MT, Wong RKH. Esophageal foreign bodies: types and techniques for removal. Curr Treat Options Gastroenterol. 2006;9(1):75–84.

Diagnosis and Management of Barrett's Esophagus

Kathryn R. Byrne and Douglas G. Adler

Introduction

Comprehensive knowledge regarding the diagnosis and management of Barrett's esophagus is essential since it is one of the most common conditions treated in every gastroenterologist's practice. Barrett's esophagus was first described in 1950 by Dr. Norman Barrett, a British thoracic surgeon. History of long-standing GERD, male gender, age >50, tobacco use, family history of esophageal cancer, and central obesity have all been identified as risk factors associated with the development of Barrett's esophagus.

Definition of Barrett's Esophagus and Screening Guidelines

Barrett's esophagus is defined by both endoscopic and histologic criteria. There must be endoscopic documentation of columnar appearing epithelium in the distal esophagus. The second component of the definition is pathologically confirmed intestinal metaplasia found on histologic evaluation

of the biopsies taken from the columnar appearing epithelium.

Screening for Barrett's esophagus is a somewhat controversial topic as there are varying recommendations and no clear approach with proven efficacy. The American Gastroenterological Society (AGA) and the American College of Gastroenterology (ACG) do not recommend endoscopic screening for the general population of patients with GERD, although in practice many patients with GERD will ultimately undergo upper endoscopy.

It is helpful to be aware of the risk factors associated with the development of esophageal adenocarcinoma from Barrett's esophagus when deciding which patients to potentially screen. Risk factors include age 50 or older, male sex, white race, the presence of a hiatal hernia, chronic GERD symptoms, elevated BMI, and intra-abdominal distribution of body fat. The AGA position statement on the management of Barrett's esophagus recommends screening patients with multiple risk factors [1]. The position of the ACG is similar in recommending screening for high-risk patients. It is also recommended by the ACG that patients with any alarm symptoms such as dysphagia, unexplained weight loss, or signs of upper GI bleeding undergo upper endoscopy for further evaluation. The American College of Physicians recommends that screening may be indicated in men over age 50 with GERD symptoms for more than 5 years, plus additional risk factors including nocturnal reflux symptoms, hiatal hernia, elevated BMI, tobacco use, and intra-abdominal distribution of fat [2].

None of the approaches to screening above has been proven in clinical trials to decrease mortality from esophageal cancer. Of note, approximately 40% of patients diagnosed with esophageal adenocarcinoma have no history of heartburn symptoms [3, 4].

The rate of progression to esophageal adenocarcinoma is approximately 0.2–0.5% per year with non-dysplastic Barrett's, approximately 0.7% per year with Barrett's with low-grade dysplasia, and approximately 7% per year with Barrett's with high-grade dysplasia [5].

Electronic supplementary material
Supplementary material is available in the online version of this chapter at 10.1007/978-3-319-49041-0_5. Videos can also be accessed at https://link.springer.com/chapter/10.1007/978-3-319-49041-0_5.

K.R. Byrne
Division of Gastroenterology, University of Utah, 30N 1900 E Room 4R118, Salt Lake City, UT 84132, USA
e-mail: Kathryn.Byrne@hsc.utah.edu

D.G. Adler (✉)
Gastroenterology and Hepatology, University of Utah School of Medicine, Huntsman Cancer Center, 30N 1900E 4R118, Salt Lake City, UT 84132, USA
e-mail: douglas.adler@hsc.utah.edu

Endoscopic Documentation and Histologic Confirmation

Barrett's esophagus was traditionally endoscopically reported as long segment (extent of intestinal metaplasia at least 3 cm above the GEJ) versus short segment (extent of intestinal metaplasia of less than 3 cm) (Figs. 5.1 and 5.2). The AGA position statement regarding the management of Barrett's esophagus recommends the use of a system such as the Prague criteria which allows the endoscopist to provide more detailed information on the extent of Barrett's esophagus in the procedure report [1, 6]. The Prague C and M criteria document the circumferential extent (the C value) of the Barrett's esophagus and also the maximum extent (the M value) of the Barrett's esophagus. The maximum extent includes the tongues and islands of columnar appearing epithelia. For example, if the GEJ is located at 40 cm (from the incisors), the proximal extent of the circumferential columnar epithelium is located at 38 cm, and there are several islands of columnar epithelium between 36 cm and 38 cm; then, the Prague criteria will be C2M4 (Diagram 1).

Diagnosis of Barrett's esophagus depends on the histologic finding of intestinal metaplasia in the biopsies of the columnar appearing epithelium. It is important to appropriately identify the GEJ (an anatomic landmark) and the z-line (squamocolumnar junction), and take biopsies for diagnosis of Barrett's in the esophagus within the segment of columnar appearing epithelium. If biopsies are taken distal to the GEJ, in the stomach proper, intestinal metaplasia of the stomach may be reported (which is not able to be distinguished histologically from intestinal metaplasia of the esophagus). Intestinal metaplasia of the stomach can be caused by chronic H. pylori gastritis, among other causes. It is important to distinguish between these two conditions as surveillance is recommended for intestinal metaplasia of the esophagus (Barrett's esophagus), however, not for intestinal metaplasia of the stomach.

Surveillance of Barrett's Esophagus

Non-dysplastic Barrett's

All patients with Barrett's esophagus, including non-dysplastic Barrett's, should be treated with PPI therapy. Once daily PPI is adequate for most patients, with twice daily dosing only necessary for endoscopic findings of esophagitis or poor control of reflux symptoms.

The ASGE Standards of Practice Committee guideline on the role of endoscopy in Barrett's esophagus incorporates recommendations for surveillance intervals [7]. For non-dysplastic Barrett's esophagus, there are multiple possible management options to consider ranging from no surveillance, proceeding with endoscopic surveillance and endoscopic therapy (primarily aimed at ablation of dysplastic Barrett's esophagus) in selected cases. Endoscopic treatment of non-dysplastic Barrett's is a controversial topic and will be further discussed in a later section. If surveillance is decided on for non-dysplastic Barrett's, then EGD is typically performed every 3–5 years with 4-quadrant biopsies every 2 cm (Fig. 5.2). The AGA medical position statement on the management of Barrett's esophagus and the ACG clinical guideline regarding diagnosis and management of Barrett's esophagus also recommend EGD every 3–5 years for non-dysplastic Barrett's surveillance.

Dysplastic Barrett's

If biopsies are indeterminate for dysplasia, then PPI therapy should be initiated (or increased in dose if already on

Fig. 5.1 a, b Endoscopic image of short-segment Barrett's esophagus

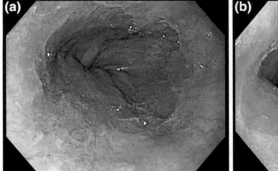
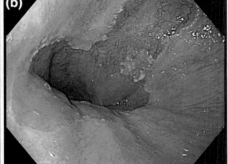

Fig. 5.2 a Endoscopic image of long-segment Barrett's esophagus. **b** Close-up image of same patient as (**a**), with narrow band imaging (NBI) applied

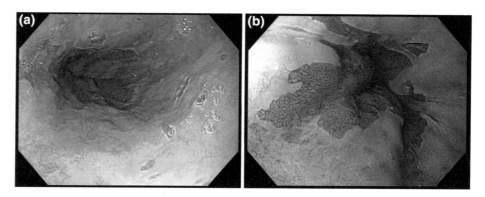

antisecretory medication), and repeat EGD with surveillance biopsies should be performed in 2–6 months to confirm or rule out the presence of dysplasia. Therapy with PPI is usually initiated at a standard dose (omeprazole 20 mg daily or equivalent) and increased only if needed based on reflux symptoms or if reflux esophagitis is present on endoscopy.

The finding of low-grade dysplasia should first be confirmed by an expert GI pathologist, and once agreed upon, repeat EGD should be performed in 6 months to confirm the presence of low-grade dysplasia and look for any signs of change (either progression or regression). Options for the management of patients with low-grade dysplasia include endoscopic eradication versus surveillance. Many patients with Barrett's esophagus with low-grade dysplasia will undergo ablative therapy, as discussed below. If patients choose to forgo ablation (for reason such as being unwilling to accept the risk of possible complications), then surveillance is a viable alternative option. If surveillance is performed, then the ASGE guidelines recommend 4-quadrant biopsies performed every 1–2 cm every 6–12 months. If surveillance is opted for, the ACG guidelines recommend 4-quadrant biopsies every 1 cm performed annually.

As with low-grade dysplasia, the finding of high-grade dysplasia should initially be confirmed by an expert GI pathologist. Surveillance is not typically performed as a first-line option for high-grade dysplasia as most of these patients undergo some type of treatment.

The Seattle protocol was initially described as a technique to differentiate high-grade dysplasia from early adenocarcinoma in patients with Barrett's esophagus [8]. The Seattle protocol continues to be widely utilized as a technique in Barrett's surveillance biopsies. In this protocol, targeted biopsies are first performed on mucosal abnormalities such as nodules. Four-quadrant biopsies are then obtained every 1 cm in the entire length of Barrett's esophagus. The ACG guidelines on diagnosis and management of Barrett's esophagus recommend biopsies every 1 cm in patients with history of any type of dysplasia, with biopsies every 2 cm in patients with no history of dysplasia.

Efficacy of Surveillance

Multiple studies have described the limited benefit of surveillance for non-dysplastic Barrett's esophagus [1, 6, 9, 10]. The cost-effectiveness of surveillance in non-dysplastic Barrett's is also controversial. The most recent AGA guidelines note that it is unclear whether endoscopic surveillance of non-dysplastic Barrett's esophagus reduces esophageal cancer incidence or mortality since no long-term trial designed to answer this question has yet been performed.

Although surveillance of non-dysplastic Barrett's esophagus is a controversial topic, it is common practice to perform surveillance as long as patients are fit-enough to ultimately undergo therapy if needed. The ACG specifically recommends that Barrett's surveillance should only be performed after counseling with patients regarding its risks and benefits [5]. The ASGE guidelines also suggest considering no surveillance in patients with non-dysplastic Barrett's esophagus.

Endoscopic Treatments: Description of Techniques and Discussion of Complications

There are two main categories of endoscopic therapies for Barrett's esophagus—mechanical treatments and ablative treatments. The mechanical treatments include endoscopic mucosal resection (EMR) and endoscopic submucosal dissection (ESD), while the most common ablative treatments include radiofrequency ablation (RFA) and cryotherapy.

Mechanical Treatments

Endoscopic Mucosal Resection (EMR)

The two most common methods of performing EMR are cap-assisted EMR and ligation-assisted EMR. Cap-assisted EMR involves submucosal injection, suction of the lesion into a cap, and then snare electrocautery. The lesion is initially lifted with a submucosal injection. The submucosal injection can be performed with saline; however, other agents can also be utilized (use of hyaluronic acid; saline with the addition of epinephrine or dye such as methylene blue). After a submucosal injection with lifting has been performed, the lesion is suctioned into a clear plastic cap affixed to the end of the endoscope and then a snare is opened and positioned within the internal ridge of the cap (various snare shapes and sizes are available). The snare is then opened and the lesion is suctioned into the cap, allowing the snare to be closed around it. Electrocautery is then utilized to remove the lesion. Cap-assisted EMR mucosectomy devices with various different cap sizes (outer diameter ranging from 12.9 to 18 mm), shape (flat circular- or oval-shaped tip), and firmness (soft or hard) are available for this technique. (Olympus America, Center Valley, Pennsylvania)

Ligation-assisted EMR is another technique utilized to perform EMR. There are several single-use band ligation devices that are available, including the Duette Multi-Band Mucosectomy device (Cook Medical Inc., Winston-Salem, North Carolina) and the Captivator EMR device (Boston Scientific, Natick, Massachusetts). Both of these devices involve attaching the ligation device to the end of the upper endoscope (very similar in structure and function to standard banding device as would be used to treat esophageal varices). The lesion is then suctioned into the banding cap (typically without prior submucosal injection) and then a band is deployed around the lesion circumferentially. The result of this process is the creation of a pseudopolyp. The included snare can then be advanced though the working channel of the endoscope through the attached device (without having to remove the device), the snare placed around the pseudopolyp (either above or below the band, whichever is technically easiest in a given situation), and then the electrocautery can be applied to remove the lesion. If necessary, for larger lesions or additional lesions, multiple bands can be utilized and the lesion can be removed in a piecemeal fashion (Fig. 5.3).

Possible complications from EMR include bleeding, perforation, and esophageal stricture formation (which are often delayed in presentation). Rates of bleeding after EMR in the literature vary widely, partially dependent on how bleeding is defined by the individual study and how aggressive the EMR procedure under evaluation is. Bleeding after esophageal EMR was evaluated in a large single-center study including 681 patients who underwent 2513 EMR procedures [11]. Clinically significant bleeding, defined in this study as any bleeding requiring endoscopic intervention, blood transfusion, or hospitalization, was only reported in 1.2% of patients.

Perforation rates after esophageal EMR are overall low with rates <0.5% for endoscopists experienced in performing EMR. The perforation risk increases when piecemeal resection is required [12–14, 23].

Stricture formation has been reported to occur in as few as 6% of patients and in as many as 88% of patients undergoing esophageal EMR for Barrett's esophagus with HGD or intramucosal carcinoma in various studies [15–19]. The higher rates of stenosis are associated with patients who have undergone EMR with more extensive resection. A study of 73 patients undergoing EMR (for Barrett's esophagus with HGD or intramucosal carcinoma) found symptomatic strictures in 25% of patients, with strictures more common if the resection area involved more than 50% of the esophageal lumen (odds ratio 4.2, 95% CI 1.3–14) [20].

The strictures caused by EMR are typically able to be effectively managed with endoscopic dilation. In a study of 136 patients undergoing esophageal EMR, a total of 37 patients (27%) developed an esophageal stricture [21]. Of note, 65% of the patients who developed a stricture also had a history of RFA treatment, so the cause of the stricture was likely multifactorial. In the group of patients that did not develop stricture, 56% had history of RFA treatment, suggesting that even EMR combined with RFA does not always

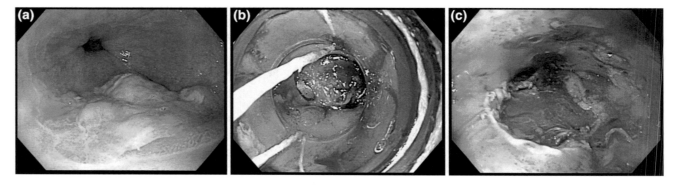

Fig. 5.3 a Intramucosal adenocarcinoma arising within Barrett's esophagus. **b** Band deployment during EMR of the intramucosal adenocarcinoma in the same patient as (**a**). **c** Status post-EMR in the same patient as (**a, b**)

lead to stricture formation. The authors note that all of the patients who developed stricture had resolution of dysphagia with endoscopic dilation. A median number of 2 dilations were needed per patient. Another study examining esophageal stricture post-EMR demonstrated similar findings with an average of 2.3 dilations required per patient [22].

Endoscopic Submucosal Dissection (ESD)

ESD is a technique that utilizes submucosal injection and then needle-knife for en bloc removal of larger (and possibly deeper) lesions. Many different types of needle-knife catheters are available for performing ESD. Overall complication rates, including perforation, are higher with ESD than with EMR. Bleeding during an ESD procedure is common and is typically able to be treated intra-procedurally with coagulation. Delayed bleeding is less common with esophageal ESD than with gastric ESD, in which rates up to 15.6% have been reported [23]. In a series of patients treated with esophageal ESD, delayed bleeding rates were reported in between 0 and 5.2% in the seven studies (with 568 cases) that provided this information [24].

Review of data from multiple series of esophageal EMR demonstrates a pooled perforation rate of 2.3% (19 of 816 cases), recognizing that most of these cases were performed by experts [25]. Almost all of these perforations were recognized during the procedure and were treated with placement of endoscopic clips. Strictures develop in approximately 12–17% of patients after esophageal ESD [26–29]. As with EMR, the stricture rate increases when more extensive and circumferential lesions are resected.

Since ESD is a technically difficult procedure with higher rates of adverse events than EMR, the utilization of ESD in the USA is limited to specialized centers with endoscopic expertise at performing this technique.

Ablative Treatments

Radiofrequency Ablation (RFA)

Radiofrequency ablation (RFA) is an endoscopic ablative therapy that delivers energy via a balloon (or catheter) with a series of closely spaced electrodes that generate a thermal injury with controlled depth and uniformity. Circumferential ablation and focal ablation are the two primary methods of performing RFA. Circumferential ablation (with an electrode-laden balloon) is typically performed in settings of more extensive areas to treat (such as long-segment Barrett's esophagus), while focal ablation (with an ablation catheter placed on the tip of the endoscope) is used to treat smaller areas. A smaller through-the-scope probe is also available for very small areas of Barrett's esophagus (Video 5.1).

Prior to performing ablation, the esophageal wall should first be irrigated with water to remove any mucus or other debris. Cleansing of the esophagus has traditionally performed using acetylcysteine; however, it has been demonstrated that water is just as effective at cleaning the esophagus [30]. The next step is careful identification of the esophageal-gastric landmarks, including the top of the gastric folds and the proximal extent of the Barrett's esophagus.

Prior to performing circumferential ablation, as the endoscope is positioned in the stomach, a stiff guidewire is placed through the working channel of the endoscope, and the endoscope is withdrawn as the wire is kept in place. The Barrx™ 360 soft sizing balloon is then advanced over the wire and connected to the Barrx FLEX generator (Medtronic, Minneapolis, Minnesota). This sizing balloon is utilized to measure the inner diameter of the esophagus prior to performing ablation. Based on the measurements from the sizing balloon, an appropriate ablation balloon catheter is selected. The BARRX™ 360 RFA balloon catheters (Medtronic, Minneapolis, Minnesota) are all 3 cm in length and are available in size diameters ranging from 18 to 31 mm.

The RFA balloon catheter is advanced over the wire and then the endoscope can be advanced adjacent to the wire and positioned proximal to the ablation balloon. With direct endoscopic visualization, the proximal edge of the balloon is positioned approximately 1 cm above the proximal extent of the Barrett's esophagus. The balloon is then inflated, and then radiofrequency energy (typically 12 J/cm^2) is activated by depressing a foot pedal attached to the generator. After the energy has been delivered, the balloon is repositioned more distally (allowing approximately 5–10 mm of overlap with the prior ablation area) and the same process repeated until the entire segment of Barrett's esophagus has been treated.

After the entire segment has been treated, the balloon catheter, wire, and endoscope are removed from the patient. A soft cap is attached to the end of the endoscope and the esophagus is then cleansed by removal of the coagulum with the soft cap combined with irrigation of the esophagus with water. After this is complete, the entire process is repeated (placement of wire, insertion of balloon catheter, and then ablation using the same settings as previously performed) as needed to treat the entire area of Barrett's esophagus.

A variety of different RFA catheters is commercially available and can be utilized to ablate smaller segments of Barrett's esophagus when non-circumferential disease is encountered. Several of the catheters (Barrx60, Barrx90, Barrx Ultra Long) can be attached to the end of the endoscope and one of the catheters (Barrx Channel) is a through-the-scope device for treatment of focal areas of Barrett's esophagus. When utilizing the attachments made to be affixed to the endoscope tip, the device is positioned at 12 o'clock on the endoscopic image. The endoscope and ablation catheter are advanced into the esophagus under direct visualization for use. The through-the-scope RFA ablation catheter is rotatable and usable under direct endoscopic visualization as well.

Once the endoscope has been advanced to the target tissue, ablation is performed by using the wheels of the endoscope to bring the ablation catheter into close contact with the mucosa in the desired treatment area. RFA energy (typically 15 J/cm^2) is then delivered by depressing a foot pedal attached to the generator. Prior to moving the electrode away from the mucosa, a second delivery of energy (at the same setting) is applied. All of the remaining areas of Barrett's esophagus are then treated in a similar fashion. As with circumferential ablation, the coagulum should then be cleansed from the esophageal wall after each treatment. This can be performed by using the tip of the electrode catheter to scrape off the coagulum. The endoscope should then be completely removed from the patient and the catheter cleansed with water. The endoscope and catheter are then reinserted and another treatment is performed in the exact same manner as previously (another two pulses of ablation at each treatment station) (Fig. 5.4).

Post-RFA treatment care typically includes high-dose PPI treatment. All patients with Barrett's esophagus should already be taking a PPI agent; however, increased acid suppression therapy may help improve esophageal healing after an ablation session. A prospective study demonstrated that effective esophageal pH control (24-h pH monitoring was utilized) was associated with improved outcomes, including reduction in Barrett's esophagus surface area and complete eradication rate, after RFA treatment [31].

As patients may experience chest pain and/or dysphagia immediately after treatment, alteration in the diet for several days after treatment is generally recommended. Dietary recommendations after RFA typically include liquids only for the first day after the procedure, a soft-consistency diet on the second day, and slow advancement as tolerated after that time. Other medications that can be considered include sucralfate suspension and pain medications if needed.

RFA treatment is generally well tolerated. There are a multitude of studies describing complication rates after RFA

for Barrett's esophagus. Overall stricture rates from RFA range between 0 and 6%, depending on the study. A multi-centered community-based study including 429 patients treated with RFA for Barrett's esophagus demonstrated a stricture rate of 1.1% of cases (2.1% of patients), with no serious adverse events (including no bleeding or perforation) [32]. In this study, the strictures resolved with a median of three endoscopic dilations. A large meta-analysis of 18 studies demonstrated that the most frequent complications from RFA include esophageal stricture (5%), chest pain (3%), and bleeding (1%) [33].

Cryotherapy

Cryotherapy is a technique that has been utilized in many different fields in medicine; however, this technology has only recently been adapted for use in endoscopy in general and Barrett's esophagus specifically. At this time, it is most commonly used for patients with refractory Barrett's esophagus who have failed or developed complications from RFA treatment (such as chest pain or stricture), or who are not candidates for RFA, or in patients who do not want to undergo RFA. Cryotherapy can also be utilized as a primary therapy for Barrett's esophagus treatment and can be used to treat esophageal cancer locally in nonsurgical candidates.

The two currently commercially available cryogens are liquid nitrogen and carbon dioxide. The destruction of the Barrett's epithelia is caused by freeze-thaw cycles using either of the cryogens. The available endoscopic systems for cryotherapy treatment include the CryoSpray Ablation system (CSA Medical, Baltimore, Maryland), Polar Wand cryotherapy (GI Supply, Camp Hill, Pennsylvania), and the Coldplay Focal Cryoballoon Ablation System (C2 Therapeutics, Redwood City, California).

Although there are different cryotherapy systems, in general a catheter is advanced through the working channel of the endoscope under direct endoscopic visualization. One system uses a cryogen-filled balloon to cool tissue; all others use a spray catheter. Administration of the cryogen is performed by depressing a foot pedal attached to the processor/pump, connected to a tank of cryogen, which

Fig. 5.4 a Initiation of RFA treatment with a BARRX90 catheter. **b** Image of the esophagus in the same patient as (**a**) after several ablation applications

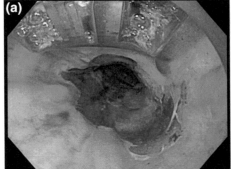 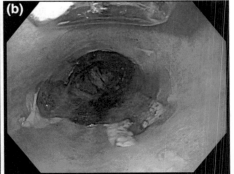

Fig. 5.5 **a** Small focus of esophageal adenocarcinoma in a patient with Barrett's esophagus undergoing cryotherapy with liquid nitrogen as cryogen. Note the spray catheter and suction tube visible in the image. Of note, the patient is not a surgical candidate. **b** Cryogen is applied and freezing begins. **c** Continued application of cryogen results in deep freezing. **d** As the freezing cycle ends, there is some diffuse, superficial freezing of tissue in the field although the focus is on the area of esophageal cancer

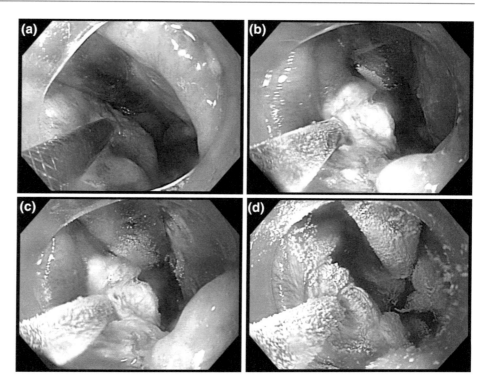

delivers the cryogen itself into direct contact with the target tissue. There are different regimens in performing cryotherapy treatment, but all involve several freeze/thaw cycles in a single endoscopic session. Three-to-four cycles per session are not uncommon (Fig. 5.5).

As cryotherapy is a more recently developed therapy for Barrett's esophagus, there are limited data with regard to outcomes when compared to that available for RFA. In general, endoscopic cryotherapy is well tolerated, but the technology has been slow to disseminate into widespread clinical practice. Also, there is no currently available method for accurate determination of dosimetry in cryotherapy, a major impediment to research in this field.

Based on numerous studies on the side effects from cryotherapy in Barrett's esophagus, the treatment is generally safe. In a series of sixty patients with Barrett's esophagus with HGD treated with cryotherapy, 2 patients (3.3%) experienced chest pain, 3 patients (5%) developed stricture, and there was 1 patient (1.7%) with GI bleeding [18]. Cryotherapy has demonstrated a favorable safety profile in multiple additional studies. A multi-center retrospective cohort study of 79 patients with esophageal cancer treated with spray cryotherapy with liquid nitrogen demonstrated no serious adverse events [34]. Ten patients developed benign strictures (12.6%); however, it was noted that 9 of the 10 patients had prior esophageal narrowing from other treatments (such as RFA). Twenty patients (25.3%) experienced chest discomfort that was treated with narcotic analgesics. A single-center retrospective study of

32 patients treated with spray cryotherapy for Barrett's esophagus with high-grade dysplasia noted esophageal stricture formation in 3 patients (9%), all of which responded to endoscopic dilation [35]. There were no serious adverse events.

Efficacy of Endoscopic Treatments

High-Grade Dysplasia/Intramucosal Carcinoma

Patients with Barrett's with HGD or intramucosal carcinoma should be all undergo treatment if they are good candidates for endoscopic therapy. Surgical esophagectomy is the historical first-line treatment for patients with Barrett's esophagus with high-grade dysplasia and/or intramucosal adenocarcinoma, and can still be discussed with patients as a potential option, especially if the disease is extensive or multifocal. Esophagectomy is the most definitive therapy as it removes the entire segment of neoplastic epithelium, a healthy margin of unaffected tissue, and regional lymph nodes. Esophagectomy, however, is a complex and extensive surgical undertaking and has high rates of morbidity, postoperative complications, and mortality, particularly in centers that do not perform high-volume number of procedures. Data from the Dutch National Registry demonstrated mortality rates from esophagectomy to be 12.1% (in centers performing 1–10 surgeries per year), 7.5% (11–20/year), and 4.9% (more than 50 per year) [25].

Most patients will prefer and select endoscopic therapy over surgical esophagectomy. If endoscopic therapy is performed, generally all mucosal irregularities (nodular mucosa) should initially be removed with EMR (endoscopic mucosal resection), and then the remainder of the Barrett's esophagus was treated with RFA, cryotherapy, or EMR. The initial EMR of any mucosal irregularities provides both therapy and staging information. Patients with submucosal depth of invasion (T1b) discovered on EMR should be referred for surgical consultation as endoscopic therapy in these patients will generally not be curative. Patients with EMR specimens revealing intramucosal cancer (T1a) will be candidates for endoscopic therapy.

Numerous studies have demonstrated the efficacy of RFA in the eradication of high-grade dysplasia/intramucosal carcinoma and intestinal metaplasia (complete eradication of Barrett's esophagus). A multi-center trial consisting of 127 patients with dysplastic Barrett's esophagus was randomized (2:1 ratio) to received RFA or a sham procedure (control). In the group of patients with high-grade dysplasia, eradication of dysplasia was achieved in 81% of patients in the RFA group, compared with 19% in the control group ($p < 0.001$) [36]. Among all patients with dysplasia, eradication of intestinal metaplasia was achieved in 77.4% of patients in the ablation group, compared with 2.3% in the control group ($p < 0.001$). The patients in the RFA group also had less disease progression (3.6 vs. 16.3%, $p = 0.03$) and fewer malignancies (1.2 vs. 9.3%, $p = 0.045$).

A systematic review including a total of 22 studies evaluated the efficacy of RFA and EMR for eradication of high-grade dysplasia and intramucosal carcinoma [37]. Eradication of dysplasia was achieved in 92% of patients after completion of RFA treatment (patients received a median of 2 RFA sessions). After medium follow-up of 21 months, the eradication of dysplasia was maintained in 94% of patients treated with RFA.

Endoscopic cryotherapy is an alternative therapy for ablation of Barrett's esophagus. Since it is a less fully developed and studied treatment for Barrett's esophagus, there is not nearly as much long-term follow-up data for cryotherapy as exists for RFA. Cryotherapy can be utilized as the first-line therapy for ablation of Barrett's esophagus and may also be used in patients that have been refractory to eradication of intestinal metaplasia with RFA or in patients having significant side effects from RFA (such as pain or stricture formation). In current practice, cryotherapy is most commonly used for patients with refractory Barrett's esophagus.

Several studies have evaluated the efficacy of endoscopic cryotherapy for treatment of Barrett's esophagus [35, 38, 39]. In a series of 32 patients with Barrett's esophagus with high-grade dysplasia treated with cryotherapy, there was complete eradication of high-grade dysplasia in 32 patients (100%) and complete eradication of intestinal metaplasia

was seen in 27 patients (84%) at 2-year follow-up. Another study of 60 patients with Barrett's esophagus with high-grade dysplasia demonstrated complete eradication of high-grade dysplasia in 52 patients (87%) and complete eradication of intestinal metaplasia in 34 patients (57%). Sixty-four patients with Barrett's esophagus with high-grade dysplasia or intramucosal adenocarcinoma were treated with cryotherapy and demonstrated eradication of high-grade dysplasia in 60 patients (94%) and eradication of intestinal metaplasia in 35 patients (55%). Cryotherapy studies have yet to elucidate the exact dosimetry and timing of this treatment, although studies are ongoing.

EMR (endoscopic mucosal resection) has been discussed above as treatment/staging for the nodular areas of Barrett's esophagus (and then treatment of the remainder of Barrett's esophagus with ablative therapies). EMR can also be utilized as a primary therapy for resection of the entire area of Barrett's mucosa. This method is not as commonly performed as there are high rates of stricture formation when circumferential EMR is performed.

Complete resection of Barrett's mucosa with EMR versus resection of mucosal abnormalities with EMR followed by ablation of the remainder of Barrett's esophagus with RFA was evaluated in a study of 47 patients with Barrett's esophagus containing HGD or intramucosal cancer [40]. The complete endoscopic resection group demonstrated eradication of neoplasia in 100% of patients and eradication of intestinal metaplasia in 92% of patients. The EMR plus RFA group demonstrated eradication of neoplasia in 96% of patients and eradication of intestinal metaplasia in 96% of patients. The eradication rates between the two groups were similar; however, the stricture rate in the EMR only group was 88 versus 14% in the EMR plus RFA group ($p < 0.001$).

Low-Grade Dysplasia

Management options for Barrett's esophagus with low-grade dysplasia include endoscopic ablative treatment versus surveillance. Currently, more patients with Barrett's esophagus and low-grade dysplasia are recommended to undergo ablative therapy as numerous recent studies have demonstrated the benefits of ablation with regard to reducing the risk of progression to malignancy. If patients are not willing to accept the potential risks of ablative therapy such as pain and esophageal stricture formation, then surveillance alone without ablative therapy remains an option, recognizing that ablation may need to be discussed in the future if the patient shows signs of progression to high-grade dysplasia or intramucosal cancer.

A multi-center randomized trial comparing surveillance versus RFA (the SURF trial) specifically evaluated patients with Barrett's esophagus with low-grade dysplasia and their risk of neoplastic progression [41]. This study included 136 patients with a diagnosis of Barrett's esophagus with low-grade dysplasia and randomized the patients (in a 1:1 ratio) to either RFA (treatment group) or endoscopic surveillance (control group). The group undergoing RFA demonstrated a marked reduced progression to HGD or adenocarcinoma during a 3-year follow-up (1.5% for the RFA group versus 26.5% for the control group; 95% CI, 14.1–35.9%; $p < 0.001$).

Another multi-center study retrospectively reviewed neoplastic progression rates in patients with Barrett's esophagus with low-grade dysplasia [42]. A total of 170 patients with confirmed Barrett's esophagus with low-grade dysplasia (45 patients who underwent RFA and 125 patients who underwent surveillance endoscopy) were reviewed and it was found that the annual rate of progression to HGD or adenocarcinoma was 0.77% in the RFA group (after mean follow-up of 889 days) and 6.6% (after a mean follow-up of 848 days) in the surveillance group. The group undergoing RFA demonstrated significantly lower risk of progression to HGD or adenocarcinoma than the surveillance group (adjusted hazard ratio = 0.06; 95% confidence interval 0.008–0.48).

Non-dysplastic Barrett's Esophagus

Endoscopic eradication therapy of non-dysplastic Barrett's esophagus is a controversial topic. In general, endoscopic therapy is not recommended for most patients with non-dysplastic Barrett's as the overall risk of progression to cancer is low. However, endoscopic therapy in select higher risk patients (young age with family history of esophageal cancer) can be considered, though there are no clear guidelines for these recommendations at this time.

The AGA medical position statement on the management of Barrett's esophagus recommends to consider endoscopic therapy in patients with non-dysplastic Barrett's who are thought to be at increased risk for progression to HGD or cancer, however notes that specific criteria to define this population have not been created as of this time. The ACG clinical guideline on management of Barrett's esophagus states that endoscopic ablative therapies should not be routinely applied to patients with non-dysplastic Barrett's esophagus. The ASGE standards of practice committee guideline note that endoscopic ablative therapies can be considered in non-dysplastic Barrett's in selected patients (such as patients with a family history of esophageal adenocarcinoma).

Non-dysplastic Barrett's esophagus can be a source of concern to patients who worry about their risk of developing cancer. Some patients with non-dysplastic Barrett's esophagus simply want to undergo ablation for peace of mind.

Surveillance After Treatment

Regardless of the treatment method, after complete eradication of intestinal metaplasia and complete eradication of dysplasia is achieved, surveillance endoscopy is recommended to evaluate for recurrence. The following recommendations from the ACG Clinical Guideline on Diagnosis and Management of Barrett's Esophagus are considered a strong recommendation, however, with low level of evidence [10].

Surveillance endoscopy for patients initially treated for Barrett's with high-grade dysplasia is recommended every three months for the first year (after eradication of both high-grade dysplasia and intestinal metaplasia), every 6 months for the second year, and then continued annually. Surveillance endoscopy for patients initially treated for Barrett's with low-grade dysplasia is recommended every 6 months for the first year (after eradication of both low-grade dysplasia and intestinal metaplasia), then continued annually.

Similar to initial surveillance endoscopy, it is generally recommended that surveillance endoscopy after eradication of intestinal metaplasia and dysplasia be performed with a careful examination of the esophagus with both white-light endoscopy and narrow band imaging. Four-quadrant biopsies are typically taken every 1 cm throughout the segment of prior Barrett's esophagus. Of note, the initial documentation of the length of Barrett's esophagus using a system such as the Prague criteria becomes very useful in the following Barrett's after treatment to know the location of the initial segment of abnormal mucosa so that it can be clearly evaluated on subsequent procedures after treatment.

Conclusion

There is general consensus among the American gastrointestinal societies regarding screening and surveillance of patients with Barrett's esophagus. Endoscopic screening should not be performed on the general population. Screening should be considered for patients at higher risk for development of esophageal cancer, including patients with long-standing GERD, male gender, age > 50, central obesity, history of tobacco use, and family history of esophageal cancer. Non-dysplastic Barrett's esophagus has a low risk of progression to esophageal adenocarcinoma, and endoscopic treatment is not generally recommended. Non-dysplastic Barrett's esophagus is most often followed with surveillance endoscopy and biopsies every 3-5 years. Patients with confirmed low-grade dysplasia, high-grade dysplasia, and intramucosal carcinoma are candidates for endoscopic therapy. The most common options for endoscopic therapy include ablative treatments (RFA and cryotherapy) and

Table 5.1 Surveillance of Barrett's esophagus

Non-dysplastic Barrett's	EGD every 3–5 years with 4-quadrant biopsies every 1–2 cm
Indefinite for dysplasia	Repeat EGD in 2–6 months to confirm or rule-out presence of dysplasia
Low-grade dysplasia	Confirm by GI pathologist. Repeat EGD in 6 months to evaluate for progression or regression. If LGD is confirmed, endoscopic treatment recommended. Alternative is surveillance every 6–12 months with 4-quadrant biopsies every 1–2 cm
High-grade dysplasia	Confirm by GI pathologist if confirmed → endoscopic treatment

mechanical treatments (EMR and ESD). It is important to note that there is risk of recurrence after complete eradication of both intestinal metaplasia and dysplasia, and patients should continue to have endoscopic surveillance after treatment is complete (Table 5.1).

References

1. American Gastroenterological Association, Spechler SJ, Sharma P, Souza RF, Inadomi JM, Shaheen NJ. American Gastroenterological association medical position statement on the management of Barrett's esophagus. Gastroenterology. 2011;140(3):1084.
2. Shaheen NJ, Weinberg DS, Denberg TD, Chou R, Qaseem A, Shekelle P. Clinical guidelines committee of the American College of Physicians. Upper endoscopy for gastroesophageal reflux disease: best practice advice from the clinical guidelines committee of the American College of Physicians. Ann Intern Med. 2012;157 (11):808.
3. Rubenstein JH, Taylor JB. Meta-analysis: the association of oesophageal adenocarcinoma with symptoms of gastro-oesophageal reflux. Aliment Pharmacol Ther. 2010;32(10):1222.
4. Lagergren J, Bergström R, Lindgren A, Nyrén O. Symptomatic gastroesophageal reflux as a risk factor for esophageal adenocarcinoma. N Engl J Med. 1999;340(11):825.
5. Nicholas J, Shaheen, Falk GW, Iyer PG, Gerson L. ACG clinical guideline: diagnosis and management of Barrett's esophagus. Am J Gastroenterol Adv. online publication, 3 November 2015.
6. Sharma P, Dent J, Armstrong D, Bergman JJ, Gossner L, Hoshihara Y, Jankowski JA, Junghard O, Lundell L, Tytgat GN, Vieth M. The development and validation of an endoscopic grading system for Barrett's esophagus: the prague C&M criteria. Gastroenterology. 2006;131(5):1392.
7. ASGE Standards of Practice Committee, Evans JA, Early DS, Fukami N, Ben-Menachem T, Chandrasekhara V, Chathadi KV, Decker GA, Fanelli RD, Fisher DA, Foley KQ, Hwang JH, Jain R, Jue TL, Khan KM, Lightdale J, Malpas PM, Maple JT, Pasha SF, Saltzman JR, Sharaf RN, Shergill A, Dominitz JA, Cash BD. Standards of practice Committee of the American Society for gastrointestinal endoscopy. The role of endoscopy in Barrett's esophagus and other premalignant conditions of the esophagus. Gastrointest Endosc. 2012;76(6):1087–94.
8. Levine DS, Haggitt RC, Blount PL, Rabinovitch PS, Rusch VW, Reid BJ. An endoscopic biopsy protocol can differentiate high-grade dysplasia from early adenocarcinoma in Barrett's esophagus. Gastroenterology. 1993;105(1):40–50.
9. Fitzgerald RC, di Pietro M, Ragunath K, Ang Y, Kang JY, Watson P, Trudgill N, Patel P, Kaye PV, Sanders S, O'Donovan M, Bird-Lieberman E, Bhandari P, Jankowski JA, Attwood S, Parsons SL, Loft D, Lagergren J, Moayyedi P, Lyratzopoulos G, de Caestecker J. British Society of gastroenterology guidelines on

the diagnosis and management of Barrett's oesophagus. Gut. 2014;63(1):7–42 Epub 2013 Oct 28.
10. Bennett C, Moayyedi P, Corley DA, DeCaestecker J, Falck-Ytter Y, Falk G, Vakil N, Sanders S, Vieth M, Inadomi J, Aldulaimi D, Ho KY, Odze R, Meltzer SJ, Quigley E, Gittens S, Watson P, Zaninotto G, Iyer PG, Alexandre L, Ang Y, Callaghan J, Harrison R, Singh R, Bhandari P, Bisschops R, Geramizadeh B, Kaye P, Krishnadath S, Fennerty MB, Manner H, Nason KS, Pech O, Konda V, Ragunath K, Rahman I, Romero Y, Sampliner R, Siersema PD, Tack J, Tham TC, Trudgill N, Weinberg DS, Wang J, Wang K, Wong JY, Attwood S, Malfertheiner P, MacDonald D, Barr H, Ferguson MK, Jankowski J. BOB CAT consortium. BOB CAT: a large-scale review and Delphi consensus for management of Barrett's Esophagus with no Dysplasia, indefinite for, or low-grade Dysplasia. Am J Gastroenterol. 2015;110(5):662.
11. Tomizawa Y, Iyer PG, Wong Kee Song LM, et al. Safety of endoscopic mucosal resection for Barrett's esophagus. Am J Gastroenterol. 2013;108:1440–7.
12. Oka S, Tanaka S, Kaneko I, et al. Advantage of endoscopic submucosal dissection compared with EMR for early gastric cancer. Gastrointest Endosc. 2006;64:877–83.
13. Konda VJ, Gonzalez Haba Ruiz M, Koons A, et al. Complete endoscopic mucosal resection is effective and durable treatment for Barretts-associated neoplasia. Clin Gastroenterol Hepatol. 2014;12:2002–10.
14. Soetikno RM, Gotoda T, Nakanishi Y, Soehendra N. Endoscopic mucosal resection. Gastrointest Endosc. 2003;57(4):567.
15. Tanaka S, Oka S, Kaneko I, et al. Endoscopic submucosal dissection for colorectal neoplasia: possibility of standardization. Gastrointest Endosc. 2007;66:100–7.
16. van Vilsteren FG, Pouw RE, Seewald S, et al. Stepwise radical endoscopic resection versus radiofrequency ablation for Barrett's oesophagus with high-grade dysplasia or early cancer: a multi-centre randomised trial. Gut. 2011;60:765–73.
17. Seewald S, Akaraviputh T, Seitz U, et al. Circumferential EMR and complete removal of Barrett's epithelium: a new approach to management of Barrett's esophagus containing high-grade intraepithelial neoplasia and intramucosal carcinoma. Gastrointest Endosc. 2003;57:854–9.
18. Peters FP, Kara MA, Rosmolen WD, et al. Stepwise radical endoscopic resection is effective for complete removal of Barrett's esophagus with early neoplasia: a prospective study. Am J Gastroenterol. 2006;101:1449–57.
19. Qumseya B, Panossian AM, Rizk C, et al. Predictors of esophageal stricture formation post endoscopic mucosal resection. Clin Endosc. 2014;47:155–61.
20. Katada C, Muto M, Manabe T, Boku N, Ohtsu A, Yoshida S. Esophageal stenosis after endoscopic mucosal resection of superficial esophageal lesions. Gastrointest Endosc. 2003;57(2):165.
21. Qumseya B, Panossian AM, Rizk C, Cangemi D, Wolfsen C, Raimondo M, Woodward T, Wallace MB, Wolfsen H. Predictors of esophageal stricture formation post endoscopic mucosal resection. Clin Endosc. 2014;47(2):155–61.

22. Konda VJ, Gonzalez Haba Ruiz M, Koons A, Hart J, Xiao SY, Siddiqui UD, Ferguson MK, Posner M, Patti MG, Waxman I. Complete endoscopic mucosal resection is effective and durable treatment for Barrett's-associated neoplasia. Clin Gastroenterol Hepatol. 2014;12(12):2002-10.e1–2.

23. Chung IK, Lee JH, Lee SH, Kim SJ, Cho JY, Cho WY, Hwangbo Y, Keum BR, Park JJ, Chun HJ, Kim HJ, Kim JJ, Ji SR, Seol SY. Therapeutic outcomes in 1000 cases of endoscopic submucosal dissection for early gastric neoplasms: Korean ESD study group multicenter study. Gastrointest Endosc. 2009;69(7):1228–35.

24. Isomoto H, Yamaguchi N, Minami H, Nakao K. Management of complications associated with endoscopic submucosal dissection/endoscopic mucosal resection for esophageal cancer. Dig Endosc. 2013;25(Suppl 1):29–38.

25. van Lanschot JJ, Hulscher JB, Buskens CJ, Tilanus HW, ten Kate FJ, Obertop H. Hospital volume and hospital mortality for esophagectomy. Cancer. 2001;91(8):1574.

26. Takahashi H, Arimura Y, Masao H, Okahara S, Tanuma T, Kodaira J, Kagaya H, Shimizu Y, Hokari K, Tsukagoshi H, Shinomura Y, Fujita M. Endoscopic submucosal dissection is superior to conventional endoscopic resection as a curative treatment for early squamous cell carcinoma of the esophagus (with video). Gastrointest Endosc. 2010;72(2):255–64 264.e1-2.

27. Mizuta H, Nishimori I, Kuratani Y, Higashidani Y, Kohsaki T, Onishi S. Predictive factors for esophageal stenosis after endoscopic submucosal dissection for superficial esophageal cancer. Dis Esophagus. 2009;22(7):626–31.

28. Ono S, Fujishiro M, Niimi K, Goto O, Kodashima S, Yamamichi N, Omata M. Predictors of postoperative stricture after esophageal endoscopic submucosal dissection for superficial squamous cell neoplasms. Endoscopy. 2009;41(8):661–5.

29. Kim JS, Kim BW, Shin IS. Efficacy and safety of endoscopic submucosal dissection for superficial squamous esophageal neoplasia: a meta-analysis. Dig Dis Sci. 2014;59(8):1862–9.

30. van Vilsteren FG, Phoa KN, Alvarez Herrero L, Pouw RE, Sondermeijer CM, van Lijnschoten I, Seldenrijk KA, Visser M, Meijer SL, van Berge Henegouwen MI, Weusten BL, Schoon EJ, Bergman JJ. Circumferential balloon-based radiofrequency ablation of Barrett's esophagus with dysplasia can be simplified, yet efficacy maintained, by omitting the cleaning phase. Clin Gastroenterol Hepatol. 2013;11(5):491.e1–498.e1.

31. Akiyama J, Marcus SN, Triadafilopoulos G. Effective intra-esophageal acid control is associated with improved radiofrequency ablation outcomes in Barrett's esophagus. Dig Dis Sci. 2012;57(10):2625.

32. Lyday WD, Corbett FS, Kuperman DA, Kalvaria I, Mavrelis PG, Shughoury AB, Pruitt RE. Radiofrequency ablation of Barrett's esophagus: outcomes of 429 patients from a multicenter community practice registry. Endoscopy. 2010;42(4):272.

33. Orman ES, Li N, Shaheen NJ. Efficacy and durability of radiofrequency ablation for Barrett's esophagus: systematic review and meta-analysis. Clin Gastroenterol Hepatol. 2013;11(10):1245.

34. Greenwald BD, Dumot JA, Abrams JA, Lightdale CJ, David DS, Nishioka NS, Yachimski P, Johnston MH, Shaheen NJ, Zfass AM, Smith JO, Gill KR, Burdick JS, Mallat D, Wolfsen HC. Endoscopic spray cryotherapy for esophageal cancer: safety and efficacy. Gastrointest Endosc. 2010;71(4):686–93.

35. Gosain S, Mercer K, Twaddell WS, Uradomo L, Greenwald BD. Liquid nitrogen spray cryotherapy in Barrett's esophagus with high-grade dysplasia: long-term results. Gastrointest Endosc. 2013;78(2):260.

36. Shaheen NJ, Sharma P, Overholt BF, Wolfsen HC, Sampliner RE, Wang KK, Galanko JA, Bronner MP, Goldblum JR, Bennett AE, Jobe BA, Eisen GM, Fennerty MB, Hunter JG, Fleischer DE, Sharma VK, Hawes RH, Hoffman BJ, Rothstein RI, Gordon SR, Mashimo H, Chang KJ, Muthusamy VR, Edmundowicz SA, Spechler SJ, Siddiqui AA, Souza RF, Infantolino A, Falk GW, Kimmey MB, Madanick RD, Chak A, Lightdale CJ. Radiofrequency ablation in Barrett's esophagus with dysplasia. N Engl J Med. 2009;360(22):2277.

37. Chadwick G, Groene O, Markar SR, Hoare J, Cromwell D, Hanna GB. Systematic review comparing radiofrequency ablation and complete endoscopic resection in treating dysplastic Barrett's esophagus: a critical assessment of histologic outcomes and adverse events. Gastrointest Endosc. 2014;79(5):718.

38. Shaheen NJ, Greenwald BD, Peery AF, Dumot JA, Nishioka NS, Wolfsen HC, Burdick JS, Abrams JA, Wang KK, Mallat D, Johnston MH, Zfass AM, Smith JO, Barthel JS, Lightdale CJ. Safety and efficacy of endoscopic spray cryotherapy for Barrett's esophagus with high-grade dysplasia. Gastrointest Endosc. 2010;71(4):680.

39. Canto MI, Shin EJ, Khashab MA, Molena D, Okolo P, Montgomery E, Pasricha P. Safety and efficacy of carbon dioxide cryotherapy for treatment of neoplastic Barrett's esophagus. Endoscopy. 2015;47(7):582.

40. van Vilsteren FG, Pouw RE, Seewald S, Alvarez Herrero L, Sondermeijer CM, Visser M, Ten Kate FJ, Yu Kim Teng KC, Soehendra N, Rösch T, Weusten BL, Bergman JJ. Stepwise radical endoscopic resection versus radiofrequency ablation for Barrett's oesophagus with high-grade dysplasia or early cancer: a multicentre randomised trial. Gut. 2011;60(6):765.

41. Phoa KN, van Vilsteren FG, Weusten BL, Bisschops R, Schoon EJ, Ragunath K, Fullarton G, Di Pietro M, Ravi N, Visser M, Offerhaus GJ, Seldenrijk CA, Meijer SL, ten Kate FJ, Tijssen JG, Bergman JJ. Radiofrequency ablation vs endoscopic surveillance for patients with Barrett esophagus and low-grade dysplasia: a randomized clinical trial. JAMA. 2014;311(12):1209–17.

42. Small AJ, Araujo JL, Leggett CL, Mendelson AH, Agarwalla A, Abrams JA, Lightdale CJ, Wang TC, Iyer PG, Wang KK, Rustgi AK, Ginsberg GG, Forde KA, Gimotty PA, Lewis JD, Falk GW, Bewtra M. Radiofrequency ablation is associated with decreased neoplastic progression in patients with Barrett's esophagus and confirmed low-grade Dysplasia. Gastroenterology. 2015;149(3):567.

Benign Strictures of the Esophagus, Stomach and Duodenum: Evaluation and Management

6

Vivek Kaul and Shivangi T. Kothari

Introduction

Benign esophageal, gastric and duodenal strictures are a significant cause of morbidity and have a variety of underlying etiologies. Clinical presentation can vary from an acute (e.g., food bolus impaction above an esophageal stricture; (Fig. 6.1) to a more chronic or subacute presentation (e.g., gastric outlet obstruction related to peptic ulcer disease). Similarly, the evaluation and management of these strictures also differs depending on the underlying cause and the clinical picture at hand. In this chapter, we will review some of the benign causes of esophageal and foregut strictures as well as discuss the best approach to evaluation and management.

Esophageal Strictures

A variety of conditions can cause benign esophageal strictures. The most commonly found and clinically significant conditions are listed in Table 6.1. In this section, we will briefly discuss the pathophysiology, epidemiology, clinical presentation and significance of the different types of benign esophageal strictures.

Electronic supplementary material
Supplementary material is available in the online version of this chapter at 10.1007/978-3-319-49041-0_6. Videos can also be accessed at https://link.springer.com/chapter/10.1007/978-3-319-49041-0_6.

V. Kaul (✉) · S.T. Kothari
Division of Gastroenterology/Hepatology, Center for Advanced Therapeutic Endoscopy, University of Rochester Medical Center & Strong Memorial Hospital, 601 Elmwood Ave, Box 646, Rochester, NY 14642, USA
e-mail: Vivek_kaul@urmc.rochester.edu

S.T. Kothari
e-mail: shivangi_kothari@urmc.rochester.edu

Peptic Strictures

Peptic strictures due to acid reflux (GERD) are the most common cause of benign esophageal strictures and represent about 70% of all such cases [1]. Clinically significant, longstanding acid exposure leads to erosive esophagitis with subsequent cicatrization leading to stricture formation and luminal narrowing (Fig. 6.2a, b). Poor esophageal motility and clearance of swallowed (or refluxed) contents and a dysfunctional lower esophageal sphincter contribute to the erosive esophagitis and stricture formation [2]. The presence of a hiatal hernia and delayed gastric emptying may also play a role in increased acid exposure and an increased risk of stricture formation. Peptic strictures are estimated to occur in about 10–20% of all patients with GERD. While peptic strictures can occur at any age, older white males are at highest risk.

The morbidity associated with peptic esophageal strictures can be significant. The most common symptoms patients report are heartburn, dysphagia, odynophagia, food impaction, weight loss and chest discomfort/pain. Persistent, refractory GERD, recurrent dysphagia, food impaction, weight loss and even aspiration pneumonia present real clinical challenges in this patient population. Barrett's esophagus frequently coexists in these patients and confers neoplastic risk over the long term as well. Atypical presentations of peptic esophageal strictures include chronic unexplained cough, regurgitation and asthma. As expected, peptic strictures are more commonly found in patients with systemic sclerosis and Zollinger–Ellison syndrome.

Esophageal Webs and Rings

Webs and rings are structural abnormalities of the esophagus that are often asymptomatic but may cause significant symptoms of dysphagia, regurgitation and aspiration. An esophageal ring is defined as a concentric, smooth, circumferential extension of normal esophageal tissue causing

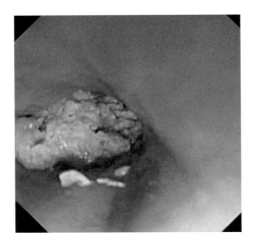

Fig. 6.1 Food bolus impaction above an esophageal stricture

Table 6.1 Causes of benign esophageal stricture

Peptic (GERD)
Webs/rings
Eosinophilic esophagitis
Radiation
Postoperative (iatrogenic)
Extrinsic compression (vascular structures)
Miscellaneous (e.g., congenital, medication related, lye/alkali ingestion)

luminal narrowing. An esophageal ring can be found anywhere along the esophagus, but it is usually found in the distal esophagus. Several theories exist regarding the pathophysiology and development of esophageal webs and rings. These include congenital defects (defects in embryologic development), autoimmune, inflammation and iron-deficiency (Plummer–Vinson syndrome)-related etiologies. In general, these are best described as congential or acquired.

Three types of lower esophageal rings exist, and they are classified as type A, B or C [3]. The most common and clinically significant ring is the "B" ring, also known as Schatzki's ring, which is primarily composed of mucosa and submucosa. The Schatzki ring is typically located at or just above the squamocolumnar junction and appears as a sharp, ring-like luminal narrowing in the distal esophagus [4, 5] (Fig. 6.3a, b).

It is postulated that GERD and esophageal dysmotility may have a role in the development of a Schatzki's ring. Other causes of lower esophageal rings include pill-induced rings, benign pemphigoid and mediastinal radiation.

Upper esophageal rings or "webs" have been described in association with the Plummer–Vinson and the Paterson–Brown–Kelly syndromes, both associated with iron-deficiency anemia and upper esophageal post-cricoid webs. Other associated features are koilonychia, cheilosis and glossitis. Pharyngeal and cervical esophageal cancers have been associated with this condition as well. Periodic screening for esophageal cancer in these patients is recommended. Upper esophageal webs have also been reported in patients with chronic graft versus host disease (GVHD) after bone marrow transplantation (Fig. 6.4a–c).

Esophageal webs have also been reported in association with some dermatologic conditions, including pemphigoid, epidermolysis bullosa, Stevens–Johnson syndrome and psoriasis. Webs may also be seen in patients with Zenker's diverticulum and esophageal duplication cysts.

Esophageal webs and rings are found in about 10–15% of routine barium studies.

Esophageal rings are most commonly found in Caucasians, and webs are more common in females. Dysphagia is the most common presentation, and it is typically described as "intermittent" and predominantly for solids. Most patients will report a history of GERD and/or a history of prior endoscopic intervention for symptoms.

Eosinophilic Esophagitis (EoE)

Approximately 10–15% of patients referred for dysphagia evaluation are found to have EoE. EoE is an inflammatory condition mediated by eosinophils, and the majority of

Fig. 6.2 Peptic stricture of the esophagus. **a** Endoscopic view of peptic stricture of esophagus and **b** barium swallow showing distal esophageal peptic stricture

(a)   **(b)**

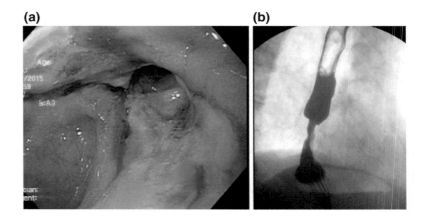

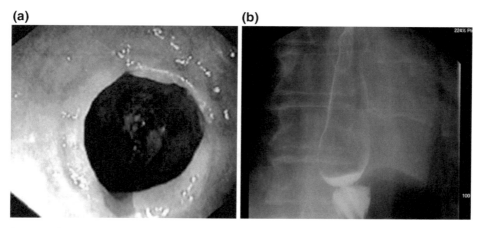

Fig. 6.3 Schatzki's ring. **a** Endoscopic view of Schatzki's ring and **b** barium swallow revealing Schatzki's ring

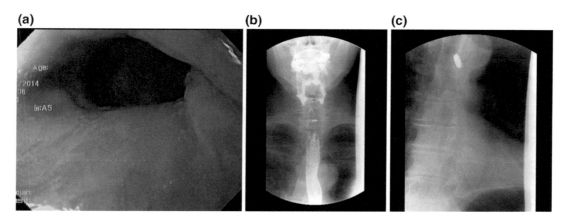

Fig. 6.4 Esophageal web. **a** Esophageal web: endoscopic image, **b** barium swallow: esophageal web and **c** barium pill hold up at esophageal web

affected adults are young men in the third and fourth decades. The most common symptoms are dysphagia, food impaction and atypical chest pain. Diagnostic criteria have been proposed for EoE which include: [6].

- Symptoms related to esophageal dysfunction
- Esophageal biopsy specimen with ≥ 15 eosinophils/high power field (hpf)
- Isolated esophageal mucosal eosinophilia that persists after a proton pump inhibitor (PPI) trial
- Secondary causes of esophageal eosinophilia excluded
- A response to treatment supports, but is not required for, diagnosis.

Patients with EoE may have a history of additional allergic or autoimmune phenomena (e.g., allergic rhinitis, asthma and eczema). The most common presenting symptoms include dysphagia and food bolus impaction, the latter typically requiring urgent endoscopic intervention. Esophageal strictures may be focal or involve a long segment of the esophagus (Fig. 6.5).

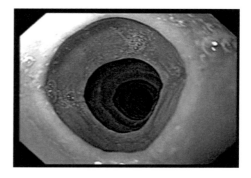

Fig. 6.5 Eosinophilic esophagitis-related stricture

Radiation-Induced Strictures

Patients undergoing brachytherapy or external beam radiation for head and neck, breast or thoracic malignancies (including esophageal malignancy) are at risk of developing radiation-induced esophageal strictures (Fig. 6.6a, b). Radiation-induced chronic ischemia leads to fibrosis and chronic

Fig. 6.6 Radiation stricture.
a Endoscopic view of radiation
stricture and **b** barium swallow
revealing radiation stricture

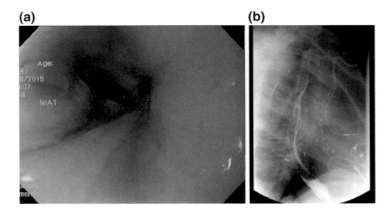

radiation esophagitis, which leads to esophageal stricturing. Neuromuscular injury from radiation exposure may also contribute to symptoms due to concomitant dysmotility.

In some cases, radiation-induced strictures can be quite complex anatomically and present a significant clinical challenge. The vast majority of such patients present with slowly progressive dysphagia and weight loss in the setting of a remote history of radiation exposure to the chest. Some patients may have odynophagia and chest discomfort as well.

Extrinsic Causes

Any cervical or mediastinal pathology or anatomic anomaly may cause an extrinsic compression of the esophagus with resultant luminal compromise and stenosis. A number of vascular abnormalities can cause focal areas of esophageal narrowing resulting in dysphagia [7, 8] (Fig. 6.7). Some examples are:

- Complete vascular ring anomalies (e.g., double aortic arch)
- Incomplete vascular ring anomalies (e.g., retroesophageal right aberrant subclavian artery and anomalous left pulmonary artery)
- In older adults, aneurysmal dilation of the thoracic aorta can compress the esophagus (dysphagia aortica).

In addition to the above, cervical spine osteophytes can also cause severe esophageal narrowing resulting in significant dysphagia, particularly in the older patient (Fig. 6.8). Inflammatory mediastinal pathology (e.g., tuberculosis, fibrosing mediastinitis) can cause traction mediated esophageal luminal distortion and narrowing which can be very difficult to manage, especially in the setting of longstanding chronic fibrosis.

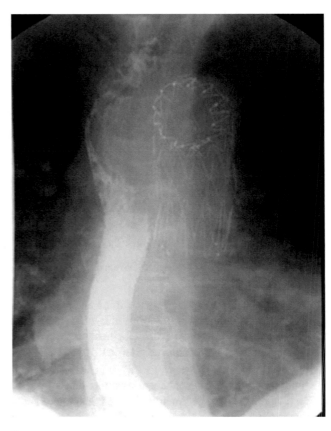

Fig. 6.7 Aortic aneurysm causing extrinsic compression of esophagus

Postoperative (Iatrogenic)

Endoscopic and surgical intervention in the esophagus can also commonly result in stricture formation. Any esophageal surgery with subsequent primary anastomosis (i.e., esophago-gastric, esophago-jejunal) whether performed for a benign or malignant condition can result in postoperative anastomotic stricture formation (Fig. 6.9a, b). The risk may be greater in

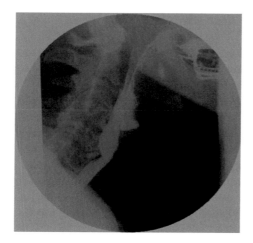

Fig. 6.8 Cervical osteophyte causing esophageal obstruction

elderly patients, those who received radiation and in patients who have repeated surgical interventions, anastomotic, leaks and local mediastinal inflammation/infection.

Endoscopic mucosal resection (EMR) or endoscopic submucosal dissection and endoluminal ablation for Barrett's and related neoplasia are also well-recognized causes of esophageal stricture formation. Both radiofrequency ablation and cryoablation of the esophagus carry about a 5–7% risk of esophageal stricture formation [9]. With endoscopic resection, the risk increases in direct proportion to the circumference of the esophagus resected, with circumferential resection carrying the highest risk of stricture formation. Most of these strictures are focal and present with dysphagia as the main symptom [10] (Fig. 6.10a–c).

Caustic Ingestion

Ingestion of a caustic substance can lead to severe esophageal injury and strictures, the degree of which depends on the nature of the ingested agent, the volume ingested and the duration of contact between the agent and the esophagus mucosa (Fig. 6.11). A majority of ingestions occur in

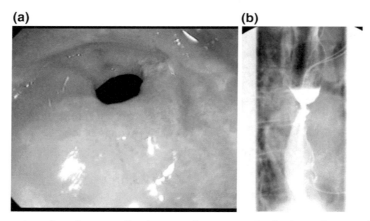

Fig. 6.9 Post-esophagectomy anastomotic stricture. **a** Esophago-gastric anastomosis: benign stricture and **b** barium swallow revealing anastomotic esophageal stricture

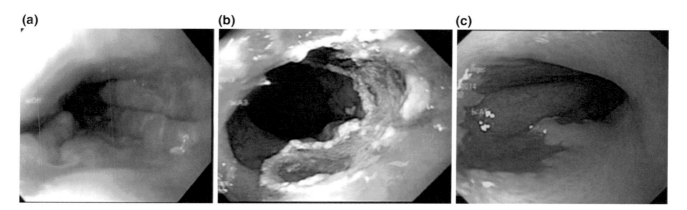

Fig. 6.10 Post-endoscopic mucosal resection (EMR) esophageal stricture. **a** Early esophageal cancer, **b** multiband EMR of early esophageal cancer and **c** post-EMR esophageal stricture

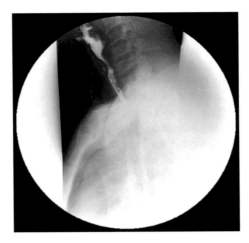

Fig. 6.11 Caustic injury-related esophageal stricture

children accidently. In adults, psychiatric illness, suicidal intent and alcoholism are common underlying reasons for ingestion, although accidental ingestion also occurs rarely in adults. Alkali causes more esophageal injury and acid causes more gastric/duodenal injury. Extensive transmural injury and inflammation can progress to severe fibrosis and stricturing over time in up to one-third of patients [11]. Patients may develop dysphagia, odynophagia and chest pain over a variable period of time from the initial injury (2 months to several years later). Patients who have experienced lye ingestion are at increased risk of development of squamous cell carcinoma of the esophagus.

Gastric and Duodenal Strictures

Gastric outlet and foregut luminal obstruction are the main presenting feature in patients who develop clinically significant strictures of the stomach and duodenum. The benign etiologies that can result in this clinical picture are listed in Table 6.2.

Table 6.2 Causes of benign gastric and duodenal strictures

Peptic ulcer disease
Crohn's disease
Caustic injury
Severe acute pancreatitis
Chronic pancreatitis
Post-surgical (iatrogenic)
Miscellaneous (annular pancreas, eosinophilic gastroenteritis, amyloidosis)

Peptic Ulcer Disease

Peptic disease remains the most common cause of inflammation and benign stricture formation in the pyloric channel and duodenum, although the overall incidence has dramatically decreased over the last several decades due to increased eradiation of H Pylori infection and H2 blocker and PPI use [12]. Local tissue inflammation and edema, when untreated, result in fibrosis and tissue deformity, resulting in luminal narrowing at the pyloro-duodenal channel which in turn causes gastric outlet obstruction. Patients present with early satiety, nausea, vomiting and chronic weight loss. They may report a history of NSAID use or a prior history of peptic ulcer disease.

Crohn's Disease

Crohn's disease of the stomach and foregut is relatively uncommon, with a reported incidence of <5% in all patient's with this disease. The vast majority of patients have concomitant disease in the lower gastrointestinal tract. Crohn's disease in the stomach and duodenum tends to involve contiguous areas in the gastro-duodenal channel, thereby leading to luminal narrowing and outlet obstruction. Stricture formation and, rarely, fistulas in this location can be problematic, and the symptoms may be insidious. Given that it is an uncommon entity, many patients may not be diagnosed accurately until there is advanced disease with significant symptomatology.

Caustic Injury

Corrosive ingestion is a well-known cause of gastric and duodenal strictures (Fig. 6.12). Patients typically become

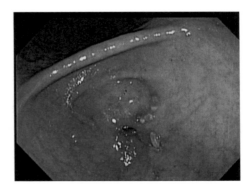

Fig. 6.12 Caustic injury-related stricture causing gastric outlet obstruction

symptomatic due to gastric outlet obstruction. In one study of 179 patients with caustic ingestion, esophageal injury was seen in 79% of patients, while gastric and duodenal injury were seen in 51 and 6%, respectively [13].

Gastric acid does not seem to be protective against injury with caustic ingestion. In another study, the rate of gastric stricture formation from post-caustic injury was 32% [14].

Pancreatitis

Both severe acute pancreatitis and chronic pancreatitis can result in significant edema, inflammation and narrowing of the pyloro-duodenal channel resulting in gastric outlet obstruction. The anatomic relationship of the pancreas with the gastric antrum and duodenal sweep results in significant alteration of the gastric outlet anatomy in the event of severe pancreatic inflammation. This mechanical obstruction further complicates the metabolic and nutritional challenges these patients already face in the wake of their pancreatic disease.

Post-surgical (Iatrogenic)

Strictures of the gastric outlet or proximal duodenum can occur in a variety of post-surgical scenarios. Patients with Roux-en-Y gastric bypass may develop stomal strictures at the gastro-enteric anastomosis. In patients who have undergone pylorus-preserving Whipple surgery, local edema and gastro-enteric anastomotic strictures may result in efferent limb outlet obstruction. In many patients, poor overall nutrition, delayed healing, local ischemia and prior radiation may contribute to stricture formation (Fig. 6.13a, b).

Evaluation and Management of Esophageal, Gastric and Duodenal Strictures

In this section, we describe the current approach to evaluation and management of the various esophageal and foregut strictures detailed above. The importance of a detailed history and review of records cannot be overemphasized. In most cases, the mainstay of investigation involves radiographic, cross-sectional imaging and endoscopic evaluation.

Depending on the anatomic location of the stricture and the patient's history and clinical presentation, one or more diagnostic tests may be needed. These are listed in Table 6.3. Similarly, depending on the location, etiology and complexity of the stricture, management may involve medical therapy or endoscopic or surgical intervention, or any combination thereof. In general, the vast majority of esophageal and foregut strictures can be managed with medical therapy and endoscopic management; surgical intervention (often viewed as a last resort) is infrequently required but provides definitive management both in the emergent (perforated viscus) or elective (refractory stricture) settings.

Radiologic Studies

For most esophageal strictures, a barium or gastrograffin swallow study is an excellent initial test to clarify the anatomy and localize the site of pathology. In the cases of

(a)   **(b)**

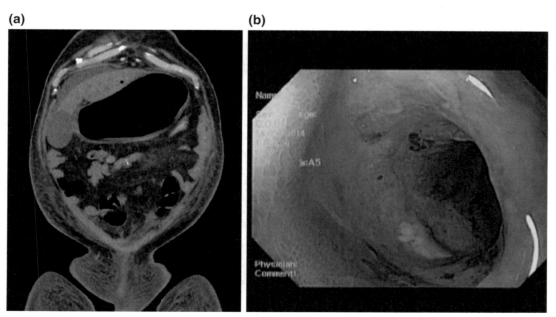

Fig. 6.13 Post-Whipple surgery ischemic ulcer causing gastric outlet obstruction. **a** CT showing gastric outlet obstruction post-Whipple surgery and **b** ischemic ulcer at anastomosis post-Whipple surgery causing gastric outlet obstruction

Table 6.3 Investigations used to evaluate benign esophageal and foregut strictures

Barium swallow
Barium swallow with 13 mm tablet
Gastrograffin swallow
Upper GI and small bowel follow through study
MR or CT enterography
Chest CT scan
Abdominal CT scan
Endoscopy/enteroscopy

extrinsic compression (osteophytes, cricopharyngeal bar, vascular impressions, etc.), a barium study will reveal the diagnosis more readily than endoscopy. In patients with radiation and caustic injury to the esophagus, barium and gastrograffin studies are extremely important to rule out complex strictures and any associated fistulas, allowing the endoscopist to more effectively plan any endoscopic intervention. Barium studies are virtually diagnostic for Schatzki's rings and esophageal webs and also provide valuable information regarding esophageal caliber in patients with EoE and caustic injury. In addition, a swallow study may also provide information regarding esophageal dysmotility, outflow obstruction and the contribution of a hiatal hernia (if present) toward a patient's symptoms. The lack of passage of a 13-mm tablet at certain luminal locations in the esophagus may provide clues regarding subtle changes in esophageal caliber that may guide endoscopic therapy (Fig. 6.14a–c).

Cross-sectional imaging (CT scan, MRI) can be useful as complementary tests in patients with benign strictures that are potentially helpful in several ways:

– Sagittal or coronal sections can delineate subtle lesions (e.g., osteophytes)
– Can rule out serious (malignant) pathology (e.g., mass lesions)
– Can confirm or rule out leaks and fistulas (e.g., in post-operative strictures)
– Can be used to evaluate for post-endoscopic therapy complications.

Endoscopy

Endoscopic evaluation is typically needed for the majority of patients who have symptomatic esophageal and foregut strictures. Since many of these patients present with significant symptoms, endoscopy with tissue sampling is a powerful tool for accurate diagnosis and for planning effective treatment. A variety of different caliber specialized endoscopes with high-definition optics are available to help navigate variable luminal diameters (5 mm–13 mm outer diameter). Tissue sampling also helps differentiate benign from malignant etiologies in almost all situations. It also helps define the criteria for EoE and certain other very specific causes of strictures (e.g., amyloidosis, eosinophilic gastroenteritis and radiation injury).

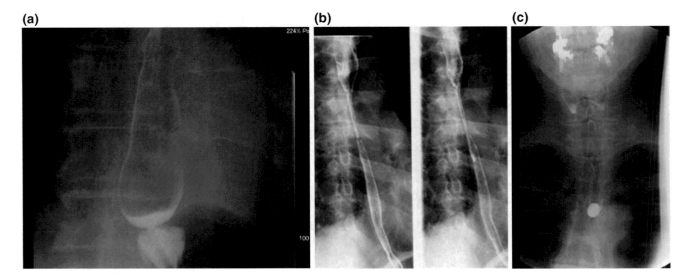

Fig. 6.14 Barium swallow and barium pill evaluation of dysphagia. **a** Barium swallow revealing Schatzki's ring, **b** Barium swallow revealing radiation stricture and **c** barium pill hold up at aortic arch causing esophageal narrowing

Table 6.4 Treatment options for esophageal and foregut strictures

Medical therapy
Oral fluticasone puff swallow (EoE)
Oral budenoside (EoE)
Proton pump therapy (GERD, EoE)
Endoscopic therapy
Balloon dilation
Bougeinage (Savary, Maloney)
Incisional (Schatzki ring, post-op stricture)
Fully covered removable stents (silicone, metal)
Surgery
Esophagectomy
Gastrectomy
Gastrojejunostomy
Other

Management of Esophageal and Foregut Strictures

Management of esophageal and foregut stricture disease is best accomplished using a stepwise and etiology-focused approach. Medical therapy, endoscopic management and surgery are the three available options for treatment. These are detailed in Table 6.4.

Medical Therapy

Patients with peptic esophageal and foregut strictures will require ongoing treatment with acid suppression. Typically, once or twice a day proton pump (PPI) therapy is initiated in these patients. NSAIDs, alcohol use and cigarette smoking are discouraged. GERD lifestyle modification is emphasized.

In patients with strictures due to EoE, a fluticasone metered dose inhaler can be used to deliver a total of 880–1760 mcg/day in adults (220 mcg × 2–4 metered dose puffs swallowed BID). Concomitant treatment with PPI is recommended in most patients. Most patients will require indefinite treatment since symptoms recur when medications are stopped. Treatment response is usually rapid (within 1–2 weeks) and side effects in general are mild/rare. Patients are advised to swallow the entire dose of the drug to reduce the risk of oral thrush. Budesonide liquid or viscous slurry has also been found useful in treating EoE. Patients should not eat or drink for at least 30 min after taking Fluticasone or Budesonide to maximize exposure to the drug.

Long-term "maintenance" treatment with either agent is frequently required since symptoms recur after cessation of medical therapy. Consultation with a food allergy specialist and consideration of an "elimination diet" are also part of the overall strategy for treating patients with EoE [6].

Endoscopic Therapy

Endoscopic treatment remains the mainstay of therapy for a vast majority of patients who have benign esophageal and foregut strictures. Modern endoscopes, high-definition imaging and novel accessories and luminal stent options have enabled endoscopic therapy to be a highly safe and effective modality for these patients. A variety of endoscopic treatment options are available depending on the nature, location, complexity of the stricture and the available expertise and resources (Table 6.4).

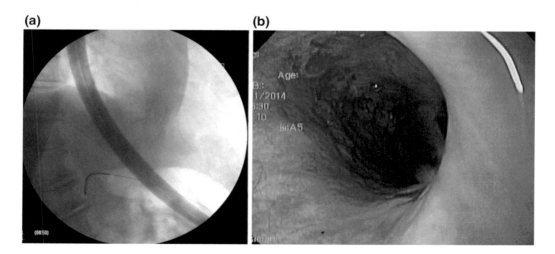

Fig. 6.15 Savary dilation of esophageal web. **a** Savary dilator over guidewire seen on fluoroscopy and **b** blood at site of cervical web post-dilation

Bougienage (Maloney and Savary Dilators)

Maloney (passed directly) and Savary (passed over the wire) are types of mechanical esophageal dilators most commonly used nowadays. Maloney dilators may be filled with mercury or tungsten, which provides weight and flexibility to the dilating catheter. The dilators are tapered and come in several graduated sizes, each with a 1–1.5 mm increment to the next size up. These dilators exert both a radial and longitudinal "shear" stress upon the stricture, moving from the proximal to the distal end of the stricture. Fluoroscopy may or may not be used with these bougie dilators (Fig. 6.15a, b).

Dilating Balloons

Through-the-scope (TTS) balloon dilation catheters are available which allow stricture dilation by providing a uniform radial expansion force throughout the length of the stricture with balloon inflation. Single size per catheter or multiple radial expansion sizes per catheter balloons are available, ranging from about 8 mm through 20 mm in maximal diameter when inflated. They are available in wire-guided or non-wire-guided configurations.

Both balloon and bougie dilation are considered equally effective, the latter is more cost-effective since the bougies are reusable after high-level disinfection (whereas the balloon catheters are disposable after single use). Bougies are not used for gastric or duodenal strictures.

For simple esophageal strictures, a Maloney dilator can be considered although many would prefer a Savary or Balloon dilation approach. Complex esophageal strictures (long strictures, tortuous anatomy, esophageal diverticulae, etc.) require dilation under direct vision using a balloon or bougie dilation over a guidewire (Savary) to prevent inad-

vertent esophageal perforation. In some cases, fluoroscopy may be necessary to ensure safe and effective dilation. As a general rule, dilation should be reserved for symptomatic patients only. It is recommended to limit the degree of dilation to three incremental sizes per session, starting with the size that initiates the first effective dilation. For balloons, the dilation is maintained for 30–60 s each. Repeat sessions of dilation may be needed in some patients with high-grade and/or complex strictures; acid suppression, and a modified diet is typically maintained during this period (Fig. 6.16a–c and Video 6.1).

The main potential complications of esophageal dilation include significant bleeding and esophageal perforation, although both are uncommon. The risk of perforation may be higher in patients with high-grade strictures in the setting of EE or radiation injury, but studies have not conclusively shown that. Most small perforations can be managed endoscopically, and most bleeding is self-limited in the absence of significant coagulopathy.

Balloon dilation of obstructing pyloric and duodenal strictures is also feasible, but typically requires multiple sessions with stepwise increase in dilation. In some cases, fluoroscopic guidance is mandatory to enable wire-guided balloon dilation, especially when the endoscope cannot traverse the stricture. Effective dilation to about 15–16 mm may provide adequate relief of symptoms of GOO (Fig. 6.17a–d). Some reports indicate a higher risk of perforation with pyloric dilation beyond this diameter [15].

Dilation of duodenal strictures using balloons may be technically more difficult and carry a higher rate of perforation. Stepwise dilation is recommended and multiple serial sessions are typically required. There should be a low threshold for obtaining a water-soluble contrast study or a CT scan for post-procedure abdominal pain or if the dilation was technically difficult or significantly traumatic.

(a)   **(b)**   **(c)**

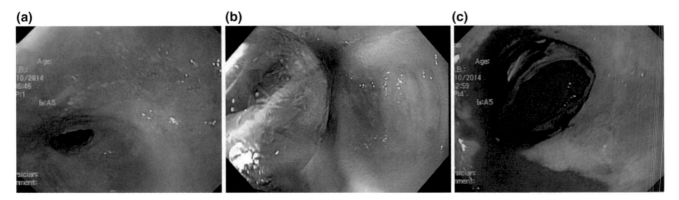

Fig. 6.16 Balloon dilation of esophageal stricture. **a** Esophageal stricture, **b** balloon dilation of esophageal stricture and **c** post-dilation blood and mucosal tear suggesting effective dilation

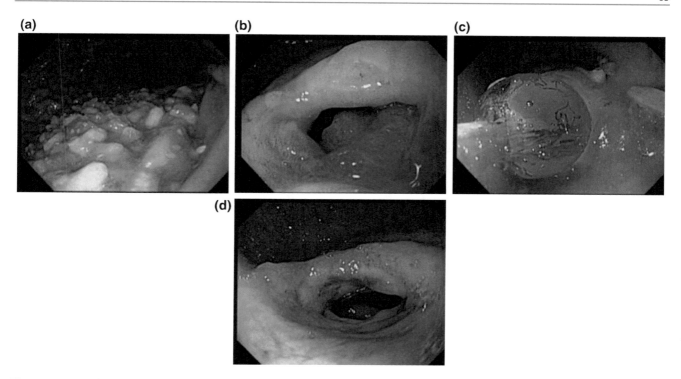

Fig. 6.17 Benign gastric outlet obstruction treated with balloon dilation. **a** Retained food in stomach from gastric outlet obstruction, **b** tight pyloric stenosis, **c** balloon dilation of pyloric stenosis and **d** post-balloon dilation image of pylorus

Fully Covered Self-Expanding Stents

Fully covered self-expanding metal (SEMS) or plastic (SEPS) stents may be used to treat benign esophageal, gastric and duodenal strictures, especially those that are "refractory" to bougienage or balloon dilation. The goal of stent placement is to restore luminal patency, allow oral nutrition, hydration and medication delivery and in some cases provide a "bridge" to surgery in a debilitated patient. Stents are particularly useful in the postoperative setting when complex anastomotic strictures may be present in conjunction with a fistula or leak.

Only fully covered SEMS or SEPS should be used to treat benign strictures, since these are endoscopically removable due to their plastic or silicon coating. Metal stents are typically made of nitinol or another alloy; the SEPS are made of polyester or silicone. SEPS, once popular, are uncommonly used in current practice.

Placement of stents is typically done using fluoroscopic guidance using an over the wire delivery catheter. A variety of lengths, diameters and flange sizes are available with different types of stent designs [16].

The overall success rates for treatment of benign strictures with fully covered stents vary depending on the

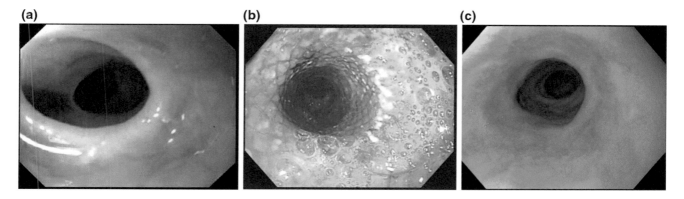

Fig. 6.18 Benign refractory esophageal stricture treated with fully covered esophageal stent. **a** Refractory esophageal stricture, **b** stent placed across esophageal stricture and **c** post-stent removal improvement of esophageal stricture seen

Fig. 6.19 Fully covered plastic esophageal stent placed under fluoroscopy and proximal end anchored with endoscopic suturing. **a** Fully covered plastic esophageal stent on fluoroscopy and **b** endoscopic sutures placed at proximal end of the fully covered plastic esophageal stent

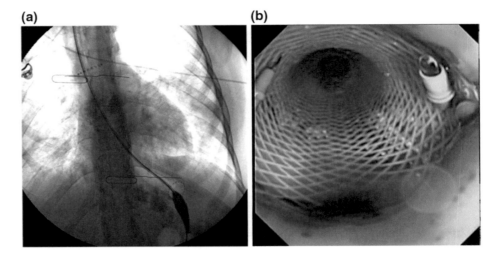

nature of the stricture, the duration of stenting and the underlying etiology. Technical success is very high, but treatment success is widely variable depending on the study (Fig. 6.18a–c) [17, 18]. With fully covered esophageal stents, the main complication is stent migration (usually distal into the stomach), which is seen in about a third of the patients. This issue can be mitigated by "anchoring" the proximal stent flange using endoscopic sutures or endoscopic clips (Fig. 6.19a, b). Some innovative stent design elements (e.g., Dog bone design and anti-migration struts) have been introduced to potentially reduce the frequency of migration [19, 20]. Chest pain after esophageal stent placement is not uncommon, but bleeding and perforation are rare.

Pyloro-duodenal stents may migrate back into the stomach, particularly if not anchored in place. Most stents that migrate into the stomach can be retrieved endoscopically. Duodenal stents may migrate further distally, which can be problematic in terms of retrieval and the potential causing small bowel obstruction.

Incisional Therapy

Refractory strictures (Schatzki rings and anastomotic strictures) can be treated with incisional therapy using needle-knife electrocautery, an insulation-tipped (IT) knife or argon plasma coagulation (APC) (Video 6.1). A proper delineation of the stricture anatomy is a critical. Circumferential radial incision of the fibrotic/stenotic rim is achieved in careful fashion, ensuring that the depth of incision is never transmural. To reduce the risk re-stenosis, concomitant balloon dilatation or intra-lesional steroids or APC treatment can be used. Short segment strictures (<1 cm) have been found to have the best outcome with this form of treatment. When compared with routine balloon dilatation, incisional therapy has equivalent results in treatment naïve cases but better long-term outcome in refractory cases [21]. Incisional treatment is not typically recommended or used for gastric or duodenal strictures.

Intra-lesional Steroid Injection

The injection of triamcinolone acetonide into the stricture immediately after endoscopic dilation may reduce local inflammation and collagen deposition, thereby increasing the efficacy of dilation and reducing the frequency or need for repeat dilations. The reports of this approach have had mixed results, with some patients responding very well and others not at all [22, 23]. Steroids are most likely to be effective if there is active inflammation, and less so in patients with severe or end-stage fibrosis. Although relatively safe, steroid injection does have the potential to increase procedure cost and duration, which needs to be weighed against any potential benefits.

Surgical Treatment

Refractory strictures that do not respond to medical and endoscopic management despite several repeat sessions of dilation may require definitive management with elective surgery. In general, surgical treatment is required for the most complex, and high-grade esophageal strictures that do not respond to aggressive endoscopic dilation or stenting and for severe pyloric and duodenal strictures that persist despite endoscopic therapy. Surgery is particularly attractive in those cases where malignancy has not been (or cannot be) conclusively ruled out, despite all efforts. In those patients, surgical intervention is both diagnostic and therapeutic and definitive. For esophageal strictures, partial or total esophagectomy with reconstruction (gastric pull-up or colonic interposition) may be required.

For pyloric strictures, a pyloroplasty or a Billroth-I or II type surgery may be offered. For duodenal strictures, options may include resection and primary anastomosis or a diverting gastrojejunostomy, depending on the location of the stricture.

Conclusion

Benign strictures of the esophagus and gastro-duodenum are commonly encountered in clinical gastroenterology practice. Radiologic studies and endoscopic evaluation are the mainstay of diagnosis. Medical therapy, endoscopic management and surgery each have a role in the management of these patients. Treatment-related complications are uncommon, and most patients have excellent long-term response to endoscopic therapy. The vast majority of patients can be managed with a combination of medical and endoscopic therapy. Patients with refractory strictures require definitive surgery. A carefully considered, thoughtful multidisciplinary team-based management plan is important to achieve the best outcome in these patients.

References

1. Richter JE. Peptic strictures of the esophagus. Gastroenterol Clin North Am 1999;28:875–91, vi.
2. Ahtaridis G, Snape WJ Jr, Cohen S. Clinical and manometric findings in benign peptic strictures of the esophagus. Dig Dis Sci. 1979;24:858–61.
3. Smith MS. Diagnosis and management of esophageal rings and webs. Gastroenterol Hepatol (N Y). 2010;6:701–4.
4. Schatzki R, Gary JE. Dysphagia due to a diaphragm-like localized narrowing in the lower esophagus (lower esophageal ring). Am J Roentgenol Radium Ther Nucl Med. 1953;70:911–22.
5. Muller M, Gockel I, Hedwig P, et al. Is the Schatzki ring a unique esophageal entity? World J Gastroenterol. 2011;17:2838–43.
6. Dellon ES, Gonsalves N, Hirano I, et al. ACG clinical guideline: evidenced based approach to the diagnosis and management of esophageal eosinophilia and eosinophilic esophagitis (EoE). Am J Gastroenterol 2013;108:679–92; quiz 693.
7. De Luca L, Bergman JJ, Tytgat GN, et al. EUS imaging of the arteria lusoria: case series and review. Gastrointest Endosc. 2000;52:670–3.
8. Bennett JR CD. Overview and symptom assessment. In: Castell DO, Richter JE, editors. The Esophagus. Philadelphia: Lippincott, Williams & Wilkins; 1999. p. 33.
9. Shaheen NJ, Sharma P, Overholt BF, et al. Radiofrequency ablation in Barrett's esophagus with dysplasia. N Engl J Med. 2009;360:2277–88.
10. Seewald S, Akaraviputh T, Seitz U, et al. Circumferential EMR and complete removal of Barrett's epithelium: a new approach to management of Barrett's esophagus containing high-grade intraepithelial neoplasia and intramucosal carcinoma. Gastrointest Endosc. 2003;57:854–9.
11. Zargar SA, Kochhar R, Nagi B, et al. Ingestion of strong corrosive alkalis: spectrum of injury to upper gastrointestinal tract and natural history. Am J Gastroenterol. 1992;87:337–41.
12. Shone DN, Nikoomanesh P, Smith-Meek MM, et al. Malignancy is the most common cause of gastric outlet obstruction in the era of H2 blockers. Am J Gastroenterol. 1995;90:1769–70.
13. Poley JW, Steyerberg EW, Kuipers EJ, et al. Ingestion of acid and alkaline agents: outcome and prognostic value of early upper endoscopy. Gastrointest Endosc. 2004;60:372–7.
14. Zargar SA, Kochhar R, Nagi B, et al. Ingestion of corrosive acids. Spectrum of injury to upper gastrointestinal tract and natural history. Gastroenterology. 1989;97:702–7.
15. Boylan JJ, Gradzka MI. Long-term results of endoscopic balloon dilatation for gastric outlet obstruction. Dig Dis Sci. 1999;44:1883–6.
16. Committee AT, Varadarajulu S, Banerjee S, et al. Enteral stents. Gastrointest Endosc. 2011;74:455–64.
17. Repici A, Hassan C, Sharma P, et al. Systematic review: the role of self-expanding plastic stents for benign oesophageal strictures. Aliment Pharmacol Ther. 2010;31:1268–75.
18. Eloubeidi MA, Lopes TL. Novel removable internally fully covered self-expanding metal esophageal stent: feasibility, technique of removal, and tissue response in humans. Am J Gastroenterol. 2009;104:1374–81.
19. Buscaglia JM, Ho S, Sethi A, et al. Fully covered self-expandable metal stents for benign esophageal disease: a multicenter retrospective case series of 31 patients. Gastrointest Endosc. 2011;74:207–11.
20. Senousy BE, Gupte AR, Draganov PV, et al. Fully covered Alimaxx esophageal metal stents in the endoscopic treatment of benign esophageal diseases. Dig Dis Sci. 2010;55:3399–403.
21. Samanta J, Dhaka N, Sinha SK, et al. Endoscopic incisional therapy for benign esophageal strictures: technique and results. World J Gastrointest Endosc. 2015;7:1318–26.
22. Kochhar R, Makharia GK. Usefulness of intralesional triamcinolone in treatment of benign esophageal strictures. Gastrointest Endosc. 2002;56:829–34.
23. Hirdes MM, van Hooft JE, Koornstra JJ, et al. Endoscopic corticosteroid injections do not reduce dysphagia after endoscopic dilation therapy in patients with benign esophagogastric anastomotic strictures. Clin Gastroenterol Hepatol. 2013;11(795–801):e1.

Shivangi T. Kothari and Vivek Kaul

Introduction

Malignant esophageal, gastric, and duodenal strictures are a significant cause of morbidity mortality. The case fatality rate for these patients is quite high, given the poor prognosis associated with these cancers. Many of these patients present at an advanced stage of malignancy, at which point management options often are limited to palliation and symptom relief. Clinical presentation can vary from an acute (e.g., food bolus impaction above an esophageal stricture and hematemesis) to a more chronic or subacute (e.g., gastric outlet obstruction (GOO) and weight loss) type of scenario. Similarly, the evaluation and management approach also differs depending on the underlying cause and the clinical picture at hand. In this chapter, we will review some of the common causes of malignant esophageal and foregut strictures as well as discuss the best approach to evaluation and management.

Esophageal Strictures

A variety of clinical conditions can cause malignant esophageal and gastro-esophageal (GE) junction strictures. They are listed in Table 7.1. The most common etiologies are intra-luminal malignancies (intrinsic) but mediastinal and thoracic (lung) malignancies can also cause infiltration into and extrinsic compression of the esophagus (Fig. 7.1a, b). In

Electronic supplementary material
Supplementary material is available in the online version of this chapter at 10.1007/978-3-319-49041-0_7. Videos can also be accessed at https://link.springer.com/chapter/10.1007/978-3-319-49041-0_7.

S.T. Kothari · V. Kaul (✉)
Center for Advanced Therapeutic Endoscopy, Division of Gastroenterology and Hepatology, University of Rochester Medical Center & Strong Memorial Hospital, Rochester, NY 14642, USA
e-mail: Vivek_kaul@urmc.rochester.edu

S.T. Kothari
e-mail: shivangi_kothari@urmc.rochester.edu

either of the cases, luminal narrowing and tumor infiltration may lead to progressive dysphagia and other symptoms (chest pain and bleeding). Dysphagia is typically the most common presenting symptom. In some patients undergoing endoscopy for Barrett's surveillance (or another indication), early lesions may be diagnosed in relatively asymptomatic patients. In this section, we will briefly review the various causes of malignant esophageal strictures.

Squamous Cell Cancer of the Esophagus (SCC)

The incidence of SCC varies widely across the globe, with countries in central Asia and the far-east (India and China) having a much higher disease burden compared to the Western world [1]. This may be directly related to increased tobacco and alcohol consumption, although genetic, familial, and environmental factors have been invoked. Achalasia and a prior history of caustic injury to the esophagus have been associated with an increased incidence of esophageal SCC. The overall incidence of SCC in the USA is on the decline.

Adenocarcinoma of Esophagus, GE Junction and Gastric Cardia

Esophageal adenocarcinoma is much more common in the USA and the Western world, compared to SCC, and is almost always found in the setting of Barrett's esophagus (BE). The overall incidence of esophageal adenocarcinoma is on the rise [2]. The presence of long-standing acid reflux, genetic factors, race (Caucasians), and high BMI has all been implicated as risk factors. Cigarette smoking increases the risk further, especially in patients with BE.

Dysphagia, weight loss, retrosternal burning or discomfort, and regurgitation of food are the usual symptoms in patients with malignant esophageal strictures. Patients may also present with gastrointestinal bleeding (melena or hematemesis) and anemia. Hoarseness and respiratory

Table 7.1 Common causes of malignant esophageal and foregut strictures

Esophagus
Esophageal cancer
– Squamous cell
– Adenocarcinoma
Gastric cardia cancer
GE junction cancer
Esophageal intramural neoplasia (GIST)
Extrinsic tumor compression
– Mediastinal tumors
– Lymphoma
– Lung cancer
– Metastatic
Gastroduodenum
Gastric cancer
Duodenal cancer
Pancreatic cancer
Metastatic cancer
Cholangiocarcinoma
Ampullary cancer

symptoms (pneumonia) may suggest laryngeal nerve involvement and/or the development of a fistula, respectively, due to locally advanced, infiltrating disease.

Mediastinal and Thoracic Malignancies

Apart from intrinsic luminal disease, esophageal strictures can also be encountered due to malignant processes that arise in the mediastinum (lymphoma) and thorax (lung cancer). These will typically cause "extrinsic" compression of the esophageal lumen leading primarily to symptoms of dysphagia, regurgitation, and chest pain as well as weight loss over a period of time due to poor nutrition (Fig. 7.2). In these patients, additional clinical signs and symptoms may coexist related to the primary pathology (e.g., superior vena cava syndrome due to lung cancer). Primary mediastinal tumors (germ cell, mesenchymal, neurogenic, and thymic origin), lymphoma, and thyroid malignancies (especially with retrosternal and substernal extension) can cause extrinsic esophageal compression and dysphagia. In addition, some of these patients may have cough, stridor, hemoptysis, and constitutional symptoms such as fever, night sweats, and weight loss. The degree and severity of the esophageal symptoms depend on the proximity of the tumor to the esophagus, tumor size, and rate of growth. Some patients can "adapt" remarkably well to a slow-growing tumor and report minimal symptoms over time.

Metastatic breast carcinoma, melanoma, and neuroendocrine tumor can also lead to a bulky mediastinal tumor burden and may cause a compressive "mass effect" on the esophagus, causing focal or complex esophageal luminal stenosis, presenting as dysphagia.

Adenocarcinoma of the lung and other primary pulmonary malignancies with associated bulky adenopathy may lead to significant esophageal compression on occasion, often presenting as dysphagia. Other symptoms such as dyspnea, hemoptysis, hoarseness, and chest pain typically also exist in patients with such advanced stage tumors.

Esophageal Intramural Neoplasia

Carcinoid tumors and gastrointestinal stromal tumors (GIST) of the esophagus are neoplastic lesions that can create luminal obstruction and stenosis depending on the size, location in the esophagus, and rate of growth. These lesions can grow in both

Fig. 7.1 a, b Malignant strictures of the esophagus: extrinsic versus intrinsic etiologies. **a** Extrinsic mass impression on esophagus from mediastinal tumor. **b** Esophageal cancer causing intrinsic luminal narrowing

(a)   **(b)**

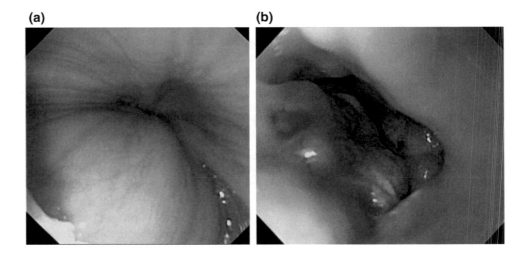

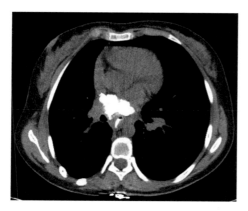

Fig. 7.2 Extrinsic compression of the esophagus caused by calcified mediastinal tumor

directions (into the mediastinum or toward the esophageal lumen) and create a mass effect, predominantly causing dysphagia and/or chest pain in most patients. Many of these tumors are "pre-malignant," although malignant features are well described, and they carry metastatic potential [3, 4].

Malignant Strictures of the Gastroduodenum

Malignant strictures of the stomach and duodenum can be due to adenocarcinoma of either organ, or secondary to obstruction of the pyloro-duodenal channel from locally advanced pancreatic cancer, ampullary cancer, cholangiocarcinoma, lymphoma, or metastatic malignancy (Table 7.1). The most common symptoms due to clinically significant malignant foregut strictures are abdominal pain,

abdominal distension, and nausea/vomiting due to GOO (Fig. 7.3a, b). Weight loss in these patients can be both dramatic and rapid. These patients may also present with anemia, gastrointestinal bleeding (melena or occult blood loss), and anorexia. In patients with pancreatic head malignancy, biliary obstruction will usually be present concomitantly with GOO. In this section, we will briefly discuss the common causes of malignant foregut (gastric and duodenal) strictures.

Malignant Gastric Strictures

Most patients with gastric adenocarcinoma present with advanced disease and even those undergoing surgery with curative intent have high rates of recurrence [5]. Tumor location in the cardia and at the GE junction as well as in the antrum predisposes the patient to luminal obstruction secondary to malignant stricture formation (Fig. 7.4a, b). Tumors in the gastric body are less likely to cause luminal obstruction, unless linitis plastica or diffuse/infiltrating gastric malignancy exists. Abdominal pain, early satiety, weight loss, anemia, and GOO are the typical clinical features seen in these patients. Any or several of these symptoms may prompt an upper endoscopy, which typically will reveal a locally advanced malignancy, especially if a stricture is encountered.

Other gastric malignancies can also present with stricture formation and a clinical picture similar to the one mentioned above (Fig. 7.5). Gastric mucosa-associated lymphoid tissue (MALT) and metastatic cancers to the

(a)   **(b)**

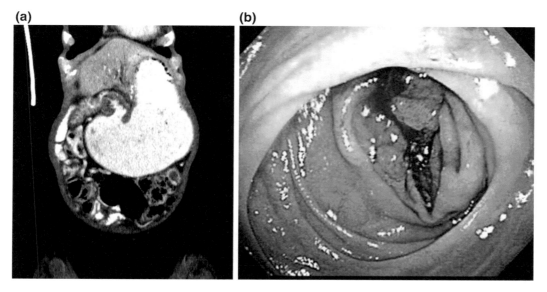

Fig. 7.3 a, b Malignant gastric outlet obstruction. **a** Gastric outlet obstruction seen on CT imaging. **b** Endoscopic view of malignant duodenal tumor causing gastric outlet obstruction

Fig. 7.4 **a**, **b** Gastric cardia
tumor and gastric cancer on CT
scan. **a** Gastric cardia cancer
endoscopic (retroflexed) view.
b Gastric cancer on CT scan

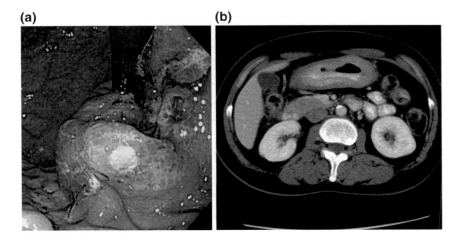

stomach can also lead to luminal narrowing, alteration of
gastric motility and GOO.

Duodenal Strictures

Malignant primary tumors that can cause duodenal strictures include adenocarcinomas, carcinoids, sarcomas, and
lymphomas. In addition, locally advanced pancreatic head
carcinoma is an important and common cause of malignant
duodenal obstruction. Ampullary cancer and cholangiocarcinoma can also produce duodenal obstruction. When this
occurs, concomitant biliary obstruction is usually present
(Fig. 7.6a–c). Metastatic tumor from other organs (e.g.,
renal cell, melanoma, and colorectal cancer) can also
occasionally present with malignant duodenal obstruction.
In these cases, the tumor compression can be either purely
extrinsic ("mass effect") or there may be gross tumor
infiltration into the duodenal lumen. These patients usually
present with GOO, abdominal discomfort, weight loss, and
anorexia.

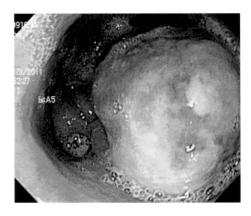

Fig. 7.5 Gastric sarcoma at GE junction causing obstruction

Evaluation and Management of Malignant Esophageal, Gastric, and Duodenal Strictures

In this section, we describe the current approach to evaluation and management of the various malignant esophageal
and foregut strictures discussed above. The importance of a
detailed history and review of records cannot be overemphasized. In most cases, the mainstay of investigation
involves radiographic (contrast studies and cross-sectional
imaging) and endoscopic evaluation.

Tissue sampling using luminal endoscopy and/or endoscopic ultrasound (EUS) is essential to make an accurate
diagnosis and to plan appropriate treatment. Depending on
the anatomic location of the stricture and the patient's history and clinical presentation, one or more diagnostic tests
may be needed in a given situation. These are listed in
Table 7.2.

Depending on the nature of the malignancy, location of
pathology, extent of disease and clinical stage, and overall
condition of the patient, several different management
options can be considered. For loco-regional disease, surgical management (with or without neoadjuvant
chemo-radiation) may be an option in patients who are
deemed fit to undergo surgery. For non-surgical candidates
(either due to comorbidity or advanced malignancy), endoscopic palliative therapy has become the first-line therapy
and provides symptomatic relief [6, 7]. Patients with
advanced disease may still be able to receive some benefits
from chemotherapy and radiation treatment concomitantly.

Radiologic Investigations

For most malignant esophageal strictures, a barium or gastrograffin swallow study is an excellent initial test to delineate the anatomy, localize the site of pathology, and

(a) **(b)** **(c)**

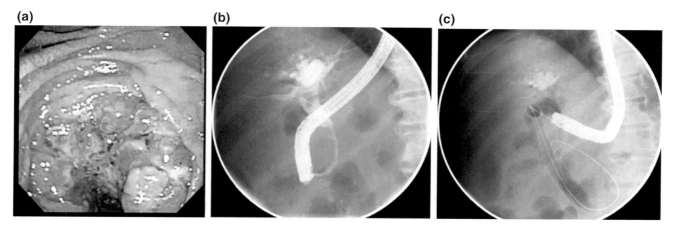

Fig. 7.6 **a–c** Pancreatic head cancer causing duodenal and biliary obstruction. **a** Pancreatic cancer causing duodenal obstruction. **b** Distal CBD stricture from pancreatic tumor invasion. **c** CBD and duodenal SEMS placed for palliation of biliary and duodenal obstruction

Table 7.2 Investigations used to evaluate malignant esophageal and foregut strictures

Barium swallow
Gastrograffin swallow
Upper GI and small bowel follow through study
MR or CT enterography
Chest CT scan
Abdominal CT scan
PET (Positron emission tomography) scan
Endoscopy/enteroscopy
Endoscopic ultrasound (±FNA)

demonstrate the extent of luminal disease. In cases of extrinsic compression (mediastinal and lung cancer, GIST tumors, etc.), the esophagram will appear as a smooth narrowing compared to the irregular mucosal detail seen with intrinsic/luminal malignancy. Barium and gastrograffin studies are extremely helpful in ruling out complex strictures and tumor or radiation-associated fistulas (Fig. 7.7a–c). This allows the endoscopist to plan the endoscopic intervention. However, many patients may be referred directly for endoscopy if the symptoms warrant it and index of suspicion for a malignancy is high, and thus may never undergo a swallow study.

Computerized tomographic scans of the chest and abdomen are routinely performed in patients with suspected malignancy as well as in those with a known malignancy. Often, these may be the initial investigations that reveal a locally advanced tumor or evidence of luminal narrowing related to a known tumor. CT scans help stage the tumor and define the axial extent of the tumor and luminal stenosis.

In the case of pyloro-duodenal strictures, CT scans can also reveal the degree of GOO and the presence and severity of gastric stasis (Fig. 7.8). This is critically important information, since pre-endoscopic nasogastric decompression in these patients can reduce the risk of aspiration and facilitate a successful intervention due to better visualization. CT scan of the chest can also help clarify the nature and extent of a mediastinal tumor invading or compressing the esophagus.

Positron emission tomography (PET-CT) is routinely used in patients with esophageal and gastroduodenal malignancy. It is helpful in delineating areas of metastatic disease that may not be easily revealed with standard imaging (Fig. 7.9). In a patient who only has evidence of loco-regional disease on standard imaging, a PET-CT revealing metastatic disease can significantly influence management decisions.

Endoscopic Evaluation

Endoscopic evaluation is the most direct tool available for investigating malignant strictures of the esophagus and foregut. In this realm, both luminal endoscopy and EUS have a significant role to play.

Endoscopy not only is impactful in obtaining an accurate tissue diagnosis, but also plays a key role in staging and treatment, as will be discussed later in this chapter. EUS is routinely used for staging esophageal and gastric malignancy, and the patient's clinical stage strongly correlates with their overall prognosis (Fig. 7.10a, b). In this context, EUS is complementary to other staging modalities (CT, PET, and MRI). EUS is less commonly used to stage duodenal malignancy, but, with the use of fine needle aspiration (FNA), it may be helpful in sampling any accessible liver lesions/regional lymph nodes and

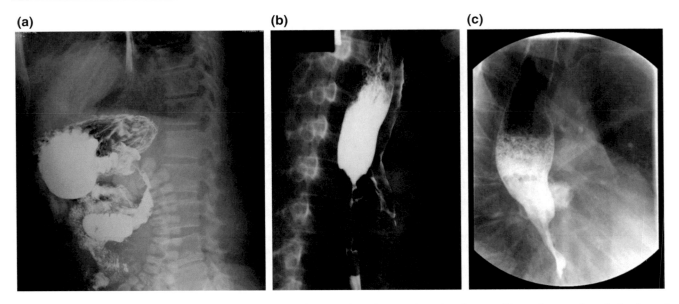

Fig. 7.7 a–c Barium study showing malignant duodenal stricture, intrinsic and extrinsic esophageal strictures. **a** Barium study delineating malignant duodenal stricture. **b** Barium study revealing malignant irregular esophageal stricture with tracheo-esophageal fistula and tracheal aspiration. **c** Smooth stricture in distal esophagus seen on barium swallow due to extrinsic compression from mediastinal mass

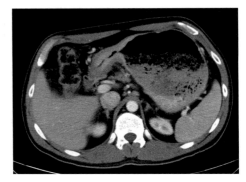

Fig. 7.8 Malignant gastric outlet obstruction on CT

also clarifying the nature of an "extrinsic" mass in the peri-duodenal area, whether pancreatic or otherwise in nature. High-definition endoscopes and high-resolution echoendoscopes allow for a detailed, direct evaluation of these malignant strictures. Specialized ultrathin upper endoscopes can traverse narrow esophageal, pyloric, and duodenal lumens and help complete a foregut examination that would otherwise not be possible using standard endoscopes.

High-quality radiologic and endoscopic diagnostic investigations set the stage for optimal management of these patients with challenging clinical problems. In the setting of a severe malignant stricture, standard endoscopes and echoendoscopes may not be able to traverse the stenosed segment and may require balloon dilation of the stenotic area to facilitate endoscope passage and complete the evaluation [8].

Management of Malignant Esophageal and Foregut Strictures

Management of malignant esophageal and foregut strictures is best accomplished using a multidisciplinary approach, typically involving discussions with (and input from) oncologists, surgeons, and radiation oncologists. Chemoradiotherapy, endoscopic management, and surgery are the three available options for treatment in these patients. These are detailed in Table 7.3.

The best treatment algorithms are the state-of-the-art, evidence-based, consensus-driven plans that ensure timely and meaningful relief of symptoms in a minimally invasive and efficient manner. This is critically important in this era of personalized cancer care and cost-conscious medicine.

Systemic Chemotherapy

This treatment approach is typically used as monotherapy in patients with advanced malignancy, for example in stage IV esophageal malignancy, and can be used in conjunction with endoscopic approaches to palliate obstructive symptoms. Chemotherapy alone has little impact on reversing the mechanical effects of a malignant esophageal or duodenal stricture, but, when used in combination with radiation, it can restore luminal patency especially in the esophagus [9].

Fig. 7.9 PET CT scan: gastric
cancer

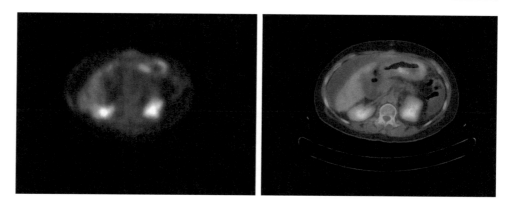

Fig. 7.10 a, b EUS evaluation
of esophageal cancer.
a Endoscopic view of distal
esophageal tumor extending into
gastric cardia. **b** EUS evaluation
of tumor revealing T3N1 stage

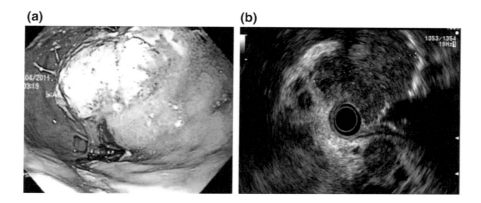

Combined chemo-radiation is commonly used as neoadjuvant treatment for those patients with locally advanced
esophageal cancer who may be candidates for surgery in the
future. In non-surgical candidates, definitive
chemo-radiation is the treatment of choice if their performance scores and medical comorbidities allow it.

In patients with proximal gastric carcinoma (GE junction
and high cardia), preoperative chemo-radiation (neoadjuvant) is routinely used. In non-cardia cancer of the stomach,
both preoperative and adjuvant treatment with chemoradiotherapy is recommended (particularly for N1 disease or T3
stage tumors), although more data are needed in this
population.

For patients who have undergone surgery for pancreatic
cancer, adjuvant chemotherapy is typically used, especially
if there is evidence of lymph node involvement. The role for
adjuvant treatment in duodenal carcinoma is more controversial, although its use has reportedly increased in the last
few decades. Neoadjuvant chemoradiotherapy for bulky or
locally advanced duodenal carcinoma has shown more pro-
mise in one recent study [10]. For patients with duodenal
carcinoid, lymphoma, or other etiologies, specific targeted
chemotherapy is indicated, the discussion of which is
beyond the scope of this review.

Radiation Therapy

Neoadjuvant chemo-radiation is more routinely used for
patients with bulky, stricturing, or locally advanced esophageal cancer. Typical protocols last about 3 months at
which point restaging determines candidacy for surgery.
Radiation treatment is particularly effective in patients with
SCC of the esophagus. For duodenal malignancies, radiation
therapy may provide pain relief and re-establish luminal
patency to some degree. It has been used both with a
pre-existing duodenal stent in place and without; however,
the role of radiotherapy alone in duodenal cancer is less
clear. In pancreatic cancer, especially in locally advanced or
"borderline resectable" cases, combined chemo-radiation is
routinely used to attempt to "downstage" the tumor in the
hopes of undergoing definitive surgery. This approach is
generally successful in about one-third of the patients [11].

Endoscopic Management

The goals of endoscopic management in patients with
malignant upper gastrointestinal stenoses are to provide
relief from obstructive symptoms, to allow the patients to

Table 7.3 Management options for malignant strictures of esophagus and foregut

Systemic chemotherapy

Radiotherapy

    Brachytherapy

    Traditional external beam

    Stereotactic

Combined chemo-radiation

    Definitive

    Palliative

Endoscopic intervention

    Laser ablation

    Photodynamic therapy

    Cryoablation

    Palliative stenting

Surgery

    Definitive

    Palliative

take oral nutrition, hydration, and medications, and to improve the patient's overall quality of life. Ablation of tumors (via laser, photodynamic therapy (PDT), cryoablation, and radiofrequency ablation) and/or recanalizing the lumen via stents are the two essential endoscopic approaches to help achieve these goals. However, definitive ablation of tumors is not often possible, especially if there is no significant intra-luminal component and/or if the stricture is primarily circumferential neoplastic infiltration with desmoplasia, especially in duodenal strictures due to pancreatic malignancy. In addition, use of endoluminal cryoablation is typically limited to the esophagus and GE junction and is discussed more fully in the chapter on BE (Fig. 7.11a, b). PDT is expensive, carries significant

morbidity, and is not widely available nor practiced. For the purpose of this review, the remainder of the discussion will focus on endoluminal stenting for malignant strictures of the esophagus and gastroduodenum.

Endoluminal Stents

In recent decades, several types of flexible and self-expandable stents have been developed. Currently available upper GI stents are almost exclusively self-expandable metal stents (SEMS) for esophageal and gastroduodenal obstruction. Self-expanding plastic stents (SEPS) are still available but have fallen out of favor. Metal stents, made of stainless steel and alloys such as nitinol, have a higher degree of flexibility and are capable of generating high radial forces to maintain stent patency and position. SEMS are currently available in partially or fully covered configurations, with the coating being made of a plastic membrane or silicone. Only partially covered or uncovered SEMS are used to palliate malignant strictures. SEMS are typically only placed in the symptomatic patient with esophageal, gastric outlet, or duodenal obstruction. The proximal flange of a stent may be "anchored" in place using endoclips or sutures (Fig. 7.12a–e and Video 7.1).

Palliative stenting of inoperable malignant obstruction remains the most common indication for esophageal and gastroduodenal stenting, although preoperative stenting of patients with esophageal cancer undergoing neoadjuvant therapy is also widely practiced. Endoscopic and fluoroscopic guidance is typically used. An atraumatic guidewire is used to traverse the stricture over which the SEMS is placed, ensuring that the entire stricture is "bridged" with the stent. Optimal placement requires that the proximal and distal flanges of the stents are placed into the normal lumen, at each end of the tumor, while bridging the entire luminal stricture.

(a)   (b)

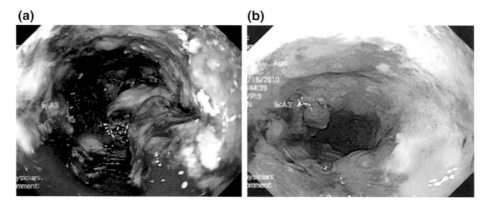

Fig. 7.11 **a**, **b** Cryoablation for palliation of esophageal cancer causing esophageal luminal obstruction despite SEMS in place. **a** Esophageal tumor causing luminal obstruction. **b** Palliation of esophageal obstruction status post-endoscopic cryotherapy of the tumor

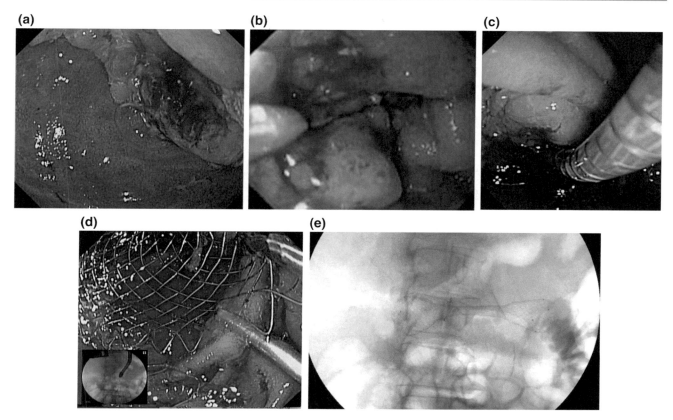

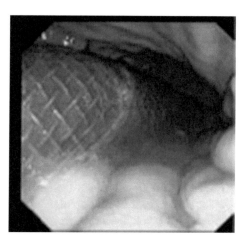

Fig. 7.12 **a–e** Enteral Stent placement for palliation of duodenal obstruction caused by duodenal adenocarcinoma. **a** Endoscopic view of the duodenal stricture. **b** Guidewire advanced across the tumor. **c** Stent advanced over the guidewire through duodenal stricture. **d** Stent placed across duodenal stricture and proximal end anchored with endoclips. **e** Fluoroscopic figure of duodenal stent in optimal position

For malignant esophageal strictures, stent placement immediately prior to chemo-radiation increases the risk for distal stent migration into the stomach, although this may not be a true complication per se and may simply be a sign that the patient is responding to their oncologic therapy, i.e., if the tumor shrinks, the stent may no longer be needed and may simply pass into the stomach (where it can remain until it is retrieved) (Fig. 7.13). On the other hand, a distally migrated stent may be left in the gastric lumen to be removed at the time of surgery (or never, in the case of a terminally ill patient).

In a patient with a malignant duodenal stricture, the presence of multiple downstream areas of obstruction (typically due to peritoneal carcinomatosis) is a relative contraindication to duodenal SEMS placement, as the endoscopist may only be opening up the most proximal stenosis but not treating the next stenosis down the line (that may or may not even be endoscopically reachable).

In patients with significantly advanced esophageal and foregut malignancy, multiple stents may be required to traverse long tracts of luminal stricturing, using the "stent overlap" technique, in an effort to provide the patent an unobstructed conduit for oral nutrition (Fig. 7.14a, b and

Fig. 7.13 Distally migrated esophageal stent (in gastric lumen)

Video 7.1). Overall, there are high technical and clinical success rates for SEMS placement in the esophagus and gastroduodenum [12, 13] (Video 7.1)

SEMS placement does carry a potential for complications. Intra-procedural complications include those related to sedation, pulmonary aspiration, stent malposition,

Fig. 7.14 **a**, **b** Complete metal
stenting of esophagus with
anchoring of proximal end of
stent with endoscopic sutures.
a Fluoroscopy image of complete
metal stenting of esophagus using
3 SEMS with "overlap"
technique. **b** Anchoring of the
proximal end of uppermost
esophageal stent with endoscopic
sutures

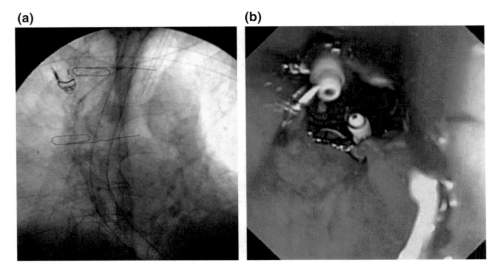

perforation, and bleeding. Late complications include stent migration, stent occlusion, fistula formation, perforation, bleeding, and occlusion.

Overall, when compared to traditional surgical bypass procedures such as gastro-jejunostomy, recent studies have shown SEMS placement as less morbid, more cost-effective, and easier on patients (especially in those with shorter life expectancy), albeit the re-intervention rates are higher when compared to surgical bypass [14]. However, SEMS placement has become the standard of care for palliation of malignant obstruction in these patients, when the local endoscopic expertise and resources allow that.

Surgical Management

In patients who are deemed surgical candidates and when the tumor stage allows it, surgical management represents the definitive option for curative treatment in patients with esophageal and gastroduodenal malignancy. It aims to provide both symptom relief and cure at the same time. However, many patients with bulky and stricturing luminal malignant disease are not immediately candidates for surgery (or never may be) and either already have more advanced disease that precludes surgery or need to undergo neoadjuvant chemo-radiation in an effort to "downstage" their tumor. The majority of these patients do not undergo curative surgery due to tumor progression despite undergoing neoadjuvant treatment.

For esophageal malignancies, the traditional or newer minimally invasive esophagectomy is the most common operation performed [15]. This may involve a "gastric pull-up" or (rarely) colonic interposition to re-establish the oro-digestive luminal conduit [16].

In the case of malignant duodenal strictures, typically a pancreaticoduodenectomy (Whipple procedure) is performed [17]. In some cases of focal or segmental obstruction in the distal duodenum, segmental resection or "enucleation" may be an option, if technically feasible. In terms of palliative surgery, a gastro-jejunostomy is the preferred operation which allows for relief of GOO and is often performed in combination with a biliary bypass to treat simultaneous biliary obstruction.

For many patients with gastric cancer, surgical intervention is preceded by neoadjuvant chemo-radiation, and followed by adjuvant therapy, depending on pathologic stage. For gastric cancer which is amenable to surgery, subtotal or total gastrectomy with a Billroth I or II, or a Roux en Y-type reconstruction are the standard operations. In terms of palliation, a gastro-jejunostomy is the usual surgical bypass that relieves GOO symptoms. Again, endoscopic SEMS placement is much preferred nowadays for luminal palliation, whenever possible.

Conclusion

Malignant strictures of the esophagus, stomach, and duodenum represent a unique challenge across different medical–surgical subspecialties. Often, these are encountered in older patients with advanced neoplasia and comorbidities. Optimization of oral nutrition and increased quality of life are frequently the major goals of management. Several options exist for accurate diagnosis, evaluation, and staging of these tumors. Excellent options exist for both curative and palliative managements of these patients. Multidisciplinary, consensus and evidence-based, cost-effective, minimally invasive management algorithms have the highest chance of yielding the best outcomes in this patient population.

References

1. Gholipour C, Shalchi RA, Abbasi M. A histopathological study of esophageal cancer on the western side of the Caspian littoral from 1994 to 2003. Dis Esophagus. 2008;21:322–7.
2. Pohl H, Sirovich B, Welch HG. Esophageal adenocarcinoma incidence: are we reaching the peak? Cancer Epidemiol Biomarkers Prev. 2010;19:1468–70.
3. Blackstein ME, Blay JY, Corless C, et al. Gastrointestinal stromal tumours: consensus statement on diagnosis and treatment. Can J Gastroenterol. 2006;20:157–63.
4. Yao JC, Hassan M, Phan A, et al. One hundred years after "carcinoid": epidemiology of and prognostic factors for neuroendocrine tumors in 35,825 cases in the United States. J Clin Oncol. 2008;26:3063–72.
5. Wanebo HJ, Kennedy BJ, Chmiel J, et al. Cancer of the stomach. A patient care study by the American College of surgeons. Ann Surg. 1993;218:583–92.
6. Piesman M, Kozarek RA, Brandabur JJ, et al. Improved oral intake after palliative duodenal stenting for malignant obstruction: a prospective multicenter clinical trial. Am J Gastroenterol. 2009;104:2404–11.
7. Ross WA, Alkassab F, Lynch PM, et al. Evolving role of self-expanding metal stents in the treatment of malignant dysphagia and fistulas. Gastrointest Endosc. 2007;65:70–6.
8. Wallace MB, Hawes RH, Sahai AV, et al. Dilation of malignant esophageal stenosis to allow EUS guided fine-needle aspiration: safety and effect on patient management. Gastrointest Endosc. 2000;51:309–13.
9. Coia LR, Soffen EM, Schultheiss TE, et al. Swallowing function in patients with esophageal cancer treated with concurrent radiation and chemotherapy. Cancer. 1993;71:281–6.
10. Kelsey CR, Nelson JW, Willett CG, et al. Duodenal adenocarcinoma: patterns of failure after resection and the role of chemoradiotherapy. Int J Radiat Oncol Biol Phys. 2007;69:1436–41.
11. Gillen S, Schuster T, Meyer Zum Buschenfelde C, et al. Preoperative/neoadjuvant therapy in pancreatic cancer: a systematic review and meta-analysis of response and resection percentages. PLoS Med. 2010;7:e1000267.
12. Sharma P, Kozarek R. Practice parameters committee of American College of G. role of esophageal stents in benign and malignant diseases. Am J Gastroenterol. 2010;105:258–73, quiz 274.
13. Cheng HT, Tsou YK, Lin CH, et al. Endoscopic metal stents for the palliation of malignant upper gastroduodenal obstruction. Hepatogastroenterology. 2011;58:1998–2002.
14. Jeurnink SM, van Eijck CH, Steyerberg EW, et al. Stent versus gastrojejunostomy for the palliation of gastric outlet obstruction: a systematic review. BMC Gastroenterol. 2007;7:18.
15. Orringer MB, Marshall B, Chang AC, et al. Two thousand transhiatal esophagectomies: changing trends, lessons learned. Ann Surg. 2007;246:363–72; discussion 372–4.
16. Mansour KA, Bryan FC, Carlson GW. Bowel interposition for esophageal replacement: twenty-five-year experience. Ann Thorac Surg. 1997;64:752–6.
17. Sohn TA, Lillemoe KD, Cameron JL, et al. Adenocarcinoma of the duodenum: factors influencing long-term survival. J Gastrointest Surg. 1998;2:79–87.

Endoscopic Appearance After Foregut Surgery

David L. Diehl and Jon D. Gabrielsen

Endoscopic Appearance After Foregut Surgery

Since the first description of successful gastric resection by Billroth in 1881, surgeons have described an ever-increasing number of ways to rearrange the anatomy of the foregut. The original methods for resecting part of the stomach and re-establishing a conduit for passage of food came from the need to surgically manage peptic ulcer disease. The Billroth I gastroduodenal anastomosis (described in 1881) and the Billroth II gastrojejunal anastomosis (1885) became common surgeries both for the management of benign disease and malignancy. After the initial understanding that such surgeries followed by creation of an anastomosis could be done with safety and low mortality, surgeons became more daring with the enteric resections that they could perform. Dr. Cesar Roux (1857–1934) described his technique of creating an anastomosis with a loop of small intestine to bypass a scarred pyloric channel. Allen Whipple described the first pancreaticoduodenectomy in 1935 which was not only a courageously aggressive pancreatic head resection, but also necessitated creating multiple anastomoses (enteric, pancreatic, and biliary).

The development of the first H2-blocking pharmaceutical agent (cimetidine in 1976, released in the USA in August of 1977) greatly reduced the need for surgical management of peptic ulcer disease [1], and the number of antrectomies with Billroth anastomoses greatly dropped. The development of proton pump inhibitors (omeprazole in 1990) further decreased the need for peptic ulcer surgery, which is now a rare undertaking. However, surgeons came up with ever more creative ways to cure with the knife, and newer anatomic (re)arrangements were described. The development of surgical approaches to the management of obesity provided yet another stimulus for novel foregut surgery. As endoscopists, we are now left to confront the various ways the "plumbing" can be rearranged, and make sense of it on the video screen (Video 8.1).

Peptic Ulcer Surgery

Excluding bariatric surgery, distal gastrectomy (aka antrectomy) is very likely the most common postoperative change that might be encountered in general endoscopy. In the history of surgical treatment of peptic ulcer disease, a number of approaches were developed. The influence of cholinergic neurons on acid secretion was discovered early. It was ascertained that the vagus nerve had an effect on cholinergic tone to the stomach and thus a considerable influence of acid secretion [2]. Truncal vagotomy was often performed as an anti-ulcer operation. Vagotomy leads to pylorospasm; thus, a pyloroplasty must be done at the same time (Fig. 8.1). An even more effective operation to reduce gastric acid was a vagotomy combined with an antrectomy, which removes the gastrin-secreting cells that reside in the antrum.

After antrectomy, the remaining mid-stomach needs to be anastomosed to the intestine. Billroth described 2 ways to do this: either the body of the stomach is sewn to the duodenal bulb directly (Billroth I), or to a loop of jejunum just past the ligament of Treitz (Billroth II) (Fig. 8.2). The mnemonic for remembering this is that a Billroth I has *one* opening from the stomach, whereas a Billroth II has *two* openings. In reality, one of the openings is actually the afferent limb, carrying pancreatic juice and bile from the

Electronic supplementary material
Supplementary material is available in the online version of this chapter at 10.1007/978-3-319-49041-0_8. Videos can also be accessed at https://link.springer.com/chapter/10.1007/978-3-319-49041-0_8.

D.L. Diehl (✉)
Department of Gastroenterology and Nutrition, Geisinger Medical Center, 100 N. Academy Ave., MC 21-11, Danville, PA 17822, USA
e-mail: dldiehl@geisinger.edu

J.D. Gabrielsen
Department of General Surgery, Geisinger Medical Center, 100 North Academy Avenue, Danville, PA 17822, USA
e-mail: jdgabrielsen@geisinger.edu

Fig. 8.1 **a** Wide open pylorus after surgical pyloroplasty. **b** Appearance of a surgical pyloroplasty done more than 60 years previously, in a 100-year old patient

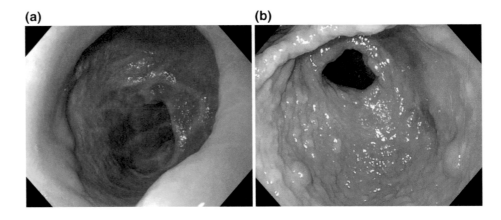

Fig. 8.2 Diagrams showing the difference between **a** Billroth I and **b** Billroth II anastomosis (*A* afferent limb, *E* efferent limb)

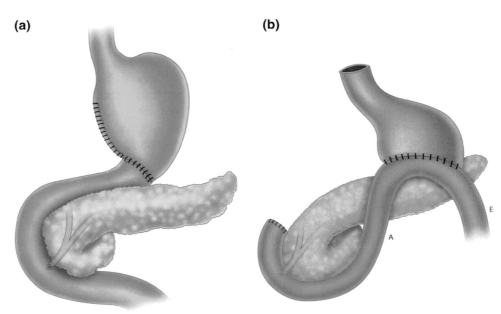

duodenum. The other is the efferent limb (the mnemonic here is the E in *Efferent* stands for *Exit*). A Billroth II anastomosis can be created in an antecolic (in front of the colon) or retrocolic fashion; however, the difference cannot usually be detected endoscopically (Fig. 8.3).

It is fortunate that in most Billroth II cases the surgeon chooses a site to anastomose the stomach to the intestine that is not too far from the ligament of Treitz. For this reason, the ampulla of Vater is typically reachable, even with a duodenoscope. The afferent limb (to be cannulated to reach the ampulla) is typically smaller and goes "down." The opening that is easier to get into is usually the efferent limb. The presence of bile is usually

another clue that you are in the afferent limb, although on occasion this is not reliable; not infrequently both limbs need to be checked in order to identify the afferent limb.

The appearance of a Billroth I anastomosis is somewhat "nondescript." Paradoxically, ERCP can be more difficult with a BI compared to a BII because the ampulla is displaced proximally, making proper orientation of the papilla sometimes quite difficult (Fig. 8.4). The papilla is easier to orient properly in patients with Billroth II anatomy, but the orientation of the CBD and PD is turned 180°/inverted (Fig. 8.5), with the bile duct being below and the pancreatic duct above.

Fig. 8.3 Endoscopic appearance of **a** Billroth I anastomosis (gastroduodenal anastomosis) and **b** Billroth II anastomosis

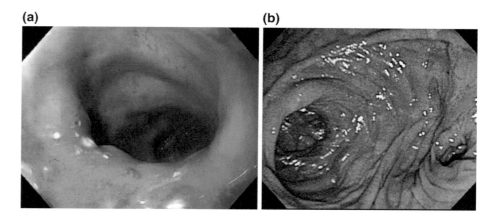

(a)　　　(b)

Fig. 8.4 Fluoroscopic appearance of ERCP scope in **a** Billroth I or **b** Billroth II anastomosis

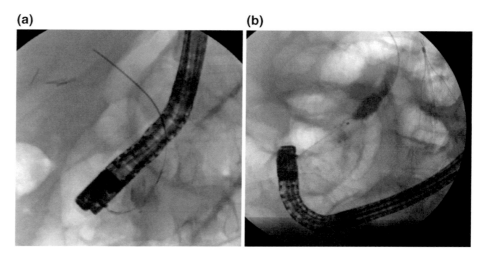

(a)　　　(b)

Fig. 8.5 Billroth II anatomy, view of ampulla with impacted stone, as seen with **a** forward-viewing endoscope and **b** side-viewing endoscope

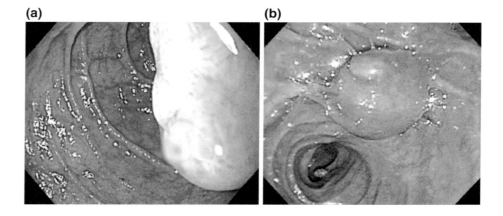

(a)　　　(b)

Rarely a "double pylorus" can be encountered (Fig. 8.6); this is not a postsurgical appearance, but basically a gastroduodenal fistula that has formed from a pre-pyloric ulcer penetrating to the duodenal bulb.

In cases of pyloric or duodenal obstruction from post-ulcer scarring, the gastric outlet can be very stenotic. Rather than resection of the stenosis, a gastrojejunostomy can be created instead. Some endoscopists have described creating a

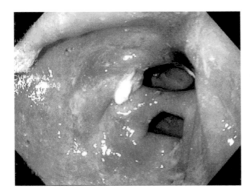

Fig. 8.6 Double pylorus; one opening is the native pyloric channel and the other is a gastroduodenal fistula caused by a peptic ulcer

Anti-reflux Surgery

There remains an important role for anti-reflux surgery despite the widespread use and effectiveness of proton pump inhibitors. Very large hiatal hernias can be very symptomatic and are not uncommonly found in patients with dysplastic Barrett's esophagus (BE). Correction of the hiatal hernia can improve symptoms, and many of these patients may be able to stop taking PPIs. Patients with regurgitation particularly benefit from a fundoplication. There is only limited long-term data of the benefit of repairing a hiatal hernia in dysplastic BE in terms of preventing recurrence or progression of the dysplasia [3]. However, it is known that after BE ablation, recurrence of dysplasia is not a rare event [4]. So theoretically, at least, HH repair may be of benefit in patients with dysplastic BE. In fact, Velanovich reported in his series of patients significant improvements in recurrence of BE and persistence of BE in patients who had a Nissen fundoplication before, at the same time as, or after ablation [5].

gastrojejunal anastomosis using the lumen opposing Axios stent (Fig. 8.7a–c). It is possible that with the refinement of this technique, it might be done more commonly than placement of a duodenal stent in cases of duodenal obstruction.

On occasion, a repeat operation is necessary after peptic ulcer surgery, particularly with the development of one of the common post-gastrectomy syndromes; this is typically conversion of a Billroth I or Billroth II to Roux-en-Y with gastrojejunostomy. The length of the Roux limb is variable, but a limb length of at least 50 cm is necessary for adequate diversion of bile away from the gastric pouch. Roux limb lengths of 50–150 cm are typically utilized, and a biliopancreatic limb of another 50–100 cm can make reaching the ampulla even more difficult than following a Billroth II, often requiring devices to assist in deep intubation or, in some cases, making endoscopic access to the ampulla impossible.

There are several different hiatal hernia repairs that have been described, and each may have benefit in specific cases. In the present day, these are almost always done laparoscopically [6]. The standard repair is a Nissen fundoplication, which is a 360° "wrap" of the fundus around the distal esophagus in association with reducing the stomach down from the mediastinum into the abdomen. A Dor fundoplication is an anterior wrap generally between 90 and 180°. This is a less robust procedure regarding control of reflux; but, it is advantageous in situations where a tighter wrap is not desired (i.e., patients with motility disorders). A Toupet fundoplication creates a 270° posterior wrap. The Hill repair recreates the angle of His and does not wrap the fundus around at all and is largely of historical significance.

(a)   **(b)**   **(c)**

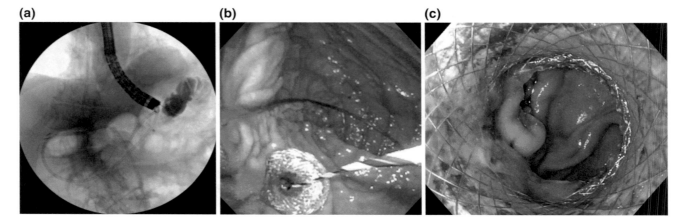

Fig. 8.7 Endoscopic gastrojejunostomy with an Axios stent. **a** Forward-viewing EUS scope used to identify jejunal loop, punctured with needle and contrast injected. **b** Immediately after Axios placement between the stomach and the jejunum. **c** View of jejunum through lumen of Axios stent

A Collis fundoplasty, or esophageal lengthening procedure, may be required in patients with foreshortened esophagus, where the stomach cannot be easily pulled down into the abdominal cavity.

There are subtle differences in endoscopic appearance of fundoplication between the different surgeries [7]. However, the Nissen is the most common done fundoplication. It has an appearance of "stacked coins" with a deep posterior groove and a shallower anterior groove (Fig. 8.8). A Dor or Toupet is similar, but the wrap does not go completely around. It may not be obvious that a patient had a Collis fundoplasty, as the surgical changes are typically covered by the wrap. As mentioned above, the proper position of a fundoplication is around the distal esophagus. Thus, endoscopically, the GEJ should be located beneath the pinch of the diaphragm/top of the fundoplication (often very close and indistinguishable from one another). If the GEJ can be seen above this level, it likely represents some degree of

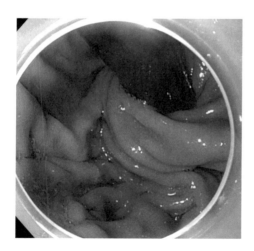

Fig. 8.8 Normal view of Nissen fundoplication with the so-called stack of coins appearance

malposition of the fundoplication which can be associated with dysphagia.

Resective Surgery for Benign and Malignant Disease

Esophagus

Esophagectomy is pursued in resectable cases of esophageal cancer (usually after neoadjuvant chemoradiation), and on occasion for benign conditions (unusual cases of dysplastic Barrett's, or end stage achalasia). In all of these cases, the stomach is "tubularized," then anastomosed to the proximal esophagus. Stricturing of the surgical anastomosis is, unfortunately, common, particularly if there has been a leak postoperatively (Fig. 8.9), and usually requires multiple frequent dilation procedures and/or esophageal stenting. Occasionally, there is Barrett's epithelium remaining after esophagectomy.

The appearance of the foregut anatomy after esophagectomy can be surprisingly similar to the normal situation, with the exception of the esophagogastric anastomosis in the chest. The entire stomach remains, although narrower, and there is an antrum and pylorus. Pyloroplasty is usually done after an esophagectomy because of concern for pylorospasm related to the obvious need for a truncal vagotomy in the process of resection. Some surgeons will choose to do Botox injection into the pylorus rather than pyloroplasty; current practices in the field are in evolution [8].

In rare cases, a colonic interposition is made to create a conduit between the upper esophagus sphincter and stomach (Fig. 8.10). In these cases, EGD for colon cancer screening and polyp surveillance will be necessary. Other unusual anatomic findings after esophagectomy may include a jejunal interposition or, uncommonly, creation of a "skin tube" (Fig. 8.11).

Fig. 8.9 a Anastomotic stricture after esophagectomy. **b** After incisional treatment with insulated tip knife; suture material is visible at 6 o'clock position

(a)   **(b)**

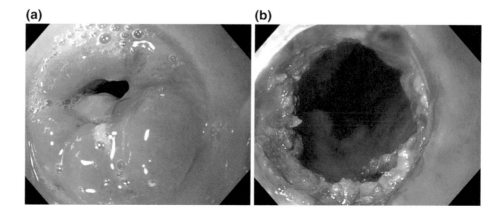

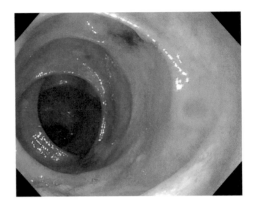

Fig. 8.10 Colonic interposition after esophagectomy

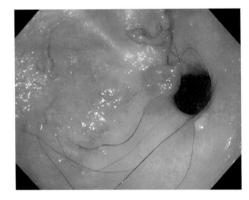

Fig. 8.11 Skin tube anastomosis from hypopharynx to gastric pull-up after esophagectomy

Stomach

The vagotomy and antrectomy that can be performed for PUD can also be utilized to treat malignancy of the distal stomach. The main difference between the two procedures is that an extended lymphadenectomy is usually done with gastrectomy for malignancy; however, this is not apparent

endoscopically. Gastric cancer in the middle of the stomach is resected with more of the stomach removed, but the anastomosis is created in a similar manner to that described above. Proximal resections, however, are often managed by total gastrectomy (rather than proximal gastrectomy), with esophagojejunal anastomosis [9]. Proximal gastrectomy seems to have a higher incidence of reflux esophagitis, anastomotic stenosis, and poor gastric emptying.

Pancreatic Head

Resection of the pancreatic head typically involves resection of adjacent duodenum. The pancreaticoduodenectomy (Whipple procedure) is a surgical *tour de force*, involving partial or complete resection of 5 structures (stomach, duodenum, gall bladder, bile duct, and head of pancreas) followed by the creation of 4 anastomoses: gastrojejunal, jejunojejunal, pancreatic duct (pancreaticojejunostomy), and bile duct (choledochojejunostomy or hepaticojejunostomy). This procedure is usually performed for pancreatic head lesions (both benign and malignant) or chronic pancreatitis, but can also be used to treat patients with duodenal malignancy.

For a period of a few years, the "pylorus-sparing Whipple procedure" was widely performed in an attempt to decrease dumping syndrome from the stomach. In this operation, the antrum and pylorus were left intact and a jejunal anastomosis created just past the pylorus. The pylorus-sparing Whipple has fallen out of favor lately because it does not seem to confer any advantage, and may lead to gastric emptying issues in some patients, although some surgeons still perform this version of the operation [10].

In many cases of Whipple resection, the afferent Roux limb may not be excessively long, making possible endoscopic access to the hepaticojejunostomy or pancreaticojejunostomy (Fig. 8.12). This access is important to treat the occasional case of pancreatic or biliary anastomotic stricture. Longer Roux limbs have to be traversed with a colonoscope,

Fig. 8.12 a Fluoroscopic appearance of forward-viewing endoscope after Whipple resection. **b** The hepaticojejunostomy is open

(a)   **(b)**

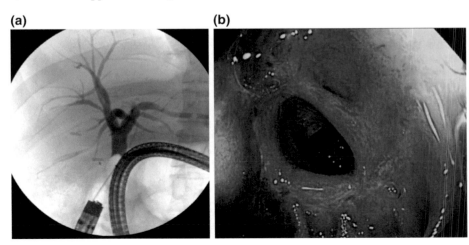

Spirus overtube, or single or double balloon forward-viewing endoscopes.

Bariatric Surgery

There has been a dramatic increase in the incidence of bariatric surgery for weight management. There are many mechanisms by which bariatric surgery works to cause weight loss, although many surgeries work via a combination of mechanical restriction of food intake and nutrient malabsorption [11]. There are a variety of surgeries that have been described, but there are clearly a few which will be most commonly seen.

Roux-Y Gastric Bypass (RYGB)

The Roux-Y gastric bypass (RYGB) has historically been the most common bariatric surgery done in the USA. In the RYGB, the stomach is partitioned with a stapler/cutter, creating a small pouch of the proximal stomach (Figs. 8.13 and 8.14). The small volume of this pouch leads to early

satiety. The pouch is drained by an end-to-side anastomosis of a Roux limb of jejunum. The anastomosis or proximal jejunum just below this point is vulnerable to ulceration (often due to ischemia) which can be made worse in post-bypass patients that continue to smoke, or take excessive amounts of NSAIDs (Fig. 8.15). Upper GI bleeding can occur at these sites, necessitating urgent endoscopy. Stricturing of the anastomosis is common but is usually managed endoscopically with through the scope balloon dilation (sometimes up to 20 mm in diameter) (Fig. 8.16).

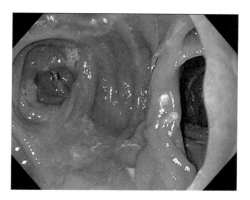

Fig. 8.14 Endoscopic appearance of gastric pouch in RYGB

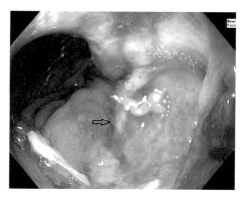

Fig. 8.15 Jejunal ulcer at anastomosis of RYGB

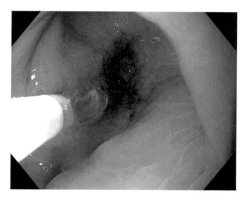

Fig. 8.16 Balloon dilation of a stenotic gastrojejunal anastomosis in RYGB

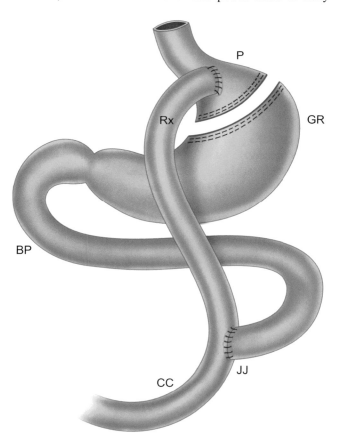

Fig. 8.13 Diagram of Roux-Y gastric bypass (RYGB), *P* pouch, *GR* gastric remnant, *BP* biliopancreatic limb, *Rx* Roux limb, *CC* common channel

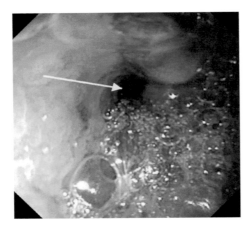

Fig. 8.17 Gastrogastric fistula after RYGB

Earlier in the history of the RYGB, the stomach was partitioned (stapled only) rather than divided (stapling plus cutting). Over time, a fistula could occur between the gastric pouch and the gastric remnant. This gastrogastric (G-G) fistula was encountered in up to half of patients. The presence of a G-G fistula is usually signaled by weight regain, loss of early satiety, or new onset of reflux symptoms (Fig. 8.17). Some surgeons may interpose omentum between the gastric pouch and gastric remnant to prevent the formation of a G-G fistula. A G-G fistula may occur after an undiagnosed small leak, or ulcer, even in the divided RYGB.

Sleeve Gastrectomy

There is an increasing use of sleeve gastrectomy, and it has now become the most commonly performed weight loss operation in the USA [11], surpassing RYGB in many centers. Sleeve gastrectomy involves resection of most of the corpus of the stomach, usually along the greater curvature. The cut edges of the stomach are sewn or stapled together

over a sizing bougie, usually 38–42 French (13–14 mm), leaving a "sleeve" of stomach. The resection typically ends 4–6 cm proximal to pylorus, so the appearance of the antrum and pylorus is normal. Endoscopically, a small pouch may be noted in the high fundus, then a narrow lumen, and finally more space in the distal antrum just before the pylorus (Fig. 8.18a, b). Weight loss is tied to increased satiety with small meal volumes and possibly changes in levels of GI hormones such as ghrelin.

Strictures may occur at the angularis after a sleeve gastrectomy. These are often managed utilizing an achalasia balloon of at least 30 mm [12]. Leaks tend to occur at the upper part of the stomach, near the angle of His. This location is a transition zone from the esophagus (which lacks serosa) to the gastric cardia and is considered somewhat of a watershed area from a blood supply standpoint, predisposing it to potential leaks. Sometimes, a "dog-ear" of stomach is left at this location surgically in an attempt to avoid the leak. This small "dog-ear" of gastric cardia/fundus represents the small pouch noted upon entering the stomach as described above.

ERCP can be more challenging after gastric sleeve creation, because the ERCP scope can only be held in "short position" along the lesser curvature (the greater curvature having been removed at the time of surgery); "long scope position," which is sometimes helpful for achieving optimal ampullary orientation to facilitate cannulation, is typically not achievable.

Biliopancreatic Diversion with Duodenal Switch (BPD/DS)

Biliopancreatic diversion with duodenal switch (BPD/DS) is another procedure that is gaining favor as a bariatric operation in patients with very high BMIs (>50), and may be better than the RYGB procedure in diabetic patients because it is a "malabsorptive" procedure. Usually, a sleeve gastrectomy is constructed, but the sleeve is wider as it is created over a slightly

Fig. 8.18 **a** Diagram of sleeve gastrectomy; *S* gastric conduit ("sleeve"), *RS* resected stomach. **b** Endoscopic appearance of the middle of sleeve gastrectomy

(a)

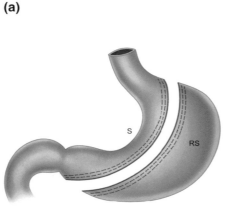

(b)

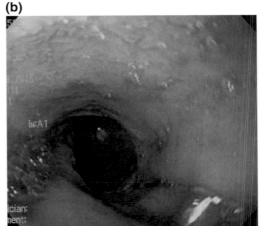

larger bougie. The small bowel is divided 250 cm proximally to the ileocecal valve. An anastomosis is created between the proximal portion of this division and the ileum 100 cm proximal to the ileocecal valve. About 3–4 cm past the pylorus, a duodenoileostomy is created between the distal portion of this division and the duodenum. Patients can lose up to 90% of excess body weight (compared to about 70% after RYGB).

Laparoscopic Band Surgery

The use of the adjustable laparoscopic band ("lap band") as a means for weight loss has lost momentum in recent years in favor of the other surgical approaches described above. Weight loss with the lap band, which restricts the amount of food that the stomach can hold, is more modest, and ongoing adjustments seem to be required in many patients. The lap band is a surgically implanted saline-filled ring that is positioned in the proximal stomach, typically 1–2 cm below the GE junction. Endoscopically, first a pouch then a narrowed segment of stomach is seen. Migration of the lap band through the wall of the stomach has been described, necessitating surgical or, rarely, endoscopic removal.

Length of Efferent Limbs of Small Bowel in Foregut Surgery

In a standard RYGB, the efferent limb of jejunum from the pouch is anastomosed to small intestine a variable distance downstream. Different surgical practices utilize varying lengths of Roux limbs; surgeons at our institution, for example, will create a Roux limb about 150 cm in length. Most surgeons create Roux limbs between 75 and 150 cm, and the length of the Roux limb has minimal, if any, impact on weight loss unless the patient has a BMI >50.

With long Roux limb lengths such as this, access to the remnant stomach is very challenging and usually impossible, even with the use of device-assisted enteroscopy (single balloon, double balloon, spiral, or other device-assisted). It may be necessary to access the gastric remnant in cases of suspected bleeding from the remaining stomach or duodenum, or to complete an ERCP. Several ways to do this have been described; a detailed description of this is beyond the scope of this chapter, but many involve surgical access to the remnant stomach.

Complications After Bariatric Surgery

Complications after bariatric surgery can be classified as immediate or delayed. Immediate complications include leak, perforation, and bleeding. Immediate leaks usually

occur at the G-J anastomosis staple line; this may be due to tension on the anastomosis and/or relative ischemia. The second most common location of a leak is usually up high on the staple line near the angle of His. This is a "watershed area" as mentioned previously, potentially predisposing it to leaks. Tension on the anastomosis can worsen blood flow to the area creating risk of ulceration and/or staple line failure. Bleeding from any staple line can occur in the immediate postoperative period or at a later date.

Long-term issues with the post-bypass anatomy can also be encountered. Strictures of the anastomosis can be seen following healing of ulcers or independent of ulceration, again likely due to blood supply/ischemia issues. Enlargement of the pouch or anastomosis is sometimes found and can often be corrected surgically or endoscopically [13]. Gastrocolic (G-C) fistulas can form in the setting of an ulcer. Patients with G-C fistulas usually have an antecolic anastomosis, since the anastomosis is often close to the colon in this configuration. Retrocolic anastomoses are less likely to develop a G-C fistula, but have other unique potential problems. For one, an opening needs to be created in the colonic mesentery to allow passage of a loop of jejunum up to the pouch. If the opening is too big, bowel can herniate through the surgically created defect and lead to a small bowel obstruction. If the opening is not big enough, the Roux limb can be "pinched" and could lead to a mechanical obstruction. In current practice, most RYGB are usually done with the antecolic approach.

Symptomatic reflux after bariatric surgery is an increasingly recognized problem [14] with treatment options more limited than in patients without altered anatomy. Most patients respond to some degree to proton pump inhibitor therapy. The Stretta device has been used with some success in these patients, and magnetic devices (similar to a magnetic bracelet) have been placed around the LES may develop a role in this patient population. It is possible to use the remnant stomach to create a partial or 360 degree fundoplication, though data regarding this is limited currently. Standard anti-reflux procedures are generally not possible, since there is so little proximal stomach left, and a "wrap" cannot be created.

Conclusions

The endoscopist must be ready to identify postsurgical anatomy. Obtaining a good surgical history is the most important component of being able to identify surgical changes, but many patients are not aware of the specific surgical details, and "figuring it out as you go" may be your only choice. Despite the striking decrease in need for peptic ulcer surgery since release of H2-blockers and PPIs, these operations may still be necessary, and Billroth II anastomoses continue to be encountered. Endoscopy on patients that have undergone a Whipple resection may be required. The ever-increasing numbers of patients who have undergone bariatric surgery represents the biggest need in understanding postsurgical anatomy of the foregut.

References

1. Fineberg HV, Pearlman LA. Surgical treatment of peptic ulcer in the United States: trends before and after the introduction of cimetidine. Lancet. 1981;317:1305–7.
2. Soll AH, Walsh JH. Regulation of gastric acid secretion. Ann Rev Phys. 1979;41:35–53.
3. Allaix ME, Patti MG. Antireflux surgery for dysplastic Barrett [sic]. World J Surg. 2015;39:588–94.
4. Corley DA. Can you stop surveillance after radiofrequency ablation of Barrett's esophagus? A glass half full. Gastroenterology. 2013;145:39–55.
5. O'Connell K, Velanovich V. Effects of Nissen fundoplication on endoscopic endoluminal radiofrequency ablation of Barrett's esophagus. Surg Endosc. 2011;25:830–4.
6. Schijven MP, Gisbertz SS, van Berge Henegouwen MI. Laparoscopic surgery for gastro-esophageal acid reflux disease. Best Pract Res Clin Gastro. 2014;28:97–109.
7. Jobe BA, Kahrilas PJ, Vernon AH, et al. Endoscopic appraisal of the gastroesophageal valve after antireflux surgery. Am J Gastro. 2004;99:233–43.
8. Cerfolio RJ, Bryant AS, Cannon CL, et al. Is botulinum toxin injection of the pylorus during Ivor-Lewis esophagectomy the optimal drainage strategy? J Thor Cardiovasc Surg. 2009;137:565–72.
9. Wen L, Chen XZ, Wu B, et al. Total vs. proximal gastrectomy for proximal gastric cancer: a systematic review and meta-analysis. Hepatogastroenterology. 2012;59:633–40.
10. Seiler CA, Wagner M, Bachmann, et al. Randomized trial of pylorus-preserving duodenopancreatectomy versus classical whipple resection—long term results. Br J Surg. 2005;92:547–56.
11. Miras AD, le Roux CW. Mechanisms underlying weight loss after bariatric surgery. Nat Rev Gastroent Hepatol. 2013;10:575–84.
12. Shnell M, Fishman S, Eldar S, et al. Balloon dilatation for symptomatic gastric sleeve stricture. Gastrointest Endosc. 2014;79:521–4.
13. Thompson CC, Chand B, Chen YK, et al. Endoscopic suturing for transoral outlet reduction increases weight loss after Roux-en-Y gastric bypass surgery. Gastroenterology. 2013;145:129–37.
14. Tutuian R. Effects of bariatric surgery on gastroesophageal reflux. Current Opin Gastroent. 2014;30:434–8.

Enteral Feeding Tubes: What Every Fellow Should Know

John C. Fang

Introduction

GI fellows rapidly discover that they must become intimately familiar with the role of feeding tubes in patients with GI disease. Gastroenterologists are frequently called upon to select which type of feeding tube is best, as well as where and how it should be placed. Enteral feeding is the preferred method of nutrition support when oral feeding is inadequate and a functional gastrointestinal (GI) tract is present. Endoscopic insertion of enteral feeding tubes was a major advance in the delivery of nutrition therapy with the first report of the percutaneous endoscopic gastrostomy (PEG) in 1980 [1]. Since that initial report endoscopic techniques for placement of nasoenteric tubes (NET), percutaneous gastrojejunostomy (PEGJ), and direct percutaneous endoscopic jejunostomy (DPEJ) have been described as well [2].

The type of enteral feeding tube selected is dependent on many factors. Ethical considerations, risk factors related to tube placement, the patient's disease state, gastric and small bowel function, short- and long-term goals, and intended length of therapy are all weighed in the decision to feed a patient via the enteral route. This is best performed by a gastroenterologist who combines the cognitive expertise in nutrition and gastroenterology together with the technical endoscopic skills to place the appropriate type of feeding tube. Communicating with and involving the patient/family, dieticians, and referring healthcare providers in the decision making process is essential for the successful delivery of enteral feedings. Gastroenterologists should also provide the appropriate post-placement care of feeding tubes to prevent complications of enteral access devices. This chapter will

cover the selection, placement and management of endoscopic feeding tubes including: nasoenteric tubes (NET), percutaneous endoscopic gastrostomy tubes (PEG), percutaneous endoscopic gastrojejunostomy tubes (PEGJ), and direct percutaneous endoscopic jejunostomy tubes (DPEJ).

Feeding Tube Types and Selection

There are several factors that assist the gastroenterologist in determining the optimal type of feeding tube to place. A clear rationale for enteral feedings, potential length of therapy and a location for enteral access placement must be determined prior to any procedure. A thorough history including the patient's current and past medical and surgical conditions (including previous upper GI surgeries) and a focused physical assessment including the anatomy and function of the upper airway, esophagus, and digestive tract is imperative in the selection of the appropriate enteral access device. Assessment of the abdominal wall for open wounds and fistula, post-surgical scars, the presence of or future requirements for ostomies, percutaneous or intraabdominal infusion devices and peritoneal dialysis catheters are all important in the evaluation for all percutaneous tubes.

The estimated duration of enteral therapy is the main factor in determining nasal tube placement versus percutaneous enterostomy. Generally, tubes used for short-term therapy (<4–6 weeks) are placed nasally or in some cases orally (often in critically ill ICU patients). These tubes include nasogastric, nasoduodenal, nasojejunal, and nasogastric-jejunal tubes and can also be placed blindly at the bedside or fluoroscopically in addition to endoscopically [3]. For longer-term placement, greater than 4–6 weeks, percutaneous endoscopic enterostomy tubes (PEG, PEGJ, DPEJ) are placed into the stomach and/or the small bowel. When long-term percutaneous access is selected, the condition of the external abdominal wall, ability to correct coagulopathies, and patient tolerance to moderate/deep sedation and anesthesia for endoscopy must also be

Electronic supplementary material
Supplementary material is available in the online version of this chapter at 10.1007/978-3-319-49041-0_9. Videos can also be accessed at https://link.springer.com/chapter/10.1007/978-3-319-49041-0_9.

J.C. Fang (✉)
Department of Gastroenterology, University of Utah,
30 N. 1900 E, SOM 4R118, Salt Lake City, UT 84132, USA
e-mail: John.fang@hsc.utah.edu

© Springer International Publishing AG 2017
D.G. Adler (ed.), *Upper Endoscopy for GI Fellows*,
DOI 10.1007/978-3-319-49041-0_9

assessed. Percutaneous feeding tubes can also be placed with local anesthesia of the abdominal wall and intravenous conscious sedation by interventional radiologists using fluoroscopic guidance in patients at high risk for endoscopic procedures.

The decision to opt for gastric or small bowel feeding is based on gastric motility, the presumed aspiration risk, alterations in gastrointestinal anatomy (i.e., post-surgical) and co-existing medical conditions. Most patients tolerate gastric feeding well with criteria for PEG feeding including a relatively normal gastric and small bowel motility and gastric anatomy acceptable to place a PEG. Patients who are unable to tolerate gastric feedings, cannot receive a PEG as a result of altered anatomy or motility, have gastric outlet or duodenal obstruction, have a gastric or duodenal fistula, or have severe gastroesophageal reflux disease should be considered for a percutaneous jejunal feeding tube (PEGJ or DPEJ). Patients with prolonged acute and chronic pancreatitis are candidates for deeper enteral feeding as well.

When there is obstruction or significant gastroparesis, the gastric port of the PEGJ (or separate PEG and DPEJ) can be used for decompression while delivering the feeding solution into the small bowel through the jejunal port [4, 5]. The use of small bowel feeding to reduce aspiration pneumonia is controversial. Meta-analyses and systematic reviews (primarily with nasogastric vs. nasoenteric tubes) are conflicting with the most recent meta-analysis showing decreased risk of aspiration pneumonia with small bowel feeding, and the most recent multi-center randomized controlled trial showing no difference in outcomes between the two [6, 7]. Retrospective studies with PEGJ (or PEG tubes for that matter) do not clearly demonstrate decreased risk of aspiration pneumonia.

The internal retention bolsters of percutaneous tubes are constructed of either solid material (silicone or polyurethane) or silicone balloons. Solid internal bolsters are more common with initial percutaneous enterostomy tube placement due to their greater longevity. Balloon-type internal bolsters are more common with standard and low profile replacement devices due to their ease in placement. These balloons generally have a lifespan of ∼6 months [8].

PEGJ tubes are available as single and two-piece devices consisting of a gastrostomy with a smaller bore extension tube that passes through the pylorus into the distal duodenum or jejunum. Most PEGJ tubes are specifically designed with separate gastric and jejunal lumens and ports allowing for both jejunal feeding and gastric decompression. If the internal bolster is of the balloon type, an additional third port is present for balloon inflation and deflation. Of note, there are no specific tubes manufactured for DPEJ so standard 14–20 F PEG kits are used for this purpose.

Feeding Tube Placement Methods

Nasoenteric Feeding Tubes (NET)

Nasoenteric feeding tubes are inserted when short-term access is indicated. These tubes can provide an opportunity to assess tolerance of enteral feedings before placement of a percutaneous enterostomy is decided upon (if longer-term access is required).

Contraindications to nasogastric or nasoenteric feeding tube placement include obstructing head, neck and esophageal pathology or injury preventing safe insertion. Plain abdominal or chest radiography after placement is often useful to confirm depth of placement, but is not mandatory. Nasoenteric feeding tubes are placed anywhere distal to the pylorus while nasojejunal tubes are, by definition, placed distal to the ligament of Treitz. Distal nasojejunal placement is reliably achieved with endoscopic techniques with >90% success rates reported [9].

Multiple methods have been described for endoscopic NET placement and familiarity and repetition with one or two techniques is often critical to successful placement. The "drag-and-pull" method has traditionally been the standard endoscopic technique employed. In this technique, an endoscopic forceps advanced through the working channel of the endoscope is used to grasp the distal end of the feeding tube or a suture attached to the end of a feeding tube, which is then dragged into position in the small bowel and released, after which the endoscope is removed. Alternatively, when using the over-the-guidewire technique, the endoscope is advanced into the small bowel and a guidewire is then passed through the working channel into the proximal jejunum. The guidewire is subsequently advanced, while the endoscope is withdrawn over the wire, maintaining position of the guidewire tip in the jejunum. Since the guidewire is traditionally passed with transoral endoscopy, an oral-nasal transfer of the guidewire must be performed. The feeding tube is then passed over the guidewire into position.

The over-the-guidewire technique can also be performed with transnasal endoscopy using a small caliber (5–6 mm diameter) endoscope to obviate the need for oral-nasal transfer and can be performed with minimal or no sedation. The smaller caliber endoscope passed orally or nasally may also be used in patients with stenosis, partial obstruction, malignancy, upper GI stents, or otherwise altered anatomy [10]. The trade off, however, is that these ultrathin endoscopes are more prone to coiling limiting the distal extent reached in the small bowel.

Coiling is problematic with each of the aforementioned techniques and several tips can facilitate successful deep enteral access. Stiffer guidewires can help prevent coiling to maximize the depth of tube placement [11]. Keeping the stomach decompressed to minimize gastric volume can also reduce coiling when advancing ultrathin endoscopes and is also important when withdrawing any type of endoscope as leaving the guidewire as straight as possible will allow deeper placement of the feeding tube. In addition, leaving the feeding tube less looped in the stomach will help prevent retrograde migration after placement. Maintaining the position of NET beyond the pylorus is often problematic because of retrograde migration, which occurs in up to 31% of patients [12]. Retrograde migration of the NET can occur at the time of initial placement as the endoscope is withdrawn or after placement if there is excessive looping of the feeding tube in the stomach.

Use of a re-closeable clip to attach the distal tip of a feeding tube to the small bowel mucosa can reduce the rate of retrograde migration. In a randomized trial comparing standard over-the-wire to clip-assisted placement (in which a feeding tube with a non-absorbable suture affixed to the tip is picked up in the stomach and then clipped to the duodenal wall) spontaneous retrograde tube migration was reduced from 4.2 to 1.4% (Fig. 9.1) [12]. The number needed to clip (treat) to avoid one repeat endoscopy was 4.8 (95% CI 3.1–11.3) [12]. Clip placement added 3 min to mean procedure time and increased mean cost per patient, which may be offset when radiographs are excluded from the clip group [12]. A systematic review identifying 5 cohort series with 41 patients did not observe any spontaneous migration of feeding tubes after clipping [13].

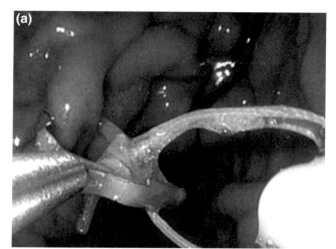

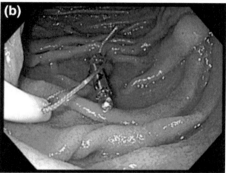

Fig. 9.1 **a** NET placement: clipping suture attached to nasoenteric feeding tube to small bowel. **b** NET placement: Nasoenteric feeding tube clipped to small bowel

Percutaneous Enterostomy Tubes

Enterostomy tubes are placed when long-term access (>4–6 weeks) is required. Routine pre-procedural testing of coagulation parameters and platelets are no longer recommended, but should be considered if there is concern for abnormal coagulation due anticoagulant medication, medical history of excessive bleeding or recent antibiotic use. Prophylactic antibiotics are administered as they have been shown to decrease peri-stomal infection rates when using endoscopic methods [14, 15]. ASGE guidelines recommend administration of IV antibiotics to all patients before PEG (and PEGJ, DPEJ) tube placement [16]. The current standard is a single dose 1 g cefazolin administered 30 min prior to the procedure.

Endoscopic placement of a percutaneous feeding tubes is considered a higher risk bleeding procedure by ASGE guidelines and has been demonstrated to have up to a 2.5% risk of severe bleeding (defined as hemorrhage requiring blood transfusion, hospital admission, or endoscopic/surgical intervention) [17]. Patients are categorized into high and low risk for thromboembolic events. Patients at low risk should have their anticoagulant agents (new oral anticoagulants (NOAC) and warfarin) stopped 2–4 half-lives before percutaneous feeding tube placement without bridging. High thromboembolic risk patients should have their anticoagulant agents held and bridged with low molecular weight or unfractionated heparin. Resumption of warfarin can occur on the same day as the procedure and when adequate hemostasis is ensured for patients on NOAC's. For antiplatelet agents, the thienopyridines (i.e., clopidogrel) should be held for at least 5–7 days before PEG placement though it is permissible to continue NSAIDs and ASA in patients with high thromboembolic risk [17]. Consultation with other relevant specialists will be important to manage these risks in specific patients. Patients can be managed with nasoenteric tubes if a relatively short NOAC treatment duration is planned. The reader is referred to comprehensive recent ASGE guideline on this topic [17].

Percutaneous Endoscopic Gastrostomy Tubes (PEG)

Percutaneous endoscopic gastrostomy (PEG) is the most common technique for obtaining long-term gastric access for enteral nutrition and is generally performed under moderate sedation [18]. There are two general indications for PEG placement; enteral feeding and gastric decompression. Absolute contraindications for endoscopic PEG placement are obstruction of the GI tract proximal to the stomach, severe coagulopathy, active peritonitis, bowel ischemia, hemodynamic instability and inability to identify a safe abdominal access site [19]. Additional relative contraindications include ascites, coagulopathy, gastric varices, active head and neck cancers, morbid obesity and neoplastic, infiltrative or inflammatory disease of the gastric or abdominal wall [20]. Reported success rates for PEG placement are greater than 95% [21]. Abnormal endoscopic findings have been identified during 10–71% of PEG procedures and have altered management in as many as 36%, showing the value of a complete EGD even in the setting of PEG placement [22]. Additional advantages of endoscopic PEG placement include the ability to perform the procedure at the bedside (i.e., in the ICU) and lack of radiation exposure.

The "pull" and "push" techniques are the most common endoscopic methods for PEG placement. The pull (or Ponsky) technique is performed much more frequently despite no documented differences in success rates or outcomes [23]. Air is insufflated into the stomach via an endoscope. The optimal site for PEG placement is determined through simultaneous endoscopic trans-illumination noted on the abdominal wall and finger indentation at the site visualized endoscopically. The abdominal wall is typically sterilized with topical agents, and a surgical drape is applied. Local anesthesia is used to reduce discomfort. A small incision is made at this site and a needle/trocar is inserted through the abdominal wall and into the stomach. A guidewire is passed through the needle/trocar and grasped endoscopically (usually with an endoscopic snare) and withdrawn through the mouth. A gastrostomy tube is then affixed to the guidewire and pulled through the esophagus into the stomach and out the abdominal wall. The gastrostomy tube is held in place by a solid "mushroom"-type internal retention device and an external bumper.

The push method is similar to the pull method except an introducer tube with a hollow central lumen is used. After the guidewire is placed, the introducer tube is threaded over the guidewire. It is then advanced over the guidewire from the mouth and pushed until it emerges from the abdominal wall. It is then grasped manually and pulled into position as described above.

Site selection and procedural technique are paramount to successful and safe PEG placement. The access site should be at least 2 cm away from the costal margin to minimize patient discomfort during respiration post-placement. The PEG site should also be >2 cm away from surgical scars as intervening bowel loops tend to adhere to scar tissue immediately deep to the scar. In addition to marking the location on the abdominal wall where trans-illumination and one-to-one finger indentation occurs, it is important to note the angle and orientation of the finger during indentation and to replicate this during the needle/trocar insertion to ensure optimal PEG placement.

The Foutch "safe tract" technique should be used when a finder needle or trocar is advanced through the abdominal wall into the stomach. Steady aspiration is applied to a saline (or 1% lidocaine) filled syringe attached to the needle to ensure that no air bubbles or blood are seen in the syringe prior to endoscopic visualization of the needle tip entering the stomach. This ensures that the needle's path does not include adjacent vessels or bowel loops [11].

A skin incision (to potentially facilitate tube passage through the abdominal wall) should be made the same size or slightly smaller than the diameter of the feeding tube. This may require extra force to pull the PEG tube through the skin, but an overly large incision violates surgical principles allowing for increased risk of infection and potentially longer and poorer healing of the site.

Patients receiving PEG tubes are at high risk of aspiration, especially during the procedure. Minimizing procedure time, dedicating an assistant to airway care and suctioning, and elevating the head of bed to 30–45° will help minimize this risk.

The risk of the post-procedural complications of peri-stomal infection, buried bumper syndrome (wherein the bumper imbeds deeply in the gastric wall and may not be identifiable endoscopically) and necrotizing fasciitis are increased when there is excessive tension between the inner and outer bumper of the PEG [19]. Keeping 0.5–1.0 cm of "play" (position off the abdominal wall) at the time of placement and at least 1 cm after stoma tract maturation can help reduce this risk. In addition, if the patient gains significant weight after tube placement (usually due to successful nutritional therapy), the external bumper will need to be additionally loosened to prevent these complications, most notably a buried bumper.

Percutaneous Endoscopic Gastrojejunostomy Tubes (PEGJ)

Percutaneous endoscopic gastrojejunostomy (PEGJ) may be performed immediately or anytime after gastrostomy tube placement. Similar to NET placement multiple methods for PEGJ placement have been described. Traditionally, a guidewire is placed through the existing gastrostomy tube, grasped endoscopically, and carried into the jejunum. The endoscope is then withdrawn leaving the guidewire in place. The jejunal extension tube is then threaded over the guidewire into the small bowel with or without fluoroscopic assistance [24, 25]. This technique, while commonly performed, frequently results in displacement of the jejunal tube back into the stomach on withdrawal of the endoscope.

The "drag-and-clip" method (similar to that described for NET) can be used to prevent this initial jejuna tube displacement and reduce feeding tube migration for the duration the clip remains in place. In this method, a jejunal feeding tube with a suture on its tip is inserted through the PEG into the stomach lumen. A re-closable clip is passed through the working channel of an endoscope and used to grasp the suture and drag the tube into the jejunum. The suture is then clipped to the jejunal mucosa, securing the feeding tube to the small bowel. Withdrawing the re-closable clip back into the working channel after grasping the suture will facilitate advancement of the endoscope while decreasing trauma on the bowel wall (Fig. 9.2). Multiple clips can also be deployed on the suture to further ensure that the position of the feeding tube is maintained. In one study, the average procedure time using a variation of this method was 21 min, employing both forceps and clips, which is less than that reported when endoclips are not used [26]. A recent retrospective study showed a 93% success rate for PEGJ placement with the use of endoclips [26]. The mean functional duration of these tube was 55 days with the primary reason for tube replacement being clogging (as opposed to displacement) [26].

Another means of placing a jejuna extension through a PEG is to place the wire into the small bowel through an ultrathin endoscope advanced directly through a PEG tube. Advancing the endoscope through the PEG itself also mitigates tube displacement upon endoscope withdrawal. This through-the-PEG placement of the jejunal extension tube uses a combination of larger diameter 24–28 Fr PEG tubes and ultrathin (5–6 mm) endoscopes, and has demonstrated good success rates and acceptable tube patency. In this method, an ultrathin endoscope is inserted through the PEG tube into the stomach and advanced deep into the small bowel. A guidewire is then advanced through the working channel of the endoscope into the jejunum. The endoscope is then exchanged over the wire while taking care to avoid looping or kinking of the wire. The jejunal extension tube is then passed over the wire and the proximal end seated on the PEG tube Y-port adapter.

This technique was 99.2% successful in a recent case series of 121 procedures [27]. Jejunal extension tube dysfunction occurred in 24% of cases, with tube kinking,

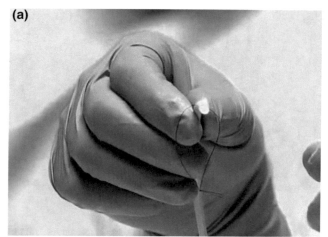

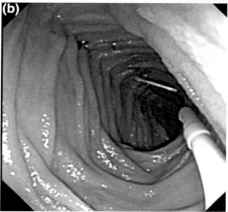

Fig. 9.2 a PEGJ placement: suture loop attached to distal end of jejunal extension tube. **b** PEGJ placement: clipping jejunal extension tube to small bowel

occlusion, and breakage as the most common problems [27]. The average lifespan of the tubes was 123.6 days, which may be partially related to the larger 12 Fr tubes used in this study [27]. Further advantages of this technique are that the jejunal extension tubes can be placed with minimal or no sedation with relatively short procedure times and without fluoroscopy. Another variation of this method uses an existing mature gastrostomy site. The PEG is removed completely and an ultrathin endoscope advanced into the jejunum and wire placed (Fig. 9.3). A one-piece gastrojejunostomy tube is then advanced over the wire as described above.

Despite high technical success rates for placement of PEGJ, the clinical success is considerably lower with reported malfunction rates of 53–84% [28]. Failure is most commonly due to retrograde migration or tube occlusion secondary to kinking or clogging of these smaller (8–12 Fr) jejunal extension tubes [28].

Technical tips to achieve maximal depth of the jejunal extension into small bowel can help optimize functional

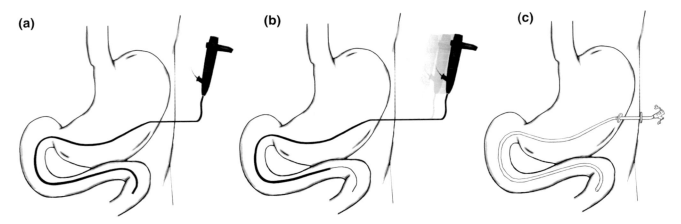

Fig. 9.3 **a** PEGJ placement through mature PEG stoma tract. Ultrathin endoscope advanced to small bowel through existing gastrostomy. **b** PEGJ placement through mature PEG stoma tract. Endoscope is withdrawn leaving wire in place in small bowel. **c** PEGJ placement through mature PEG stoma tract. PEGJ tube advanced over wire into small bowel and wire is withdrawn

success. The antrum should be considered for the gastrostomy insertion site as this allows a shorter and straighter track to the small intestine for the jejunal extension tube [11]. Directing the puncture of the stomach with the needle/trocar angled toward the pylorus will also help achieve this goal. Minimizing dead space (i.e., excessive intra-gastric length of the tube) reduces coiling and allows maximal length of jejunal placement beyond the pylorus [11]. Cutting the external length of the PEG short (<10 cm) also allows maximal length of the jejunal tube by minimizing its length outside the body [11]. Using an extension tube of longer length will also allow for a deeper and more stable position in the jejunum. Finally, it is important that the jejunal extension tube should be advanced far enough into the small bowel to minimize looping in the stomach (not advancing far enough) without creating excess tension (advancing too far), both of which can lead to retrograde migration. While fluoroscopy is not absolutely required for PEGJ placement, the authors have found it useful to reduce looping in the stomach and achieve more distal (and stable) placement.

Direct Percutaneous Endoscopic Jejunostomy Tubes (DPEJ)

DPEJ is indicated for jejunal feeds when an existing PEG is not present, for persistent dysfunction of PEGJ tubes and, most importantly, when expertise in placing a DPEJ exists. DPEJ tubes have greater durability as the larger bore tubes clog less and do not migrate or kink as frequently when compared to PEGJ [28, 29]. DPEJ may also reduce aspiration in high-risk patients [30]. DPEJ, however, is performed much less frequently than PEGJ, at least in part due to the perceived risk and need for greater technical expertise. Direct percutaneous jejunostomy is considerably more difficult technically than percutaneous gastrostomy despite similar methods. Success rates are lower and complications rates are higher when compared to PEG tubes [5: 4–8]. Success rates for endoscopic jejunostomy range from 68 to 100% [31].

Direct percutaneous endoscopic jejunostomy (DPEJ) is a modification of the pull PEG technique. A pediatric colonoscope or enteroscope is advanced into the small bowel. Transillumination and finger palpation is performed over the jejunum instead of the stomach. A sounding needle and/or trocar is passed through the anterior abdominal wall into the jejunum. An insertion wire is advanced through the trocar and grasped. The procedure is then completed as per the pull type PEG (Figs. 9.4, 9.5, video 9.1) [32, 33]. Both single balloon enteroscopy (SBE) and double balloon enteroscopy (DBE) allow for deeper intubation of the small bowel, compared to standard push enteroscopy, increasing the likelihood of reaching an appropriate site for DPEJ insertion. A recent study showed successful DPEJ placement in 10/10 patients using the DBE under general anesthesia (GA) after failed conventional placement with a pediatric colonoscope using conscious sedation [34]. In another study, Despott et al. also reported successful DPEJ tube placement by DBE under GA in nine of the ten consecutive cases, with failure in one case secondary to inadequate trans-illumination [35]. The mean procedure time was 35 min, and no procedure-related complications were reported [35]. Similarly, in yet another study single balloon enteroscopy (SBE) demonstrated success in 11 of 12 DPEJ procedures attempted with conscious sedation [36]. Initial

Fig. 9.4 a DPEJ placement.
b DPEJ placement. From Ref.
[28]. With permission from
Elsevier

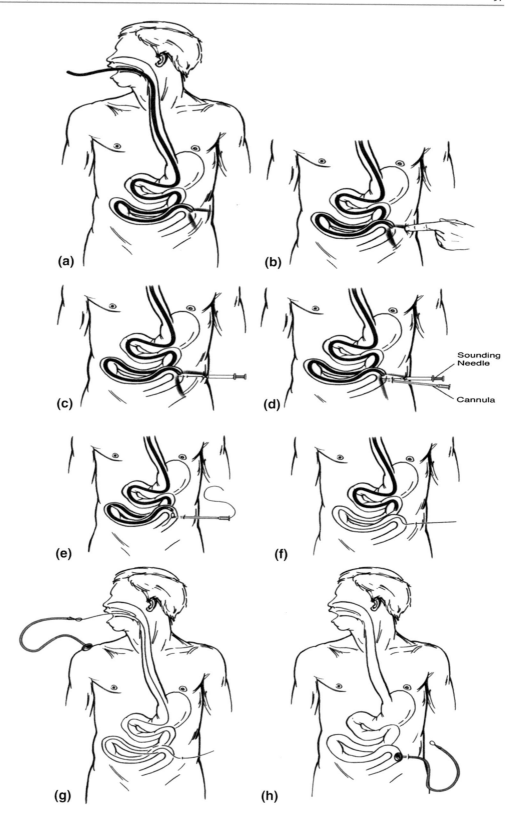

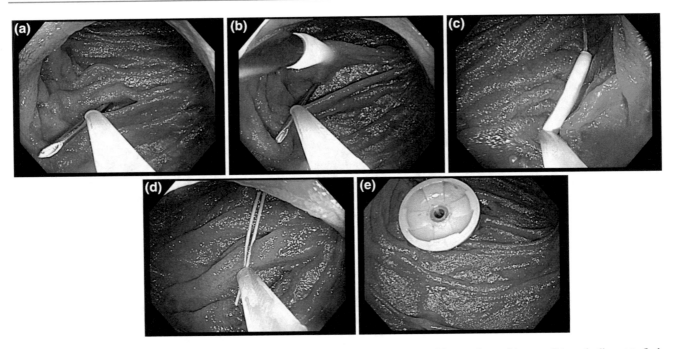

Fig. 9.5 **a** DPEJ placement: finder needle snared to stabilize small bowel. **b** DPEJ placement: Trocar advanced into small bowel adjacent to finder needle. **c** DPEJ placement: Snare transferred to trocar/wire. **d** DPEJ placement: Trocar removed and wire snared. **e** DPEJ placement: Final position

data suggest that balloon assisted enteroscopy is a safe and effective innovation for DPEJ.

Despite the similarity in the technique of PEG and DPEJ placement, DPEJ is a considerably more difficult procedure. Several technical tips can help identify a safe access site and stabilize the small bowel to increase success. Using the trans-illumination function on the light processor maximizes potential for localizing an access site [30]. Surgical scars do not need to be avoided (as opposed to this case when placing a PEG tube, where they are usually avoided). In patients undergoing DPEJ placement, scars may represent ideal sites to attempt to access the small bowel as they are often where adhesions fix small bowel loops to the anterior abdominal wall [28]. Once an access site has been identified, it is important to stabilize the small bowel. The finder needle is inserted into the jejunum and grasped with the endoscopic snare to anchor the jejunum to the abdominal wall [37]. The trocar is then passed through the abdominal wall and into the small bowel at a location adjacent to the finder needle, and the snare is transferred off the needle to the trocar to minimize bowel movement and the risk of interposed bowel (Fig. 9.5). Glucagon or hyoscine may also be administered to reduce intestinal peristalsis. Consideration should be given to general anesthesia for all DPEJ placements given prolonged procedure times (compared with the time required for PEG tube placement) with increased aspiration risk while patients are supine [28].

Post-Procedure Management

Skin Care

Regardless of the tube type or insertion technique, all patients require appropriate stomal hygiene. Good stomal hygiene is often important for reducing or even preventing aspiration pneumonia in ventilator dependent patients or those with a depressed level of consciousness. Patients and caregivers may use mild soap and water to cleanse the stoma site for percutaneous tubes. The area should be rinsed and dried thoroughly. Routine use of antibiotic ointments or hydrogen peroxide at the tube site is not recommended. Dressings can be applied if there is drainage from the stoma site; however, they should not be placed with excessive tension which can promote infection and buried bumper syndrome.

Prevention of Clogging

All tubes are prone to clogging. Common causes of clogging include suboptimal flushing, not flushing between each medication administration, accumulation of pill fragments, and high protein/fiber formulas [24, 25]. Feeding tubes should, in general, not be used to check residuals.

Compliance with good, intermittent flushing protocols is essential to reduce the rate of feeding tube clogging. Water should be used as the flush fluid of choice although other agents can help to keep tubes patent for longer periods of time. Two reports have demonstrated benefit to the prophylactic use of pancreatic enzymes to prevent tubes occlusion compared to standard H_2O flushes [38, 39]. Medications in liquid form are less likely to clog than crushed pills and should be used if available. Whether a medication is in pill or liquid form, each medication should be given separately with a water flush before and after each medication [40].

Exchange/Removal of Enterostomy Tubes

Enterostomy tubes can be safely removed after the stoma tract has matured, usually >2 weeks after insertion. In patients receiving steroid medication, the immunosuppressed, significant obesity, or other risk factors for poor wound healing, 4–6 weeks is often required for the tract to mature fully. Premature removal of enterostomy tubes may result in the stomach falling away from the abdominal wall, allowing gastric contents to leak into the peritoneum. If this occurs, tube replacement with the assistance of endoscopy, interventional radiology, or surgery is required.

Although not typically supplied as part of the initial tube placement, low profile skin level *replacement* devices for PEG, PEGJ or DPEJ tubes are an excellent option for patients who are concerned about cosmetic appearance. These devices can also be more comfortable for the patient who is active, sleeps in the prone position, or who only needs intermittent therapy. Because of the need to attach a feeding connector to the skin level device, some degree manual dexterity or caregiver assistance is needed. Low profile devices are usually placed as an exchange tube for a pre-existing tube; however, low profile PEG's can also be inserted at the time of initial tube placement [41].

After stoma tract maturation, a standard profile or low profile replacement tube can be placed at the bedside without endoscopy or fluoroscopy. Removal of a PEG with a solid silicone mushroom internal bolster is accomplished at the bedside using simple traction. The exposed gastric tubing is firmly grasped and pulled forcefully with the patient in the supine position while using the other hand to brace the abdominal wall. For devices held in place with an internal balloon, the balloon is deflated and the tube is then gently removed. The length of the existing stoma tract is measured before choosing and placing the correct size of a new, low profile device. Skin level tubes are held in place with an inflated internal balloon or a deformable solid silicone internal retention bolster. Correct tube position can be checked after replacement by aspiration of gastric contents or auscultation of insufflated air. However, these methods are not fully reliable and if there is any concern for misplacement correct tube position should be confirmed with fluoroscopic or endoscopic imaging.

Complications of Feeding Tubes

Nasoenteric Feeding Tubes (NET)

Post-procedural complications include inadvertent tube dislodgement, tube malfunction, tube occlusion, tube feeding aspiration and sinus infection. Dislodgement occurs in 25–41% of cases [42–44]. The use of a nasal bridle has been clearly shown to decrease the tube dislodgment rate. A recent report decreased the incidence of accidental dislodgement from 36 to 10% using a magnet-based system to place the nasal bridle [45]. Malfunction of nasoenteric tubes by various means including breaking, cracking or kinking of the tube; these events have been reported to occur in 11–20% of patients [43, 44]. When accurately diagnosed by sinus needle puncture and aspiration, sinusitis occurs ~12% of patients with nasoenteric tubes [46]. This is believed secondary to obstruction of physiologic sinus drainage by the nasoenteric tube itself.

Tube occlusion is a frequent problem (20–45%) often requiring tube replacement [44, 47, 48]. Risk factors for tube occlusion include; increasing tube length, decreasing tube caliber, inadequate water flushing, frequent medication delivery and use of the tube to measure residual volumes [48]. When feeding tubes become clogged, simple flushing with water can relieve the obstruction in about one-third of the patients [49]. If flushing fails to clear the tube, the installation of pancreatic enzymes can reopen an additional 50% of occluded tubes [49, 50]. Mechanical dislodgement may also be achieved using an endoscopic cytology brush, an ERCP catheter or a commercial corkscrew device [51]. Finally, replacing a nasoenteric feeding tube can be undertaken as the last resort.

Percutaneous Enterostomy Tubes (PEG, PEGJ, DPEJ)

Complications of enterostomy tubes can be divided into procedural and post-procedural events. Procedure-related complications and mortality are uncommon (1.5–4% and 0–2% of the time respectively) and include intraprocedural aspiration, hemorrhage, perforation of the GI lumen and prolonged ileus [52]. Risk factors for aspiration include placement of the tube with the patient in the supine position, advanced age, the need for sedation and neurologic impairment [53].

Pneumoperitoneum as a result of the percutaneous procedure is common and in the absence of peritoneal signs is of no clinical consequence [54]. This can be significantly decreased by use of CO_2 for insufflation during endoscopy [55]. Infusion of water-soluble contrast with fluoroscopic imaging is the test of choice if peritonitis is suspected. The procedural and long-term mortality rate directly related to PEG placement is very low despite the up to 50% annual mortality in patients receiving gastrostomy tubes [54]. This very high rate is a function of the significant co-morbidities of the patients rather than the procedure or the feeding tube itself.

The overall post-procedure complication rate of percutaneous enterostomy tubes ranges from 4.8 to 10.8% [52]. Minor post-procedural complications are two to three times more common than major ones (Table 9.1). Peristomal infection is the most common complication of gastrostomy placement [18, 56]. The majority of infections are mild. In rare cases necrotizing fasciitis with high morbidity and mortality can develop. Prophylactic antibiotics before placement, early recognition of wound infections, treatment with antibiotics, local wound care and debridement, if necessary, are the keys to successful management [18, 20, 57].

Leakage around the gastrostomy site is a common and under-recognized problem facing nutrition support providers [58]. Risk factors include infection, excessive cleansing with irritant solutions (H_2O_2, betadine), and excessive tension and lateral tension on the external portion of the feeding tube (usually from external tubing). Prompt treatment of infection, loosening of the outer bumper and stabilizing the gastrostomy tube to prevent tension or torsion on the tube will usually address these issues [51].

Skin care is an important adjunct to management of peristomal leakage. Stoma adhesive powders, powdered absorbing agents or zinc oxide can be applied to the site to prevent and treat skin irritation and breakdown. Foam dressings rather than gauze dressings can help to reduce local skin irritation caused by gastric contents (foam lifts the drainage away from the skin, whereas gauze tends to trap it). Local fungal skin infections may also be associated with leakage and can be treated with topical antifungal agents. It should be stressed that wound and ostomy nurses are an invaluable resource in the management of leaking gastrostomy sites.

Buried bumper syndrome results from growth of the gastric mucosa over the internal bumper and migration of the bumper itself out of the gastric or bowel lumen. Risk factors include excessive tension between the internal and external bumpers, poor wound healing and significant weight gain (leading to thickening of the gastric wall) [59–61]. Treatment is based on maintaining the stoma tract while restoring the internal bumper entirely within the stomach lumen [62, 63].

Inadvertent percutaneous feeding tube removal before stoma maturation should be addressed urgently. If a replacement tube is not immediately available, a suitably sized Foley or "red rubber" catheter can be used to keep the tract open until a replacement tube can be placed. In patients prone to pulling on their tubes (often due to confusion or mental illness), the use of an abdominal binder, placing mittens on the patients hands, cutting down the external tube length to 6–8 cm, or switching to a low profile device can reduce the risk of future removal [52].

Complications of gastrojejunal tubes and jejunal tubes are similar to gastrostomy tubes described above. Gastrojejunal feeding tubes are also complicated by frequent (up to 70%) malfunction, migration and/or occlusion of the smaller jejunal extension tube [64, 65]. Additional complications of direct jejunostomy tubes include jejunal volvulus and/or small bowel perforation [66]. Although often recommended by expert opinion, there is no clear evidence that more distal feeding with jejunal tubes markedly decreases a patient's aspiration risk. However, as stated earlier, recent data suggest that jejunal feeding may be associated with decreased risk of aspiration pneumonia [67–69].

Table 9.1 Major and minor complications of PEG tube placement

Reported frequency (%)	
Major complications	
Aspiration	0.3–1.0
Hemorrhage	0–2.5
Peritonitis/necrotizing fasciitis	0.5–1.3
Death (related to PEG placement)	0–2.1
Minor complications	
Peristomal infection	5.4–30
Peristomal leakage	1–2
Buried bumper	0.3–2.4
Inadvertent removal	1.6–4.4
Fistuluous tracts (after PEG removal)	0.3–6.7

Ethical Issues

There are significant ethical, religious and legal issues in addition to the medical concerns in evaluating patients for feeding tubes. Enteral feeding tube placement may not be appropriate in patients with either poor quality of life or a very short life expectancy. There are specific patient populations in which percutaneous feeding tubes have not been shown to improve outcomes. Feeding tube placement has not been shown to improve outcomes (pneumonia, pressure ulcers, nutritional status) or mortality in patients with advanced dementia or end-stage malignancy [70–75].

Enteral nutrition is a medical therapy and therefore can be refused by a competent, informed patient or their surrogate [76, 77]. In addition to the procedural risks, a discussion about realistic post-procedure goals and expectations from enteral feeding can increase patient and caregiver satisfaction with their decision. Inappropriate feeding tube placement can be avoided if the patient and family members understand that in the final stages of a terminal illness decreased oral intake is not associated with hunger or discomfort [78].

Conclusions

Enteral feeding remains the feeding route of choice in the presence of a functional gastrointestinal tract. Success depends on the placement of the appropriate access device, placed in the correct location of the gastrointestinal tract by skilled endoscopists. Proper care and maintenance of these enteral access devices with early recognition and management of their complications is critical to successful enteral nutrition therapy. This is best performed by a gastroenterologist who combines the cognitive expertise in nutrition together with the endoscopic skills to place the appropriate type of feeding tube. In this regard, the gastroenterologist is part of the multidisciplinary team consisting of the patient/family, dieticians, and primary and sub-specialty care providers for the successful delivery of enteral nutrition in the hospital or outpatient setting.

References

1. Gauderer MW, Ponsky JL, Izant RJ Jr. Gastrostomy without laparotomy: a percutaneous endoscopic technique. J Pediatr Surg. 1980;15(6):872–5.
2. ASGE Standards of Practice Committee, Jain R, Maple JT, Anderson MA, Appalaneni V, Ben-Menachem T, Cecker GA, Fanelli RD, Fisher L, Fukami N, Ikenberry SO, Jue T, Khan K, Krinsky ML, Malpas P, Sharaf RN, Dominitz JA. The role of endoscopy in enteral feeding. Gastrointest Endosc. 2011;74(1):7–12.
3. Vanek V. Ins and outs of enteral access. Part 1: short-term enteral access. Nutr Clin Prac. 2002;17(1):275–83.
4. Vanek V. Ins and outs of enteral access. Part 2: long-term access-esophagostomy and gastrostomy. Nutr Clin Prac. 2003;18(1):50–74.
5. Vanek V. Ins and outs of enteral access. Part 3: long-term access-jejunostomy. Nutr Clin Prac. 2003;18(1):201–20.
6. McClave SA, Taylor BE, Martindale RG, Warren MM, Johnson DR, Braunschweig C, McCarthy MS, Davanos E, Rice TW, Cresci GA, Gervasio JM, Sacks GS, Roberts PR, Compher C, The Society of Critical Care Medicine, The American Society for Parenteral and Enteral Nutrition. Guidelines for the provision and assessment of nutrition support therapy in the adult critically ill patient: society of critical care medicine (SCCM) and American Society for parenteral and enteral nutrition (A.S.P.E.N.). JPEN J Parenter Enteral Nutr. 2016;40(2):159–211.
7. Davies AR, Morrison SS, Bailey MJ, Bellomo R, Cooper DJ, Doig GS, Finfer SR, Heyland DK. ENTERIC study investigators, ANZICS clinical trials group. A multicenter, randomized controlled trial comparing early nasojejunal with nasogastric nutrition in critical illness. Crit Care Med. 2012;40(8):2342–8.
8. Heiser M, Malaty H. Balloon-type versus non-balloon-type replacement percutaneous endoscopic gastrostomy: which is better? Gastroenterol Nurs. 2001;24(1):58–63.
9. Fang JC, Hilden K, Holubkov R, DiSario JA. Transnasal endoscopy vs. fluoroscopy for the placement of nasoenteric feeding tubes in critically ill patients. Gastrointest Endosc. 2005;62(5):661–6.
10. Zhang L, Huang YH, Yao W, Chang H, Guo CJ, Lin SR. Transnasal esophagogastroduodenoscopy for placement of nasoenteric feeding tubes in patients with severe upper gastrointestinal diseases. J Dig Dis. 2012;13(6):310–5.
11. Palmer LB, McClave SA, Bechtold ML, Nguyen DL, Martindale RG, Evans DC. Tips and tricks for deep jejunal enteral access: modifying techniques to maximize success. Curr Gastroenterol Rep. 2014;16(10):409.
12. Hirdes MM, Monkelbaan JF, Haringman JJ, van Oijen MG, Siersema PD, Pullens HJ, Kesecioglu J, Vleggaar FP. Endoscopic clip-assisted feeding tube placement reduces repeat endoscopy rate: results from a randomized controlled trial. Am J Gastroenterol. 2012;107(8):1220–7.
13. Schrijver AM, Siersema PD, Vleggaar FP, Hirdes MM, Monkelbaan JF. Endoclips for fixation of nasoenteral feeding tubes: a review. Dig Liver Dis. 2011;43(10):757–61.
14. ASGE Standards of Practice Committee, Banerjee S, Shen B, Baron TH, Nelson DB, Anderson MA, Cash BD, Dominitz JA, Gan SI, Harrison ME, Ikenberry SO, Jagannath SB, Lichtenstein D, Fanelli RD, Lee K, Can Guilder T, Stewart LE. Antibiotic prophylaxis for GI endoscopy. Gastrointest Endosc. 2008;67(6):791–8.
15. Lipp A, Lusardi G. Systemic antimicrobial prophylaxis for percutaneous endoscopic gastrostomy. Cochrane Database Syst Rev. 2013;14(11):CD005571.
16. ASGE Standards of Practice Committee, Khashab MA, Chithadi KV, Acosta RD, Bruining DH, Chandrasekhara V, Eloubeidi MA, Fanelli RD, Faulx AL, Fonkalsrud L, Lightdale JR, Muthusamy VR, Pasha SF, Saltzman JR, Shaukat A, Wang A, Cash BD. Antibiotic prophylaxis for GI endoscopy. Gastrointest Endosc. 2015;81(1):81–9.
17. ASGE Standards of Practice Committee, Acosta RD, Abraham NS, Chandrasekhara V, Chathadi KV, Early DS, Eloubeidi MA, Evans JA, Faulx AL, Fisher DA, Fonkalsrud L, Hwang JH, Khashab MA, Lightdale JR, Muthusamy VR, Pasha SF, Saltzman JR, Shaukat A, Shergill AK, Wang A, Cash BD, DeWitt JM.

The management of antithrombotic agents for patients undergoing GI endoscopy. Gastrointest Endosc. 2016;83(1):3–16.

18. Gossner L, Keymling J, Hahn E, Ell C. Antibiotic prophylaxis in percutaneous endoscopic gastrostomy (PEG): a prospective randomized clinical trial. Endoscopy. 1999;31(2):119–24.

19. Rahnemai-Azar AA, Rahnemaiazar AA, Naghshizadian R, Kurtz A, Farkas DT. Percutaneous endoscopic gastrostomy: indications, technique, complications and management. World J Gastroenterol. 2014;20(24):7739–51.

20. Jain NK, Larson DE, Schroeder KW, Burton DD, Cannon KP, Thompson RL, MiMagno EP. Antibiotic prophylaxis for percutaneous endoscopic gastrostomy. A prospective, randomized, double-blind clinical trial. Ann Intern Med. 1987;107(6):824–8.

21. Duszak R Jr, Mabry M. National trends in gastrointestinal access procedures: an analysis of medicare services provided by radiologists and other specialists. J Vasc Interv Radiol. 2003;14 (8):1031–6.

22. Wolfsen HC, Kozarek RA, Ball TJ, Patterson DJ, Botoman VA Jr, Ryan JA. Value of upper endoscopy preceding percutaneous gastrostomy. Am J Gastroenterol. 1990;85(3):249–51.

23. Ponsky J, Gauderer M. Percutaneous endoscopic gastrostomy: a non-operative technique for feeding gastrostomy. Gastrointest Endosc. 1981;27(1):9–11.

24. DiSario J, Baskin W, Brown R, DeLegge MH, Fang JC, Ginsberg GG, McClve SA. Endoscopic approaches to enteral nutritional support. Gastrointest Endosc. 2002;55(7):901–8.

25. DeLegge M, Patrick P, Gibbs R. Percutaneous endoscopic gastrojejunostomy with a tapered tip, nonweighted jejunal feeding tube: improved placement success. Am J Gastroenterol. 1996;91 (6):1130–4.

26. Udorah MO, Fleischman MW, Bala V, Cai Q. Endoscopic clips prevent displacement of intestinal feeding tubes: a long-term follow-up study. Dig Dis Sci. 2010;55(2):371–4.

27. Donnelly MC, McKay R, Barber D, McKinlay AW, Leeds JS. Outcomes after through-the-PEG tube placement of jejunal extensions: a case series from a single center. Gastrointest Endosc. 2014;80(2):349–53.

28. Fang J. Percutaneous access for enteral nutrition. Techn Gastrointest Endosc. 2007;9(3):176–82.

29. Zhu Y, Shi L, Tang H, Tao G. Current considerations of direct percutaneous endoscopic jejunostomy. Can J Gastroenterol. 2012;26(2):92–6.

30. Murphy JM, Fang JC. Direct percutaneous endoscopic jejunostomy: who, when, how, and what to avoid. Pract Gastroenterol. 2014;9(1):24–36.

31. Itkin M, DeLegge MH, Fang JC, McClave SA, Kundu S, d'Othee B, Martinez-Salazar GM, Sacks D, Swan TL, Towbin RB, Walker TG, Wojak JC, Zuckerman DA, Cardella JF. Multidisciplinary practical guidelines for gastrointestinal access for enteral nutrition and decompression from the society of interventional radiology and American Gastroenterological Association (AGA) Institute, with endorsement by Canadian Interventional Radiological Association (CIRA) and Cardiovascular and Interventional Radiological Society of Europe (CIRSE). Gastroenterology. 2011;141(2):742–65.

32. Varadarajulu S, DeLegge M. Use of a 19-gauge injection needle as a guide for direct percutaneous endoscopic jejunostomy tube placement. Gastrointest Endosc. 2003;57(7):942–5.

33. Shike M, Latkany L, Gerdes H, Bloch A. Direct percutaneous endoscopic jejunostomies for enteral feeding. Gastrointest Endosc. 1996;44(5):536–40.

34. Song LM, Baron TH, Saleem A, Bruining DH, Alexander JA, Rajan E. Double-balloon enteroscopy as a rescue technique for failed direct percutaneous endoscopic jejunostomy when using

35. Despott EJ, Gabe S, Tripoli E, Konieczko K, Fraser C. Enteral access by double-balloon enteroscopy: an alternative method of direct percutaneous endoscopic jejunostomy placement. Dig Dis Sci. 2011;56(2):494–8.

36. Aktas H, Mensink PB, Kuipers EJ, van Buuren H. Single-balloon enteroscopy-assisted direct percutaneous endoscopic jejunostomy. Endoscopy. 2012;44(2):210–2.

37. Paski SC, Dominitz JA. Endoscopic solutions to challenging enteral feeding problems. Curr Opin Gastroenterol. 2012;28 (5):427–31.

38. Sriram K, Jayanthi V, Lakshmi RG, George VS. Prophylactic locking of enteral feeding tubes with pancreatic enzymes. JPEN J Parental Enteral Nutr. 1997;21(6):353–6.

39. Bourgault AM, Heyland DK, Drover JW, Keefe L, Newman P, Day AG. Prophylactic pancreatic enzymes to reduce feeding tube occlusions. Nutr Clin Prac. 2003;18(5):398–401.

40. Lord L. Restoring and maintaining patency of enteral feeding tubes. Nutr Clin Prac. 2003;18(1):422–6.

41. Pattamanuch N, Novak I, Loizides A, Montalvo A, Thompson J, Rivas Y, Pan D. Single-center experience with 1-step low-profile percutaneous endoscopic gastrostomy in children. J Pediatr Gastroenterol Nutr. 2014;58(5):616–20.

42. Damore LJ II, Andrus CH, Herrmann VM, Wade TP, Kaminski DL, Kaiser GC. Prospective evaluation of a new through-the-scope nasoduodenal enteral feeding tube. Surg Endosc. 1997;11(5):460–3.

43. Lee S, Mathiasen R, Lipkin C, Margulies DR. Endoscopically placed nasogastrojejunal feeding tubes: a safe route for enteral nutrition in patients with hepatic encephalopathy. Am Surg. 2002;68(2):196–200.

44. McClave S, Sexton L, Spain D, Adams JL, Owens NA, Sullins MB, Blandford BS, Snider HL. Enteral tube feeding in the intensive care unit: factors impeding adequate delivery. Crit Care Med. 1999;27(7):1252–6.

45. Gunn S, Early B, Zenati M, Ochoa J. Use of a nasal bridle prevents accidental nasoenteral feeding tube removal. JPEN J Parenter Enteral Nutr. 2009;33(1):50–4.

46. Brandt CP, Mittendorf EA. Endoscopic placement of nasojejunal feeding tubes in ICU patients. Surg Endosc. 1999;13(12):1211–4.

47. Patrick P, Marulendra S, Kirby D, DeLegge M. Endoscopic nasogastric-jejunal feeding tube placement in critically ill patients. Gastrointest Endosc. 1997;45(1):72–6.

48. Bosco JJ, Gordon F, Zelig MP, Heiss F, Horst DA, Howell DA. A reliable method for the endoscopic placement of a nasoenteric feeding tube. Gastrointest Endosc. 1994;40(6):740–3.

49. Marcuard S, Stegall K, Trogdon S. Clearing obstructed feeding tubes. JPEN J Parental Enteral Nutr. 1989;13(1):81–3.

50. Stahlfeld K, Hiltner L. Clogged feeding tube management now that viokase is unavailable. JPEN J Parental Enteral Nutr. 2011;35(1):11.

51. McClave S. Managing complications of percutaneous and nasoenteric feeding tubes. Tech Gastrointest Endosc. 2001;3(1):62–8.

52. Lynch C, Fang J. Prevention and management of complications of PEG tubes. Pract Gastroenterol. 2004;28:66–76.

53. Safadi B, Marks J, Ponsky J. Percutaneous endoscopic gastrostomy. Gastrointest Endosc Clin N Am. 1998;8(1):551–68.

54. Wojtowycz MM, Arata JA Jr, Micklos TJ, Miller FJ Jr. CT findings after uncomplicated percutaneous gastrostomy. Am J Roentgenol. 1988;151(2):307–9.

55. Murphy CJ, Adler DG, Cox K, Sommers DN, Fang JC. Insufflation with carbon dioxide reduces pneumoperitoneum after percutaneous endoscopic gastrostomy (PEG): a randomized controlled trial. Endoscopy International Open. Forthcoming. 2016.

conventional push enteroscopy (with video). Gastrointest Endosc. 2012;76(3):675–9.

56. James A, Kapur K, Hawthorne A. Long-term outcome of percutaneous endoscopic gastrostomy feeding in patients with dysphagic stroke. Age Ageing. 1998;27(6):671–6.

57. Akkersdijk WL, van Bergeijk JD, van Egmond T, Mulder CJ, van Berge Henegouwen GP, van der Werken C, van Erpecum KJ. Percutaneous endoscopic gastrostomy (PEG): comparison of push and pull methods and evaluation of antibiotic prophylaxis. Endoscopy. 1995;27(4):313–6.

58. Lin H, Ibrahim H, Kheng J, Terris DJ. Percutaneous endoscopic gastrostomy: strategies for prevention and management of complications. Laryngoscope. 2009;111(10):1847–52.

59. Segal D, Michaed L, Guimber D, Ganga-Zandzou PS, Turck D, Gottrand F. Late-onset complications of percutaneous endoscopic gastrostomy in children. Pediatr Gastroenterol Nutr. 2001;33 (4):495–500.

60. Venu R, Brown R, Pastika B, Erikson LW Jr. The buried bumper syndrome: a simple management approach in two patients. Gastrointest Endosc. 2002;56(4):582–4.

61. Walton G. Complications of percutaneous endoscopic gastrostomy in patients with head and neck cancer—an analysis of 42 consecutive patients. Ann R Coll Surg Engl. 1999;81(4):272–6.

62. Ma MM, Semlacher EA, Fedorak RN, Lalor EA, Duerksen DR, Sherbaniuk RW, Chalpelsky CE, Sadowski DC. The buried gastrostomy bumper syndrome: prevention and endoscopic approaches to removal. Gastrointest Endosc. 1995;41(5):505–8.

63. Boyd J, DeLegge M, Shamburek R, Kirby D. The buried bumper syndrome: a new technique for safe, endoscopic PEG removal. Gastrointest Endosc. 1995;41(5):508–11.

64. DiSario J, Foutch P, Sanowski R. Poor results with percutaneous endoscopic gastrojejunostomy. Gastrointest Endosc. 1990;36(3):257–60.

65. DeLegge M, Duckworth PF Jr, McHenry L Jr, Foxx-Orenstein A, Craig RM, Kirby DF. Percutaneous endoscopic jejunostomy: a dual center safety and efficacy trial. JPEN J Parental Enteral Nutr. 1995;19(3):239–43.

66. Maple J, Baron T, Petersen B. The frequency, severity, and spectrum of adverse events associated with direct percutaneous endoscopic jejunostomy (DPEJ). Gastrointest Endosc. 2005;61(5): AB80.

67. Metheny N, Stewart B, McClave S. Relationship between feeding tube site and respiratory outcomes. JPEN J Parental Enteral Nutr. 2011;35(3):346–55.

68. Hsu C, Sun S, Lin S, Kang S, Chu K, Lin C, Huang H. Duodenal versus gastric feeding in medical intensive care unit patients: a prospective, randomized, clinical study. Crit Care Med. 2009;37 (6):1866–72.

69. Panagiotakis P, DiSario J, Hilden K, Ogara M, Fang J. DPEJ prevents aspiration in high-risk patients. Nutr Clin Prac. 2008;23 (2):172–5.

70. Finucaine TE, Christmas C, Travis K. Tube feeding in patients with advanced dementia. A review of the evidence. JAMA. 1999;282(14):1365–81.

71. Gillick MR. Rethinking the role of tube feeding in patients with advanced dementia. N Eng J Med. 2000;342(3):206–10.

72. Cervo F, Bryan L, Farber S. To PEG or not to PEG. Geriatrics. 2006;62(6):30–5.

73. Sampson E, Candy B, Jones L. Enteral tube feeding for older patients with advanced dementia. Cochrane Database Syst Rev. 2009;15(2):CD007209.

74. Sanders DS, Carter MJ, D'Silva J, James G, Bolton RP, Bardhan KD. Survival analysis in percutaneous endoscopic gastrostomy feeding: a worse outcome in patients with dementia. Am J Gastroenterol. 2000;95(6):1472–5.

75. Teno JM, Gozalo P, Mitchell SL, Kuo S, Fulton AT, Mor V. Feeding tubes and the prevention of healing or pressure ulcers. Arch Intern Med. 2012;172(9):697–701.

76. Truog RD, Cist AF, Brackett SE, Burns JP, Curley MA, Danis M, DeVita MA, Rosenbaum SH, Rothenberg DM, Sprung CL, Webb SA, Wlody GS, Hurford WE. Recommendations for end-of-life care in the intensive care unit: the ethics committee of the society of critical care medicine. Crit Care Med. 2001;29 (12):2332–48.

77. Beauchamp TL, Childress JF. Principles of biomedical ethics. Oxford (England): Oxford University Press; 2001.

78. Ritchie CS, Wilcox CM, Kvale E. Ethical and medicolegal issues related to percutaneous endoscopic gastrostomy placement. Gastrointest Endosc Clin N Am. 2007;17(4):805–15.

Complications of Upper Endoscopy and Their Management

C. Andrew Kistler, Aaron Martin, Jeremy Kaplan, Joseph Yoo, and Ali A. Siddiqui

Introduction

Esophagoduodenoscopy (EGD) is one of the most frequently utilized procedures by gastroenterologists. In 2009, there were close to 7 million EGD procedures performed in the USA [1].

Although upper endoscopy is considered one of the safest gastroenterology procedures, it is still associated with complications that must be anticipated and therefore managed appropriately. The overall complication rates have been reported between 1 in 200 and 1 in 10,000 with mortality rates ranging from 0 to 1 in 2000 [2]. These wide ranges are attributable to differences in study populations, reporting techniques, definitions of complications, and timing of follow-up reporting.

Before an upper endoscopy is conducted, both technical- and patient-related factors must be taken into account in attempts to minimize the risk of complications. The ASGE 2015 Quality Indicators for GI Endoscopic Procedures Guidelines clearly state that an EGD should not be performed unless the results will affect the overall management of the patient [3]. If the results of an EGD would not affect this management, then the EGD should not be performed or should be reconsidered.

EGD can be used to evaluate and treat numerous conditions including acute and chronic upper gastrointestinal bleeding (UGIB), gastroesophageal reflux disease (GERD), dysphagia, peptic ulcer disease (PUD), celiac disease, diarrhea, screening and surveillance of Barretts esophagus (BE), abnormal imaging, foreign body, and/or caustic ingestion [3].

Potential *contraindications* to upper endoscopy are relatively few but should be reviewed prior to performing an endoscopy as to limit the risk of complications: Some potential contraindications include a lack of informed consent, anesthesia-related contraindications, and a known perforated viscus (except if the upper endoscopy is indicated for potential correction/closure of the perforation). A thorough checklist of potential bad outcomes should be reviewed prior to the upper endoscopy in order to minimize complications: patient informed consent, anesthesia evaluation, dietary history, medication history (especially including anticoagulation, antibiotics and sedatives), concurrent medical history, hemodynamics, patient positioning, availability of staff and endoscopic products and supplies, recent laboratory and imaging studies, and potentially challenging anatomy [3].

EGDs have both diagnostic and therapeutic modalities, each of which carry their own unique benefits and risks of complications; their management will be discussed in this chapter.

Complications of Diagnostic Upper Endoscopy

Complications of upper endoscopy can be secondary to sedation/analgesia, the endoscopic procedure itself, or as a result of therapeutic interventions performed during the procedure. Complications occurring during diagnostic upper gastrointestinal (UGI) endoscopy are rare and have been reported at a rate of <0.2% per endoscopy when no therapeutic interventions are performed [4–6]. The majority of complications associated with diagnostic endoscopy are cardiopulmonary adverse events, infection, bleeding, and perforation. Here we will review the complications of diagnostic upper endoscopy, their respective management, and the use of routine pre-procedural testing to prevent them.

Electronic supplementary material

Supplementary material is available in the online version of this chapter at 10.1007/978-3-319-49041-0_10. Videos can also be accessed at https://link.springer.com/chapter/10.1007/978-3-319-49041-0_10.

C. Andrew Kistler · A. Martin · J. Kaplan · J. Yoo · A.A. Siddiqui
Division of Gastroenterology and Hepatology, Thomas Jefferson University, Philadelphia, PA, USA

A.A. Siddiqui (✉)
Department of Gastroenterology, Thomas Jefferson University Hospital, 132 S. 10th StreetMain Bldg, Suite 585, Philadelphia, PA 19107, USA
e-mail: aas138@jefferson.edu

© Springer International Publishing AG 2017
D.G. Adler (ed.), *Upper Endoscopy for GI Fellows*,
DOI 10.1007/978-3-319-49041-0_10

Cardiopulmonary Adverse Events (Table 10.1)

Most UGI endoscopies in the USA and Europe are performed using sedation and/or analgesia. Cardiopulmonary complications related to sedation and analgesia are the most common complications of diagnostic UGI endoscopy, comprising approximately 60–70% of all adverse events associated with UGI endoscopy [7–9]. The reported rate of significant cardiopulmonary adverse events during diagnostic endoscopies varies widely in the literature ranging from 1 in 170 to 1 in 10,000 endoscopies [2, 4, 7–10]. This variation is largely due to differences in event reporting, varying skill levels of endoscopists, and the definition of adverse events used. Cardiopulmonary adverse events range from minor changes in the heart rate or oxygen saturation to more severe events such as aspiration pneumonia, myocardial infarction, stroke, cardiopulmonary arrest, and death. Sharma et al. identified several independent predictors of cardiopulmonary adverse events that included: advanced age (>60 y/o), increased American Society of Anesthesia (ASA) classification (particularly an ASA >3), procedures performed in the inpatient setting, and involvement of a trainee in the procedure [7].

Infection

Infectious adverse events associated with UGI endoscopy can be from an endogenous source (usually as a result of the procedure itself) or from an exogenous source (secondary to poor reprocessing of endoscopic devices). Infectious complications of UGI endoscopy are rare. The mechanism of endogenous infection is thought to be the result of normal GI flora gaining access to the circulation through areas of mucosal trauma or instrumentation during an endoscopic procedure.

A number of studies have examined the rate of bacteremia following UGI endoscopy. These studies drew blood cultures before and after an endoscopy was performed in an effort to identify bacteremia. The reported rate of bacteremia following diagnostic UGI endoscopy has been reported as 1–8% [11–14]. Bacteremia observed in these studies was usually transient, and the rate of clinically significant infectious symptoms or sequelae (e.g., endocarditis, meningitis, or abscess formation) was extremely low [15]. The current American Heart Association (AHA) and ASGE guidelines do not recommend the use of prophylactic antibiotics to prevent endocarditis in patients undergoing diagnostic UGI endoscopies [16, 17].

Infections from an exogenous source are exceedingly rare and have nearly all occurred as a result of a breach in the current guidelines for cleaning and disinfecting endoscopic equipment. A 2003 review published in *Gastrointestinal Endoscopy* identified 317 reported episodes of pathogen transmission over a 36-year period. Pathogens most frequently identified in these studies include *Pseudomonas, Salmonella, H. Pylori, and Hepatitis B* [18]. Recent concerns regarding dissemination of carbapenem-resistant *Enterobacteriaceae* (CRE) infections during GI procedures have predominantly been limited to ERCP procedures but could theoretically be transmitted by any endoscope [19]. The inherent complexity of the duodenoscope design used during ERCP is one of the primary factors leading to challenges with appropriate CRE disinfection [19]. As a traditional upper endoscope does not have this same level of complexity, transmission of CRE infection during an EGD is much less likely to occur [20].

Bleeding (Table 10.2)

Bleeding is a rare complication of diagnostic UGI endoscopy. Mallory–Weiss tears have been reported following <0.5% of upper endoscopies, usually as a result of the patient having coughing or retching during the examination [21, 22]. Most of these tears do not result in clinically significant bleeding. Management of Mallory–Weiss tears involves admission to the hospital for observation, intravenous fluids, and serial hemoglobin testing. Thrombocytopenia and coagulopathies have been shown to increase the risk of bleeding. There is no agreed upon platelet count recommended prior to performing a diagnostic UGI endoscopy. Some studies have suggested that upper GI endoscopy is safe in patients with platelet counts >20,000/mL [4,

Table 10.1 Risk factors for cardiopulmonary adverse events during endoscopic procedures[7]	Bleeding	Perforation
Gastric polypectomy	6–7.2% [95–97]	0–0.45% [9, 98]
EMR:		
Esophagus	1.2% [101]	0.5–5% [102, 106]
Gastric	0–11.5% [102–105]	1% [108]
ESD:		
Esophageal	4.5–15.6% [108, 115]	2.3% [108, 118, 119]
Gastric		4.5% [108, 118, 119]

Table 10.2 Reported bleeding and perforation rates for various upper endoscopic resection techniques

Risk factors	Odds ratios [95% CI]
Age > 60 years old	1.8 [1.6–1.9]
ASA classification:	
III	1.8 [1.6–2.0]
IV	3.2 [2.5–4.1]
V	7.4 [3.2–17.6]
Inpatient procedures	1.5 [1.3–1.7]
Involvement of trainee	1.3 [1.2–1.4]

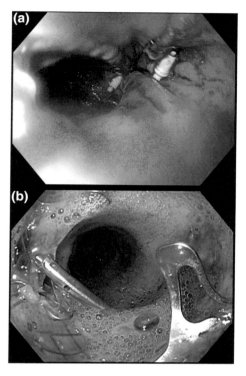

Fig. 10.1 An esophageal perforation caused by balloon dilation of a stricture (**a**) is treated by placement of a fully covered self-expanding metal stent (**b**). The stent is anchored to the esophageal wall using an Over-The-Scope Clip

23]. Video 10.1 demonstrated control of hemostasis with endoscopic hemoclips due to biopsy of an antral submucosal mass after unroofing.

Perforation (Table 10.2)

While an UGI endoscopy is the most common cause of esophageal perforation, its incidence as a result of a diagnostic UGI endoscopy is overall very rare. The risk of esophageal perforation during diagnostic UGI endoscopy has been reported as <0.04% [8, 9]. Risk factors associated with esophageal perforation include anterior cervical osteophytes, Zenker's diverticulum, upper gastrointestinal malignancies, and esophageal diverticula. The morality rate of esophageal perforation is reported between 2 and 36% [2]. Early identification of esophageal perforations is essential and has been shown to reduce the morbidity and mortality associated with this complication [24, 25]. The most frequent symptom of esophageal perforation includes neck, chest, or abdominal pain [26–28]. Other frequently reported signs and symptoms include fever, dyspnea, crepitus, and leukocytosis [26]. If esophageal perforation is suspected, initial diagnostics should include thoracic and cervical radiographs, which may reveal mediastinal or subcutaneous air dissection. However, studies have shown that radiographic findings may not be present immediately following perforation [29]. In patients with a high suspicion of esophageal perforation with a normal X-ray, further confirmatory testing with a gastrografin esophagram should be performed. If no site of perforation is identified but clinical suspicion remains high, a dilute barium esophagram or CT scan of the chest should be performed [30, 31]. The management of esophageal perforations depends on the clinical status of the patient and the size/involvement of the perforation. Most perforations can be medically managed with intravenous antibiotics, avoidance of oral intake, and parenteral nutrition [32]. Surgical intervention should be considered for patients who develop sepsis, those with pleural space involvement, and patients who do not improve with medical management [2]. Case

reports and studies describing the use of endoscopically placed stents (Fig. 10.1) and clips to treat esophageal perforations have been published, and these techniques are coming into more widespread use [33–35].

Prevention of Adverse Events: The Use of Routine Testing Prior to Endoscopy

Routine pre-endoscopy laboratory testing is the practice of ordering a set panel of tests on every patient undergoing an endoscopy regardless of the patient's history, physical, and/or preexisting medical conditions. Routine laboratory testing is often used in an attempt to prevent adverse events that may arise during endoscopy. The use of routine laboratory testing prior to endoscopy has not been validated as an effective way to prevent complications. Many studies have shown that routine laboratory testing rarely influences periprocedural management and that the cost of screening and the expense of following-up on these results outweigh their benefit [36, 37]. The American Society of Gastrointestinal Endoscopy (ASGE) recommends against routine pre-endoscopy testing in healthy patients. They recommend screening patients based on their history, physical, and preexisting medical conditions [37].

Complications of Therapeutic Upper Gastrointestinal Endoscopy

In addition to being an important diagnostic tool, the upper endoscopy procedure has become a widely adopted therapeutic modality for a wide range of GI conditions. As expected, more invasive therapeutic maneuvers during EGD also carry additional complications.

Complications of Dilation with Upper Endoscopy

The overall rate of reported adverse events associated with UGI dilation with endoscopy is between 0.1 and 0.4% [2, 4, 38]. The most common adverse events associated with UGI dilation are perforation, bleeding, aspiration, and bacteremia. The type and frequency of adverse events differ depending on the condition being treated. The most devastating adverse event associated with UGI dilation is esophageal perforation. Esophageal perforation in this setting is associated with a high mortality rate of 4–20% [25, 39].

Dilation of Esophageal Strictures

The most common adverse events associated with dilation of esophageal strictures are bleeding and perforation. The incidence of perforation with dilation of esophageal strictures is low; however, it is largely dependent on the technique used and the etiology of the stricture. The rate of perforation with the dilation of benign esophageal stricture has been reported between 0.1 and 0.3% [4, 40–43]. The rates of adverse events appear to be lower with wire-guided or pneumatic dilation as opposed to that performed with blind passage dilators [42]. Certain stricture types and etiologies that are associated with a higher risk of perforation include complex strictures (angular, tortuous, or long), strictures from caustic ingestion or eosinophilic esophagitis, and malignant or radiation-induced strictures [2].

Dilation for Achalasia

Pneumatic dilation of the lower esophageal sphincter is a frequently used treatment modality for achalasia. Endoscopic balloon dilation in this setting can only be called an aggressive maneuver, with balloons being inflated to 30–40 mm in diameter. The most severe complication of endoscopic balloon dilation for achalasia is perforation [44]. Perforation following pneumatic dilation for achalasia was reported to be 2% in a recent meta-analysis by Katzka et al. Most perforations examined in this study were managed medically with nasogastric decompression, intravenous antibiotics, and nothing by mouth. Only 1% of esophageal perforations required surgical intervention [45].

Dilation for Benign Gastric Outlet Obstruction (GOO)

The most common etiology of benign GOO is PUD. Conservative management with acid suppression, avoidance of NSAIDs, and H Pylori eradication when applicable is the first-line therapy. Endoscopic balloon dilation should be attempted only in patients who fail medical therapy. Perforation rates of pneumatic dilation for benign causes of GOO have been reported from 1.1 to 8.0% [46–49]. The risk of perforation is increased with active ulceration at the site of obstruction and dilation with balloons greater than 15 mm in diameter [47, 50].

Complications of Foreign Body Retrieval

Ingestion of foreign bodies is the second most common endoscopic emergency behind GI hemorrhage [51]. The type of foreign body ingested often varies based upon patient demographics. Fish and chicken bones, as well as impacted meat boluses, are typically seen in adults, while coins and toys are often seen in pediatric populations [52–54]. Intentional ingestion of various potentially obstructive foreign objects can also be seen in psychiatric patients and prisoners [55, 56]. Ingested foreign bodies can cause significant morbidity and mortality when they become impacted in the esophagus. Specific complications resulting from ingested foreign bodies include inflammation, mucosal laceration, perforation, hemorrhage, and even death [51, 57].

Though complications resulting from the endoscopic retrieval of foreign bodies are rare, they can be difficult to distinguish from the complications that result from ingestion of the foreign body itself. This is demonstrated by the fact that the most commonly reported complications of endoscopic retrieval of foreign bodies are superficial mucosal laceration ($\leq 2\%$), GI hemorrhage ($\leq 1\%$), and perforation ($\leq 0.8\%$) [2]. Factors that have been shown to increase the risk of complications resulting from endoscopic intervention include presentation greater than 24 h after the onset of symptoms, sharp foreign objects, and the presence of multiple objects [51, 55, 58]. Sharp and irregular objects, in particular fish bones and chicken bones, significantly increase the risk of perforation [2, 54].

Special consideration should be given to include careful examination of the cervical esophagus as well as to technique when removing boluses of food or sharp foreign objects in order to minimize the risk of aspiration and perforation. During routine upper endoscopy, passing through the upper esophageal sphincter quickly and reaching the middle esophagus are a common practice. However, in cases when foreign body obstruction is suspected, extra care should be taken to prevent secondary injury to the esophagus, as foreign bodies located at the level of the cervical esophagus are often difficult to remove due to a limited working space for the endoscope [51, 56]. This is compounded by the fact that the majority of foreign bodies are found in the upper esophagus [51, 55, 56, 59, 60]. Currently, the ASGE guidelines regarding the management of food or meat boluses by piecemeal extraction recommends consideration of using an esophageal overtube and/or endotracheal intubation in order to minimize the risk of aspiration [2]. The ASGE has previously advocated against pushing the bolus into the stomach without first examining the esophagus distal to the obstruction by passing the endoscope around the bolus. However, 2 large published series using the push technique reported no perforations, and this technique may minimize the risk of aspiration [55, 56]. Tools such as an overtube or rubber hoods attached to the end of an endoscope are tools that can be used to help minimize the risk of perforation during removal of sharp or pointed objects. Additionally, removing foreign objects so that the sharp end is trailing also helps to minimize the risk of perforation [2, 52, 56].

After endoscopic retrieval of a foreign body, the mucosa should be carefully assessed for complications such as mucosal lacerations, bleeding, and especially perforation [2, 55]. In cases where retrieval was difficult, patients should be watched closely for signs and symptoms of perforation and should be considered for immediate radiographic contrast studies or chest radiograph to detect any evidence of mediastinal air [55, 61]. While the majority of mucosal injuries and bleeding can be managed either conservatively or with standard endoscopic hemostasis techniques, surgery may sometimes be indicated for more serious complications such as perforation [2, 61]. Perforation, when recognized immediately during endoscopy with no evidence of mediastinal contamination, can sometimes be treated with removable plastic or covered metal esophageal stents or with endoscopic clips [35, 61]. These strategies can be especially beneficial in patients who are not good surgical candidates or in patients with an underlying esophageal neoplasm [35, 61, 62]. Perforation, when foreign body induced, recognized later by signs and symptoms such as fever, tachycardia, chest or abdominal pain, and crepitus involving the soft tissue surrounding the neck can be treated with surgery if endoscopic options fail or are not felt to be appropriate [55, 61].

Complications of Percutaneous Endoscopic Gastrostomy (PEG) Placement

Percutaneous endoscopic gastrostomy (PEG) was first introduced in 1980 as a means to provide long-term enteral nutritional support to patients with a functional gastrointestinal system, without the need for surgical laparotomy [63]. Currently, PEG continues to be one of the most

common endoscopic procedures worldwide [64]. It is generally considered to be a safe procedure, with an overall rate of adverse events reported to be between 4.9 and 10.3%, and a rate of serious adverse events reported in 1.5–9.4% of cases [2, 64]. Minor complications of PEG placement include tube occlusion, tube migration causing gastric outlet obstruction, granuloma formation, pneumoperitoneum, and peristomal leakage and/or pain. Major complications include aspiration pneumonia, bleeding, internal organ injury, gastric perforation, "buried bumper syndrome," wound infection, necrotizing fasciitis, and tumor seeding of the stoma [2, 65, 66]. Death resulting from PEG placement is very rare, and according to one meta-analysis of 4194 PEG procedures, PEG-procedure-related mortality was reported to be only 0.53% [65, 66].

Several different strategies for PEG placement have been developed since it was first introduced, such as the "pull" technique, the "push" technique, and the introducer technique. The "pull" technique is currently reported to be the most common technique, though no significant differences in complication and efficacy rates has been reported between the different methods [67, 68]. Tumor seeding of the stoma is a rare complication seen in patients with head and neck or esophageal cancer, with only 22 cases reported [69]. Though hematogenous spread is possible, the exact mechanism of this phenomenon is not well established. It is generally believed that direct seeding of the gastrostomy site can occur when the PEG tube comes into contact with head and neck cancer during the "push" or "pull" technique [64]. For cases of PEG placement in patients with head and neck cancer, greater consideration for the introducer technique can be given as opposed to the more commonly used "push" or "pull" techniques [65].

Peristomal wound infection is the most common infectious complication following PEG placement. According to a meta-analysis of 10 randomized clinical trials, the pooled rate of peristomal wound infection was 26% [2, 64, 70]. Patients undergoing PEG placement are considered to be at higher risk of developing infections as the patient population often have significant underlying comorbidities, poor nutritional intake, and advanced age [71]. Minor infections can often be treated with topical antiseptics and local wound care, while more serious wound infections require systemic antibiotics [64]. A single dose of an intravenous cephalosporin- or penicillin-based antibiotic administered 30 min before the procedure is currently recommended as it has been shown in multiple randomized, controlled trials to be effective in reducing the occurrence of peristomal wound infections [2, 64, 70–73]. In areas where MRSA is endemic, pre-procedure screening of patients for colonization with MRSA, and subsequent decontamination if positive, has been shown to be beneficial in reducing the rate of MRSA wound infections following PEG placement [64, 71, 74, 75].

Necrotizing fasciitis is a rare but potentially life-threatening infectious complication of PEG placement [76, 77]. It is characterized by the necrosis of abdominal fascia due to a rapidly progressing infection along the fascial planes. Two main risk factors in the development of necrotizing fasciitis are traction and pressure on the PEG tube; therefore, maintaining a distance of 1–2 cm between the external bumper and the abdominal wall can help prevent this complication [64, 78]. Additional risk factors for development of necrosis after PEG placement include diabetes mellitus, atherosclerosis, alcoholism, malnutrition, immunosuppression, and older age [2, 64, 77, 79]. Development of necrotizing fasciitis is an emergency and requires immediate surgical consultation for consideration of wide surgical debridement, broad-spectrum empiric antibiotics, and intensive care support [64].

Buried bumper syndrome is another major complication that can occur as early as 3 weeks following PEG placement [80, 81]. It is characterized by ischemic necrosis of the gastric wall, believed to be caused by excessive traction on the internal bumper and migration of the tube out of the gastric lumen and toward the abdominal wall [2, 64]. Buried bumper syndrome is preventable by checking tube position regularly, leaving a small distance between the external bumper and the skin, and rotating the PEG tube 180–360° daily [64]. Treatment involves removal and replacement of the PEG tube, either endoscopically, surgically, or by external traction of the tube [64, 82, 83]. A case of "buried bumper syndrome" is demonstrated in Fig. 10.2.

Other major complications of endoscopic PEG tube placement include aspiration pneumonia, bleeding, and injury to internal organs. Aspiration directly related to the procedure of PEG placement is reported to be between 0.3 and 1.0%, though it can be difficult to determine whether the aspiration event occurs during the procedure itself or later during feeding via the PEG tube [2, 65, 84, 85]. The risk factors for aspiration include supine position, advanced age, need for sedation, and neurologic impairment. Aspiration risk can be reduced by avoiding over sedation, minimizing air insufflation, and thoroughly aspirating gastric contents before PEG placement [86]. Bleeding can occur either from traumatic erosions of the esophageal or gastric mucosa, as well as from puncturing gastric or abdominal wall vessels, including the gastric artery and splenic or mesenteric veins [2, 64, 65]. Fortunately, acute hemorrhage is a rare complication and occurs in less than 1% of procedures [2, 64, 65]. Bleeding can usually be managed by applying direct pressure over the abdominal wound, though endoscopic or surgical exploration may be necessary in some cases [64]. Correcting coagulation disorders and stopping anticoagulants prior to PEG placement as much as possible are recommended to decrease the risk of significant bleeding [87].

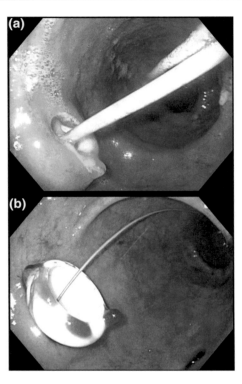

Fig. 10.2 Patient with a "buried bumper" of his PEG tube. The old PEG tube is removed and replaced with a new PEG tube under wire-guided assistance

Injuries to internal organs and gastric tears or lacerations are also rare complications of PEG placement, occurring in less than 0.5–1.8% of cases, though elderly patients may have a slightly increased risk of injury to bowels due to laxity of the colonic mesentery [65, 88]. Generally, injury to the colon or small bowel is more common than injury to the spleen or liver [64]. Injury to internal organs often warrants surgical intervention, though specific management has not been well studied [2, 64, 89]. Diagnosis of injury to internal organs can often be complicated by the fact that benign, transient (up to 72 h) pneumoperitoneum is reported to occur in 12–38% of patients undergoing uncomplicated PEG, therefore limiting the reliability of plain films in the diagnosis of suspected perforation of visceral organs [2, 64, 88, 90, 91]. In such cases, using a water-soluble oral contrast with computed tomography (CT) scan is a useful alternative in the diagnosis of possible defects in gastrointestinal integrity [64].

Development of gastrocolocutaneous fistulas may result if a loop of bowel is inadvertently perforated during PEG placement, or even over time via erosion into adjacent loops of. Asymptomatic or chronic gastrocolocutaneous fistulas can similarly be diagnosed using computed tomography (CT) with water-soluble contrast, and management of these cases includes simple removal of the tube [2, 65]. Surgery is required only in rare cases where a fistula persists after removal of the tube [65]. Using proper technique for PEG placement minimizes the risk of injury to internal organs and includes measures such as adequate gastric trans-illumination, finger indentation, and use of the "safe-tract" method during PEG placement [2, 92].

After successful PEG placement, inadvertent dislodgment of the PEG tube has been reported to occur in 1.6–4.4% of cases [65]. If dislodgement occurs before a mature tract is able to develop (usually 7–10 days), a free intra-abdominal perforation can result as the stomach separates from the anterior abdominal wall. If identified immediately, endoscopic placement of a new tube either via the same opening in the abdominal wall, or near the original site, is appropriate as pulling the stomach back against the anterior abdominal wall will seal the perforation [2, 65]. If tube dislodgement is identified late in a patient with an immature tract, management should include placement of a nasogastric Salem sump tube, broad-spectrum antibiotics, and new PEG placement within 7–10 days, as long as the patient does not show signs of peritoneal inflammation [65]. Patients who have a mature tract that experience tube dislodgement can have a new PEG tube placed safely through the same tract without the need for endoscopy [64].

Complications of Therapeutic Endoscopy

Complications of Polypectomy

While upper GI endoscopy is a routinely performed procedure with a relatively low risk of mortality and adverse events, therapeutic interventions increase the incidence of complications including bleeding, pain, dysphagia, and perforation [4, 5, 8–10, 93]. Snare polypectomy of gastric polyps is frequently performed in order to assess polyp histology for diagnosis [94]. Bleeding is the most common complication with an incidence of 6–7.2% [95–97]. In comparison with colonic polypectomy, gastric polypectomy demonstrates a much higher rate of bleeding (1% vs. 7%, respectively) [98]. Suggested risk factors for post-polypectomy bleeding include large size (greater than 8 mm) and sessile appearance [99]. Bleeding is often effectively controlled with injection of 5–15 mL of 1:10,000 diluted epinephrine followed by bipolar electro-cauterization or hemoclip application [99]. Closure of a gastric polyp defect after polypectomy of a gastric adenoma is demonstrated in Fig. 10.3.

Endoscopic Mucosal Resection (EMR)

EMR is increasingly being used to remove benign and early malignant lesions of the GI tract. Initially developed for the removal of sessile or flat neoplasms confined to the mucosa and submucosa, EMR may involve submucosal injection or ligation assistance to lift the lesion and aid in resection [100]. Bleeding represents the most common adverse event

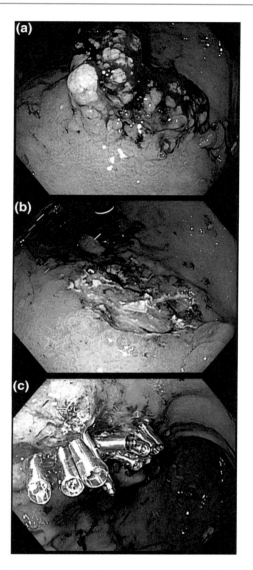

Fig. 10.3 A large gastric adenoma was removed using hot snare polypectomy (**a**). The ulcerated defect and bleeding from an endoscopic mucosal resection site were closed using endoscopic clips (**b, c**)

associated with EMR. A single-center study including 681 patients who underwent 2513 EMRs of the esophagus showed a rate of significant bleeding of 1.2%. The authors defined significant bleeding as a drop in hemoglobin greater than 2 mg/dl from baseline, bleeding requiring therapeutic intervention or blood transfusion, and/or bleeding at a later time requiring rehospitalization. In the 8 cases of post-EMR bleeding, seven were treated successfully with epinephrine injection, clips, and thermal coagulation. One patient required surgery for adequate hemostasis. Factors including patient age, length of Barrett's esophagus, number of EMR performed, and use of anticoagulants were all analyzed, and none of which were found to correlate with post-EMR bleeding. Bleeding occurred at a mean time of 2.5 days following the EMR procedure [101].

Like esophageal EMR, EMR of gastric and duodenal lesions may also be complicated by intra-procedural bleeding with reported rates of 0–11.5% [102–104]. Bleeding following gastric tumor EMR occurred in approximately 5% of patients based on a retrospective study of 472 patients [105]. Bleeding can be effectively controlled with hemostatic clipping, even in cases of spurting blood vessel from the EMR site [102].

EMR of the esophagus may also be complicated by perforation with reported rates ranging from 0.5 to 5% [102, 106]. The rate of perforation appears to be correlated with physician experience. A multicenter randomized clinical trial comparing endoscopic resection to radiofrequency ablation for Barrett's esophagus with high-grade dysplasia or early cancer demonstrated a perforation rate of 5% in the first 120 esophageal EMRs performed by 6 physicians who were provided with structured training [107]. A prospectively maintained database of patients with Barrett's esophagus reported no EMR-related perforations in the study period possibly related to operator experience [101].

Perforations due to EMR of the stomach and duodenum appear to be uncommon. A systematic review demonstrated the risk of perforation after EMR to be 1% [108]. A prospectively maintained database of patients who underwent endoscopic resection of duodenal adenomas or laterally spreading tumors demonstrated a duodenal perforation rate after EMR to be 2% [109]. Perforation rates of the duodenum due to EMR have been shown to be related to physician experience. Perforations can be effectively closed using endoscopic clips in cases in which the perforation was recognized at the time of occurrence. In delayed perforations, the patients should be managed with surgical repair [109]. Closure of a gastric perforation using an Over-The-Scope Clip (OTSC) is shown in Fig. 10.4.

Stenosis may occur in 6–88% of patients following EMR of the esophagus [106, 107, 110–113]. Larger mucosal resections and circumferential EMR are associated with higher rates of stenosis. Strictures are typically amenable to esophageal dilation [107, 113].

Complications of Endoscopic Submucosal Dissection (ESD)

ESD is a technique of endoscopic resection that allows for en bloc removal of lesions in the epithelium. Intra-procedural bleeding is common and may be treated with coagulation current via the ESD knife or with hemostatic forceps [114]. Occurring in 4.5–15.6% of cases, post-procedure bleeding is a known complication, which occurs more frequently with gastric resections as compared to esophageal resections [108, 115]. Risk factors for delayed bleeding include lesion size greater than 40 mm and resumption of antithrombotic therapy [116]. A meta-analysis of 6 studies demonstrates a reduced incidence of delayed

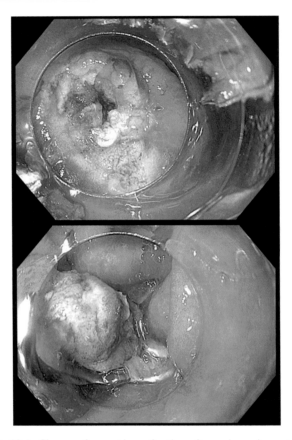

Fig. 10.4 Closure of a gastric perforation after endoscopic mucosal resection of a polyp with an Over-The-Scope Clip (OTSC; Ovesco Endoscopy GmbH, Tuebingen, Germany)

bleeding after gastric ESD in patients treated with a proton pump inhibitor compared to those treated with an H_2 receptor antagonist [117].

A meta-analysis of gastric ESD reports a perforation rate of 4.5%, while a review of a series of studies of esophageal ESD reports a pooled rate of perforation of 2.3% [108, 118, 119]. It should be noted that a meta-analysis comparing adverse event rates for ESD and EMR for superficial esophageal cancers demonstrated a significantly higher rate of perforation in the ESD group [120]. Treatment of perforations may be non-operative with the use of clip closure. A Japanese study of 10 years of ESD/EMR gastric perforations describes successful closure of perforations in 98% of cases [121].

Like EMR, ESD may be complicated by post-ESD strictures, which most often occur in the esophagus. Reported rates of stricture formation are 12–17% with greater circumference of resection and length of resection being known risk factors [122–125]. Reported treatments include serial dilation, intra-lesional steroid injection, topical steroid application, radial electroincision, and prophylactic placement of self-expandable metal stents [126–128].

Complications of Endoscopic Eradication Therapy (EET) and Coagulation With an increasing incidence of esophageal adenocarcinoma in the Western world, there has been heightened interest in EET in the treatment of Barrett's esophagus [4]. Also, hemostasis during upper endoscopy is increasingly accomplished by both contact and non-contact thermal devices.

Complications of Argon Plasma Coagulation (APC)

APC is a non-contact thermocoagulation modality often used to eradicate mucosal lesions. Randomized trials with APC report bleeding rates as high as 4%, esophageal perforation rates as high as 2% and strictures in up to 6% of patients, all of which appears to be higher than other ablative modalities [129–132]. However, a Cochrane randomized control trial comparing APC and multipolar electrocoagulation for the treatment of Barrett's esophagus demonstrated no serious adverse events [129]. More commonly reported are events of upper GI discomfort including pain, dysphagia, and nausea [129].

APC may also be used in cases of gastrointestinal bleeding and adenoma eradication. There have been case reports of pneumoperitoneum following APC [133]. Pneumoperitoneum following APC may not be a sign of perforation and may simply be due to argon gas passing through the GI tract wall into the abdomen. APC-induced ulcers may result in gastrointestinal bleeding [134]. A large series of 2193 sessions of APC in 1062 patients demonstrated a perforation rate of 0.2% [135].

Complications of Photodynamic Therapy (PDT)

PDT is another ablative modality that uses porfimer sodium with a photosensitizing agent. Similar to APC, the most commonly reported adverse event is chest discomfort and photosensitivity. A randomized, multicenter study conducted over 5 years reported resolution of all cases of photosensitivity [136]. Another study reported pleural effusions and fever in patients who underwent PDT [137]. Of the ablative modalities, PDT appears to have the highest incidence of post-procedure esophageal strictures with rates up to 35%. However, after being followed for 5 years post-treatment for any complications, none of the study patients reported any long-term adverse events [136].

Complications of Radiofrequency Ablation (RFA)

RFA is commonly used in the ablation of Barrett's esophagus. RFA involves the delivery of a preset amount of radiofrequency energy via a balloon, resulting in circumferential superficial tissue destruction [138, 139]. RFA may be associated with chest discomfort in up to 2% of patients, which resolves within 1 week of the procedure [140]. Superficial lacerations from the procedure were reported in

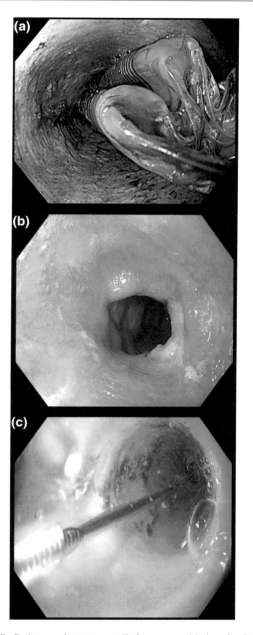

Fig. 10.5 Patient underwent a radiofrequency ablation for Barrett's esophagus (**a**). Patient developed a esophageal stricture (**b**) four weeks later. This was treated successfully with balloon dilation (**c**)

6% of patients in a single trial [141]. Hemodynamically significant bleeding is relatively rare, occurring in less than 2% of procedures [140, 142]. A multicenter study of 429 patients who underwent RFA reported no serious adverse events. Strictures were seen in 1.8% of the participants with other trials reporting a stricture rate of 2–8% [140–142]. These strictures are easily treated using endoscopic balloon dilation (Fig. 10.5). Esophageal perforation successfully treated with an endoprosthesis has been reported [143].

Complications of Cryotherapy

Cryotherapy in which liquid nitrogen is applied to an area of Barrett's esophagus is a relatively novel idea. Initially reports demonstrate that the procedure is relatively well tolerated. In a study of 333 treatments performed on 98 patients, there were no serious adverse events. Two percentage of patients reported chest discomfort, which resolved after a brief treatment course with narcotics. Strictures were seen in 3% of patients, all of whom underwent successful esophageal dilation thereafter [144]. Perforation was reported in 1 patient who had Marfan's syndrome [145].

Complications of Enteral Stenting of the Upper Gastrointestinal Tract

Esophageal, gastric, and duodenal stenting have become common procedures for the management of benign and malignant strictures [35, 146, 147]. Esophageal stents are also used to treat benign esophageal perforations and anastomotic leaks [148]. Features and design of these stents are variable with complication rates frequently correlating with design specifics of the stent [149]. Historically, the use of rigid esophageal stents carried a complication rate of 20% and a mortality rate of 9%, respectively. Complications with these older devices included bleeding, fistula formation, stent migration, food impaction, and tissue overgrowth [150]. These devices are now obsolete and are not commercially available.

With the advent of self-expandable metal stents (SEMS), complication rates have significantly dropped leading to the demise of rigid stents [151]. SEMS may be partially covered or fully covered. Partially covered stents are more frequently subject to tissue ingrowth and, to a lesser extent, overgrowth, while fully covered stents are more likely to migrate as they cannot embed in the mucosa [152–155]. Significant immediate adverse events following SEMS placement may occur in 2–12% of patients and include aspiration, respiratory compromise, stent mal-positioning, and perforation [156–159]. Most post-procedure adverse events are self-limiting and include chest pain and nausea [156, 160]. More significant adverse events include tumor overgrowth, stent migration, luminal perforation, and bleeding. Stents may migrate and tumor overgrowth may occur in up to 27% of patients [159, 161]. A Swedish study of 152 patients who underwent SEMS placement for esophageal strictures reported transient chest/pharyngeal discomfort in all patients, stent migration in 5%, perforation in 1%, and stent occlusion in 10% [160]. Stents placed across the esophagogastric junction may result in increased rates of gastroesophageal reflux [162]. Patients with stents that cross the esophagogastric junction are often placed on prophylactic acid suppression medication to good effect.

Stent placement is also a well-established palliative treatment modality for malignant gastric outlet obstruction [163]. Nonetheless, gastroduodenal stents are frequently placed in older patients who often have multiple comorbidities [164]. Severe early adverse events including bleeding and perforation are reported in 1–5% of patients [163, 165, 166]. A prospective study of 108 patients with malignant gastric outlet obstruction who underwent stent placement reported no procedure-related mortality. The most common adverse event was stent occlusion, which was reported in 14.8% of patients. It must be noted that the stent used in this study was uncovered. Other reported adverse events were GI bleeding (3.7%) and stent migration (1.9%) [164]. Precautions must be taken to avoid aspiration during placement of the stent as this represents a significant periprocedural complication [167].

Complications of Upper Endoscopy Performed for Evaluation of Upper Gastrointestinal Bleeding

Gastrointestinal bleeding (GIB) is one of the most common diagnoses leading to hospitalization in the USA. GIB is the principal diagnosis in up to 182 per 100,000 adults [168] and in the top 10 GI diagnoses within a hospitalization and causes of GI mortality [1]. Upper GIB has traditionally been described as bleeding within the gastrointestinal tract proximal to the ligament of Treitz. Upper endoscopy is frequently used to diagnose and potentially treat the source of UGIB. Based on source of bleeding and intervention performed, the complications and management can vary widely.

Complications of Endoscopic Variceal Hemostasis

Acutely bleeding esophageal varices (EV) or gastric varices (GV) are a common indication for performing an EGD and carry a relatively high mortality if not intervened on in a timely manner. Prior to performing an EGD in a patient who potentially has bleeding EV or GV, certain steps should be considered prior to starting the endoscopy in order to minimize complications.

Patients should be stabilized in an intensive care unit or other monitored setting with appropriate intravenous access in order to maximize hemodynamic stability. Goal hemoglobin concentration is typically 7–8 g/dL [169, 170]. Caution must be used to not over-resuscitate a cirrhotic patient with blood products or crystalloid solutions since this may lead to increased portal pressures resulting in increased risk of rebleeding and mortality [170].

Additional blood products should be available before, during, and after the endoscopy. Fresh-frozen plasma (FFP) and/or platelets can be administered in patients with significant coagulopathy. The data regarding the use of recombinant factor VIIa (rFVIIa) in cirrhotic patients with UGIB are somewhat controversial and need further elucidation before its use can be definitively recommended [170].

Intravenous or oral fluoroquinolone (norfloxacin 400 mg po bid or ciprofloxacin 500 mg bid) or intravenous ceftriaxone 1 g daily should be administered to the cirrhotic patient with or without ascites with suspected UGIB for seven days. This short-term antibiotic prophylaxis in cirrhotic patients with or without ascites reduces all-cause mortality, mortality secondary to infection, rebleeding events, hospitalization length, and over bacterial infection rate [169–171]. Cirrhotics that are hospitalized have been demonstrated to have a bacterial infection rate of 20%, and up to 50% can develop an infection while hospitalized with a GIB [170, 172]. Aside from bacterial peritonitis, these patients also are at more risk of respiratory infections, UTIs, and bacteremia [170]. The use of the EGD procedure without the proper antibiotic prophylaxis and/or treatment doses could potentially lead to the complication of increased risk of infection.

If an acute esophageal variceal bleed (EVB) is suspected, intravenous octreotide should be initiated with a bolus dose of 50 μg followed by an infusion of 50 μg/h. If the source of the UGIB is confirmed to be from bleeding EV, then octreotide should be continued for 3–5 days post-EGD [170].

The use of a high-dose IV infusion of proton pump inhibitor should be considered if other etiologies of UGIB outside of an acute variceal bleed are possible or until confirmation of EVB during EGD.

EGD should be performed within 12 h of admission [170]. In addition to the medical management mentioned above, endotracheal intubation (EIT) should be considered prior to performing an EGD. The 2014 ASGE guidelines for endoscopic management of variceal hemorrhage suggest that "intubation of patients before endoscopy to prevent aspiration during the procedures, especially in patients with encephalopathy" [169]. Similarly, AASLD guidelines state that "intubation may be required for airway protection prior to endoscopy" [170]. Despite these statements, the data are not entirely clear on benefits of prophylactic intubation prior to emergent endoscopy, in both variceal and non-variceal UGIB. Some clinical studies actually suggest an increased risk of aspiration pneumonia in patients prophylactically intubated prior to EGD [173].

Despite maximal medical and endoscopic management, variceal bleeding may not be controlled during initial or rebleeding episodes. Patients who survive an episode of acute variceal hemorrhage have a median rebleeding rate in untreated patients of approximately 60% with 1–2 years of initial bleed with a mortality of 33% [170]. The risk of rebleeding is multifactorial and may occur as a complication of EGD. Endoscopic and/or pharmacological treatments may not control variceal bleeding on initial or recurrent episodes

in up to 10–20% of patients [170]. In these situations, TIPS should be considered as a salvage therapy, and surgical consultation may be warranted [170].

Complications of Endoscopic Variceal Sclerotherapy (EVS)

EVS is successful in controlling active EVB in more than 90% of patients [169]; however, its use has been primarily supplanted by esophageal variceal ligation (EVL) based on its adverse event profile.

The most common sclerosing agents used during an EGD include ethanolamine oleate, cyanoacrylate, polidocanol, absolute alcohol, sodium tetradecyl sulfate [2]. No agent has been shown to be more efficacious or safer [2]. Overall adverse event rate with EVS ranges from approximately 35 to 78% along with a mortality rate between 1 and 5% [174, 175]. Minor, temporary complications that may be encountered in the first 24–48 h post-EVS include: low-grade fevers, chest pain, and dysphagia [169, 176]. These transient symptoms typically do not require any treatment and are managed conservatively with symptomatic control.

Injecting the sclerosing agent can be technically challenging as the sclerosing agent needs to be injected directly into the varix, compared with banding where the band can be placed in the vicinity of the bleeding varix. Placement of the sclerosing agent into the surrounding tissue can lead to further complications and tissue damage.

Esophageal ulcerations are sometimes deemed a "complication" of EVS or EVL (Fig. 10.6); however, they are expected phenomena after successful endoscopic treatment of bleeding EV. EVS-associated esophageal ulcers are deeper and heal slower compared with those secondary to post-EVL [177]. The severity of these ulcers may also be worsened when EVS is repeated within 1 week of the initial session [178, 179]. These ulcers cannot be prevented with agents such as sucralfate, H2 receptor antagonists, although PPIs may promote ulceration healing [180]. Post-EVS ulcers can bleed in up to 20% of patients, during which traditional endoscopic treatments can be performed for hemostasis, such as clipping [176].

EV rebleeding rates are generally higher in patients treated with EVS compared to EVL. Rebleeding rates range from approximately 33% [181] to 42% [170]. This higher rate of rebleeding may be due to an increase in portal pressure observed in patients treated with EVS but not EVL [182]. Immediate bleeding may occur in up to 6% of patients [183] and can be treated with endoscopic clipping and banding; however, repeat injection of sclerosing agents should be used with caution and may put the patient at increased risk of further complications. Delayed bleeding occurs in between 19 and 24% [184] of patients and can be treated with repeat endoscopy (endoscopic clipping, banding) and the appropriate pharmacological

---

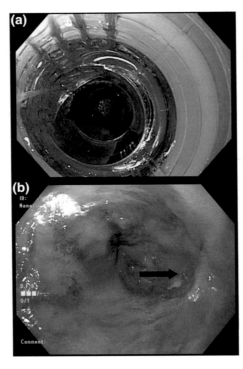

Fig. 10.6 Banding of an esophageal varix (**a**) that led to a superficial ulcer on surveillance endoscopy 3 weeks after the initial banding (**b**)

treatment such as high-dose IV PPI infusions. Delayed bleeding can occur from post-EVS ulcers, esophagitis, or recurrent esophageal variceal bleed. Intramural hematoma occurs in up to 1.6% of patients undergoing EGD with EVL and typically resolve spontaneously and requires no intervention [185].

Esophageal strictures occur in up to 20–26% of patients undergoing EGD with EVS and potentially is associated with total number of EVS sessions and volume/type of sclerosant used [185–188]. EVS-induced strictures will typically improve with dilation [169].

Perforation has been reported in 0.5–5% of patients undergoing EGD with EVS [185] and is typically initially managed conservatively. Depending on the patient's clinical status, they may require further advanced endoscopic procedures such as placement of esophageal stents or surgical consultation and intervention.

Aspiration pneumonia occurs in up to 5% of patients but usually during emergent procedures [187, 188] and is typically medically managed with antibiotics and respiratory support as needed.

A rare yet still important complication of EVS includes the possible extension of thrombus into the portal and mesenteric venous system causing mesenteric or splenic infarction; however, there are limited reports of this [189–192]. Among the available sclerosing agents, alcohol and cyanoacrylate have been reported to cause systemic emboli to the spleen, portal vein, and lung [192–194].

Transient bacteremia has been reported anywhere from 0 to 53% of patients undergoing EGD with EVS [176, 195]. Prophylactic antibiotics are recommended if the patients are acutely bleeding; however, patients undergoing elective EVS are not recommended to have prophylactic antibiotics administered [170]. Patients with potential transient bacteremia should be watched closely, and further management would be dictated by their clinical status.

Complications of Endoscopic Variceal Ligation

Endoscopic variceal ligation (EVL) is preferred over EVS secondary to improved safety profile and superior efficacy [169, 170]. The overall complication rate for EVL is about 14% [170]. The most common adverse events are transient and include dysphagia and chest discomfort and are managed conservatively and will typically stop within 24–48 h post-EVL. If other more serious causes of chest discomfort have been ruled out, this post-EVL chest discomfort can be treated with a 50:50 mixture of lidocaine–antacid mixture or similar compounds. These patients can also initially be placed on a clear liquid diet until the discomfort dissipates. Post-EVL patients should not typically complain of fever or findings consistent with mediastinitis; therefore, these findings should be closely investigated for another etiology if present.

Rebleeding rates after EVL can be between 21.7% [181] and 32% [170]. Early rebleeding can be re-treated endoscopically with additional EVL. After initial hemostasis, EVL sessions can be repeated at approximately 7- to 28-day intervals until variceal obliteration, which typically requires 2–4 sessions. Once eradicated, an EGD is usually repeated every 3–6 months or as per the treating physician.

Esophageal ulcers are expected after successful EVL. These ulcers are typically less severe than those found post-EVS. Post-EVL ulcers are limited to the mucosa and heal quicker (less than 3 weeks), unlike EVS-related ulcers which are often deeper [2, 177]. PPIs have been shown to help heal these ulcers, but not prevent them [170, 196]. Bleeding from post-EVL esophageal ulcers can occur in up to 14% of patient and can be treated with standard endoscopic modalities such as clipping [169]. Risk factors for EVL-associated ulcer bleeding include high platelet ratio index (APRI) score, esophagitis, and prior variceal bleeding [197].

Esophageal strictures occur in only 0–2% of patients following EVL and are usually due to excessive scarring and have been treated with endoscopic dilation [174, 185, 187]. Perforation is exceedingly rare during EVL, with rates less than 1% [174, 185]. Initially perforations are managed conservatively with making the patient nothing by mouth, and administering IV fluid and antibiotics. Repair of the

Table 10.3 Comparison of endoscopic variceal sclerotherapy (EVS) and endoscopic variceal ligation (EVL) complication rates

	Endoscopic variceal sclerotherapy (EVS)	Endoscopic variceal ligation (EVL)
Overall complication rate	35–78% [174, 175]	14% [170]
Mortality rates in acute bleeding case	24.6%–32% [174, 181]	22.8% [181]
Rebleeding rates	33–42% [170]	21.7–32% [170]
Post-therapy bleeding rates	Up to 20% [176]	Up to 14% [169]
Esophageal strictures	20–26% [185–188]	0–2% [174, 185, 187]
Esophageal perforation	0.5–5% [185]	<1% [174, 185]
Aspiration pneumonia	≤5% [187, 188]	<1% [187, 200]
Transient bacteremia	0–53% [176, 195]	3–6% [195]

esophageal perforation with endoscopic stenting is an option along with surgical consultation.

There is some controversy on whether EVL or EVS contributes to increased portal hypertensive gastropathy (PHG) and gastric varices (GV) as a result of increased gastric blood flow [198, 199]; however, many of these studies are limited by sample size and patient population. Therefore, there are no formal guidelines on how to treat post-EVL PHG aside from typical treatments.

Aspiration pneumonia after EVL has been reported in 1% of patients [187, 200] and is medically managed with antibiotics and respiratory support if necessary. Bacterial peritonitis has been reported in 4% of patients undergoing EVL [187, 200]. Management includes appropriate antibiotics, evaluation of ascitic fluid for spontaneous bacterial peritonitis and initiation of secondary prophylaxis with an antibiotic upon completion of treatment doses and duration. Transient bacteremia has been reported in 3–6% [195] of patients undergoing EVL, which is significantly less than with EVS.

A comparison of endoscopic variceal sclerotherapy (EVS) and endoscopic variceal ligation (EVL) complication rates is illustrated in Table 10.3.

Complications of Endoscopic Non-variceal Hemostasis

Major adverse events associated with upper endoscopy-directed non-variceal hemostasis are less than 0.5% [2, 201]. There are a series of general steps to assist in preventing complications. Intravenous metoclopramide or erythromycin administered 20–120 min before upper endoscopy decreased the need for a repeat endoscopy to determine the site and cause of bleeding by approximately 45% [201]. This reduction in the need for repeat endoscopy could hypothetically reduce the risk of exposing the patient to unnecessary procedure-related risks in the future. As with acute variceal bleeding, endotracheal intubation should be considered prior to upper endoscopy although the data are not definitive with respect to its benefits [202, 203].

Continuous infusion of a high-dose proton pump inhibitor for 72 h should be considered in patients with an acute peptic ulcer bleed as it significantly reduces rebleeding rates and mortality in patients with ulcers with high-risk stigmata (active bleeding, adherent clot, non-bleeding visible vessel) treated endoscopically [201].

Injection of 1:10,000 dilutions of epinephrine has been associated with hypertension, arrhythmias, tachycardia, of which there appears to be dose dependence based on the volume injected [204]. However, these effects are typically transient and have limited clinical significance. Rare reports of tissue necrosis, worsening of bleeding or perforation after injection with cyanoacrylate, polidocanol, ethanol, or thrombin during EGD have been documented [2]. Multipolar electrocautery or heater probe has perforation rates up to 2% [2] but can increase to up to 4% when repeated heater probe treatments are applied within 24–48 h of the initial EGD. Induction or exacerbation of bleeding occurs in up to 5% of thermal hemostasis cases [205].

Although generally of similar risk, dual therapy (epinephrine with endoscopic clipping, another injection agent or thermal probe) in patients with high-risk stigmata may have a higher risk of certain adverse events when compared to monotherapy including perforation, necrosis, and thrombosis when sclerosing agents were used with epinephrine [205, 206].

There have been no reported adverse events from the use of endoscopic clips for hemostasis in non-variceal upper GIB [205, 207].

Conclusions

The upper endoscopy procedure will undoubtedly continue to be one of the most common procedures conducted by gastroenterologists in the present and future. As there are more advances and innovations in the endoscopic technology readily available to gastroenterologists, EGDs may have their diagnostic and therapeutic roles further expanded. As these roles expand, there will be a need for hypervigilance in identifying, limiting, and treating complications that may not have been previously reported or anticipated.

References

1. Peery AF, Dellon ES, Lund J, Crockett SD, McGowan CE, Bulsiewicz WJ, et al. Burden of gastrointestinal disease in the United States: 2012 update. Gastroenterology. 2012;143 (5):1179–87 (e1–3).
2. Committee ASoP, Ben-Menachem T, Decker GA, Early DS, Evans J, Fanelli RD, et al. Adverse events of upper GI endoscopy. Gastrointest Endosc. 2012;76(4):707–18.
3. Park WG, Shaheen NJ, Cohen J, Pike IM, Adler DG, Inadomi JM, et al. Quality indicators for EGD. Am J Gastroenterol. 2015;110(1):60–71.
4. Silvis SE, Nebel O, Rogers G, Sugawa C, Mandelstam P. Endoscopic complications. Results of the 1974 American Society for gastrointestinal endoscopy survey. JAMA. 1976;235(9):928–30.
5. Wolfsen HC, Hemminger LL, Achem SR, Loeb DS, Stark ME, Bouras EP, et al. Complications of endoscopy of the upper gastrointestinal tract: a single-center experience. Mayo Clin Proc. 2004;79(10):1264–7.
6. Zubarik R, Eisen G, Mastropietro C, Lopez J, Carroll J, Benjamin S, et al. Prospective analysis of complications 30 days after outpatient upper endoscopy. Am J Gastroenterol. 1999;94 (6):1539–45.
7. Sharma VK, Nguyen CC, Crowell MD, Lieberman DA, de Garmo P, Fleischer DE. A national study of cardiopulmonary unplanned events after GI endoscopy. Gastrointest Endosc. 2007;66(1):27–34.
8. Quine MA, Bell GD, McCloy RF, Charlton JE, Devlin HB, Hopkins A. Prospective audit of upper gastrointestinal endoscopy in two regions of England: safety, staffing, and sedation methods. Gut. 1995;36(3):462–7.
9. Sieg A, Hachmoeller-Eisenbach U, Eisenbach T. Prospective evaluation of complications in outpatient GI endoscopy: a survey among German gastroenterologists. Gastrointest Endosc. 2001;53 (6):620–7.
10. Froehlich F, Gonvers JJ, Fried M. Conscious sedation, clinically relevant complications and monitoring of endoscopy: results of a nationwide survey in Switzerland. Endoscopy. 1994;26(2):231–4.
11. O'Connor HJ, Hamilton I, Lincoln C, Maxwell S, Axon AT. Bacteraemia with upper gastrointestinal endoscopy–a reappraisal. Endoscopy. 1983;15(1):21–3.
12. Shull HJ Jr, Greene BM, Allen SD, Dunn GD, Schenker S. Bacteremia with upper gastrointestinal endoscopy. Ann Intern Med. 1975;83(2):212–4.
13. Mellow MH, Lewis RJ. Endoscopy—related bacteremia. Incidence of positive blood cultures after endoscopy of upper gastrointestinal tract. Arch Intern Med. 1976;136(6):667–9.
14. Baltch AL, Buhac I, Agrawal A, O'Connor P, Bram M, Malatino E. Bacteremia after upper gastrointestinal endoscopy. Arch Intern Med. 1977;137(5):594–7.
15. Nelson DB. Infectious disease complications of GI endoscopy: Part I, endogenous infections. Gastrointest Endosc. 2003;57 (4):546–56.
16. Wilson W, Taubert KA, Gewitz M, Lockhart PB, Baddour LM, Levison M, et al. Prevention of infective endocarditis: guidelines from the American Heart Association: a guideline from the American Heart Association Rheumatic Fever, Endocarditis, and
Kawasaki Disease Committee, Council on Cardiovascular Disease in the Young, and the Council on Clinical Cardiology, Council on Cardiovascular Surgery and Anesthesia, and the Quality of Care and Outcomes Research Interdisciplinary Working Group. Circulation. 2007;116(15):1736–54.
17. Asge Standards of Practice C, Banerjee S, Shen B, Baron TH, Nelson DB, Anderson MA, et al. Antibiotic prophylaxis for GI endoscopy. Gastrointest Endosc. 2008;67(6):791–8.
18. Nelson DB. Infectious disease complications of GI endoscopy: Part II, exogenous infections. Gastrointest Endosc. 2003;57 (6):695–711.
19. Muscarella LF. Risk of transmission of carbapenem-resistant enterobacteriaceae and related "superbugs" during gastrointestinal endoscopy. World J Gastrointest Endosc. 2014;6(10):457–74.
20. ASGE Press Release: Transmission of CRE bacteria through endoscopic retrograde cholangiopancreatography (ERCP) [press release]. Feb 2015.
21. Penston JG, Boyd EJ, Wormsley KG. Mallory-Weiss tears occurring during endoscopy: a report of seven cases. Endoscopy. 1992;24(4):262–5.
22. Montalvo RD, Lee M. Retrospective analysis of iatrogenic Mallory-Weiss tears occurring during upper gastrointestinal endoscopy. Hepatogastroenterology. 1996;43(7):174–7.
23. Chu DZ, Shivshanker K, Stroehlein JR, Nelson RS. Thrombocytopenia and gastrointestinal hemorrhage in the cancer patient: prevalence of unmasked lesions. Gastrointest Endosc. 1983;29 (4):269–72.
24. Abbas G, Schuchert MJ, Pettiford BL, Pennathur A, Landreneau J, Landreneau J, et al. Contemporaneous management of esophageal perforation. Surgery. 2009;146(4):749–55 (discussion 55–6).
25. Brinster CJ, Singhal S, Lee L, Marshall MB, Kaiser LR, Kucharczuk JC. Evolving options in the management of esophageal perforation. Ann Thorac Surg. 2004;77(4):1475–83.
26. Hasimoto CN, Cataneo C, Eldib R, Thomazi R, Pereira RS, Minossi JG, et al. Efficacy of surgical versus conservative treatment in esophageal perforation: a systematic review of case series studies. Acta Cir Bras. 2013;28(4):266–71.
27. Pettersson G, Larsson S, Gatzinsky P, Sudow G. Differentiated treatment of intrathoracic oesophageal perforations. Scand J Thorac Cardiovasc Surg. 1981;15(3):321–4.
28. Larsen K, Skov Jensen B, Axelsen F. Perforation and rupture of the esophagus. Scand J Thorac Cardiovasc Surg. 1983;17 (3):311–6.
29. Panzini L, Burrell MI, Traube M. Instrumental esophageal perforation: chest film findings. Am J Gastroenterol. 1994;89 (3):367–70.
30. Bladergroen MR, Lowe JE, Postlethwait RW. Diagnosis and recommended management of esophageal perforation and rupture. Ann Thorac Surg. 1986;42(3):235–9.
31. Madanick RD. Medical management of iatrogenic esophageal perforations. Curr Treat Options Gastroenterol. 2008;11(1):54–63.
32. Altorjay A, Kiss J, Voros A, Bohak A. Nonoperative management of esophageal perforations. Is it justified? Ann Surg. 1997;225(4):415–21.
33. Siersema PD, Homs MY, Haringsma J, Tilanus HW, Kuipers EJ. Use of large-diameter metallic stents to seal traumatic nonmalignant perforations of the esophagus. Gastrointest Endosc. 2003;58(3):356–61.
34. Qadeer MA, Dumot JA, Vargo JJ, Lopez AR, Rice TW. Endoscopic clips for closing esophageal perforations: case report and pooled analysis. Gastrointest Endosc. 2007;66(3):605–11.
35. van Heel NC, Haringsma J, Spaander MC, Bruno MJ, Kuipers EJ. Short-term esophageal stenting in the management

of benign perforations. Am J Gastroenterol. 2010;105(7):1515–20.

36. Richman DC. Ambulatory surgery: how much testing do we need? Anesthesiol Clin. 2010;28(2):185–97.

37. Committee ASoP, Pasha SF, Acosta R, Chandrasekhara V, Chathadi KV, Eloubeidi MA, et al. Routine laboratory testing before endoscopic procedures. Gastrointest Endosc. 2014;80 (1):28–33.

38. Lew RJ, Kochman ML. A review of endoscopic methods of esophageal dilation. J Clin Gastroenterol. 2002;35(2):117–26.

39. Vogel SB, Rout WR, Martin TD, Abbitt PL. Esophageal perforation in adults: aggressive, conservative treatment lowers morbidity and mortality. Ann Surg. 2005;241(6):1016–21 (discussion 21–3).

40. Mandelstam P, Sugawa C, Silvis SE, Nebel OT, Rogers BH. Complications associated with esophagogastroduodenoscopy and with esophageal dilation. Gastrointest Endosc. 1976;23(1):16–9.

41. Pereira-Lima JC, Ramires RP, Zamin I Jr, Cassal AP, Marroni CA, Mattos AA. Endoscopic dilation of benign esophageal strictures: report on 1043 procedures. Am J Gastroenterol. 1999;94(6):1497–501.

42. Hernandez LV, Jacobson JW, Harris MS. Comparison among the perforation rates of Maloney, balloon, and savary dilation of esophageal strictures. Gastrointest Endosc. 2000;51(4 Pt 1):460–2.

43. Piotet E, Escher A, Monnier P. Esophageal and pharyngeal strictures: report on 1,862 endoscopic dilatations using the Savary-Gilliard technique. Eur Arch Otorhinolaryngol. 2008;265 (3):357–64.

44. Chuah SK, Hsu PI, Wu KL, Wu DC, Tai WC, Changchien CS. 2011 update on esophageal achalasia. World J Gastroenterol. 2012;18(14):1573–8.

45. Katzka DA, Castell DO. Review article: an analysis of the efficacy, perforation rates and methods used in pneumatic dilation for achalasia. Aliment Pharmacol Ther. 2011;34(8):832–9.

46. Solt J, Bajor J, Szabo M, Horvath OP. Long-term results of balloon catheter dilation for benign gastric outlet stenosis. Endoscopy. 2003;35(6):490–5.

47. Lau JY, Chung SC, Sung JJ, Chan AC, Ng EK, Suen RC, et al. Through-the-scope balloon dilation for pyloric stenosis: long-term results. Gastrointest Endosc. 1996;43(2 Pt 1):98–101.

48. Kozarek RA, Botoman VA, Patterson DJ. Long-term follow-up in patients who have undergone balloon dilation for gastric outlet obstruction. Gastrointest Endosc. 1990;36(6):558–61.

49. Rana SS, Bhasin DK, Chandail VS, Gupta R, Nada R, Kang M, et al. Endoscopic balloon dilatation without fluoroscopy for treating gastric outlet obstruction because of benign etiologies. Surg Endosc. 2011;25(5):1579–84.

50. Lam YH, Lau JY, Fung TM, Ng EK, Wong SK, Sung JJ, et al. Endoscopic balloon dilation for benign gastric outlet obstruction with or without Helicobacter pylori infection. Gastrointest Endosc. 2004;60(2):229–33.

51. Lin HH, Lee SC, Chu HC, Chang WK, Chao YC, Hsieh TY. Emergency endoscopic management of dietary foreign bodies in the esophagus. Am J Emerg Med. 2007;25(6):662–5.

52. Ginsberg GG. Management of ingested foreign objects and food bolus impactions. Gastrointest Endosc. 1995;41(1):33–8.

53. Webb WA. Management of foreign bodies of the upper gastrointestinal tract. Gastroenterology. 1988;94(1):204–16.

54. Goh BK, Chow PK, Quah HM, Ong HS, Eu KW, Ooi LL, et al. Perforation of the gastrointestinal tract secondary to ingestion of foreign bodies. World J Surg. 2006;30(3):372–7.

55. Webb WA. Management of foreign bodies of the upper gastrointestinal tract: update. Gastrointest Endosc. 1995;41 (1):39–51.

56. Mosca S, Manes G, Martino R, Amitrano L, Bottino V, Bove A, et al. Endoscopic management of foreign bodies in the upper gastrointestinal tract: report on a series of 414 adult patients. Endoscopy. 2001;33(8):692–6.

57. Schwartz GF, Polsky HS. Ingested foreign bodies of the gastrointestinal tract. Am Surg. 1976;42(4):236–8.

58. Singh B, Kantu M, Har-El G, Lucente FE. Complications associated with 327 foreign bodies of the pharynx, larynx, and esophagus. Ann Otol Rhinol Laryngol. 1997;106(4):301–4.

59. Athanassiadi K, Gerazounis M, Metaxas E, Kalantzi N. Management of esophageal foreign bodies: a retrospective review of 400 cases. Eur J Cardiothorac Surg. 2002;21(4):653–6.

60. Al-Qudah A, Daradkeh S, Abu-Khalaf M. Esophageal foreign bodies. Eur J Cardiothorac Surg. 1998;13(5):494–8.

61. Triadafilopoulos G, Roorda A, Akiyama J. Update on foreign bodies in the esophagus: diagnosis and management. Curr Gastroenterol Rep. 2013;15(4):317.

62. Schmidt SC, Strauch S, Rosch T, Veltzke-Schlieker W, Jonas S, Pratschke J, et al. Management of esophageal perforations. Surg Endosc. 2010;24(11):2809–13.

63. Gauderer MW, Ponsky JL, Izant RJ Jr. Gastrostomy without laparotomy: a percutaneous endoscopic technique. J Pediatr Surg. 1980;15(6):872–5.

64. Rahnemai-Azar AA, Rahnemaiazar AA, Naghshizadian R, Kurtz A, Farkas DT. Percutaneous endoscopic gastrostomy: indications, technique, complications and management. World J Gastroenterol. 2014;20(24):7739–51.

65. McClave SA, Chang WK. Complications of enteral access. Gastrointest Endosc. 2003;58(5):739–51.

66. Wollman B, D'Agostino HB, Walus-Wigle JR, Easter DW, Beale A. Radiologic, endoscopic, and surgical gastrostomy: an institutional evaluation and meta-analysis of the literature. Radiology. 1995;197(3):699–704.

67. Hogan RB, DeMarco DC, Hamilton JK, Walker CO, Polter DE. Percutaneous endoscopic gastrostomy–to push or pull. A prospective randomized trial. Gastrointest Endosc. 1986;32(4):253–8.

68. Kozarek RA, Ball TJ, Ryan JA Jr. When push comes to shove: a comparison between two methods of percutaneous endoscopic gastrostomy. Am J Gastroenterol. 1986;81(8):642–6.

69. Brown MC. Cancer metastasis at percutaneous endoscopic gastrostomy stomata is related to the hematogenous or lymphatic spread of circulating tumor cells. Am J Gastroenterol. 2000;95 (11):3288–91.

70. Jafri NS, Mahid SS, Minor KS, Idstein SR, Hornung CA, Galandiuk S. Meta-analysis: antibiotic prophylaxis to prevent peristomal infection following percutaneous endoscopic gastrostomy. Aliment Pharmacol Ther. 2007;25(6):647–56.

71. Committee ASoP, Khashab MA, Chithadi KV, Acosta RD, Bruining DH, Chandrasekhara V, et al. Antibiotic prophylaxis for GI endoscopy. Gastrointest Endosc. 2015;81(1):81–9.

72. Jain NK, Larson DE, Schroeder KW, Burton DD, Cannon KP, Thompson RL, et al. Antibiotic prophylaxis for percutaneous endoscopic gastrostomy. A prospective, randomized, double-blind clinical trial. Ann Intern Med. 1987;107(6):824–8.

73. Sturgis TM, Yancy W, Cole JC, Proctor DD, Minhas BS, Marcuard SP. Antibiotic prophylaxis in percutaneous endoscopic gastrostomy. Am J Gastroenterol. 1996;91(11):2301–4.

74. Thomas S, Cantrill S, Waghorn DJ, McIntyre A. The role of screening and antibiotic prophylaxis in the prevention of percutaneous gastrostomy site infection caused by methicillin-resistant Staphylococcus aureus. Aliment Pharmacol Ther. 2007;25(5):593–7.

75. Horiuchi A, Nakayama Y, Kajiyama M, Fujii H, Tanaka N. Nasopharyngeal decolonization of methicillin-resistant

Staphylococcus aureus can reduce PEG peristomal wound infection. Am J Gastroenterol. 2006;101(2):274–7.

76. Evans DA, Bhandarkar DS, Taylor TV. Necrotising fasciitis—a rare complication of percutaneous endoscopic gastrostomy. Endoscopy. 1995;27(8):627.

77. Haas DW, Dharmaraja P, Morrison JG, Potts JR 3rd. Necrotizing fasciitis following percutaneous endoscopic gastrostomy. Gastrointest Endosc. 1988;34(6):487–8.

78. Chung RS, Schertzer M. Pathogenesis of complications of percutaneous endoscopic gastrostomy. A lesson in surgical principles. Am Surg. 1990;56(3):134–7.

79. Cave DR, Robinson WR, Brotschi EA. Necrotizing fasciitis following percutaneous endoscopic gastrostomy. Gastrointest Endosc. 1986;32(4):294–6.

80. Rino Y, Tokunaga M, Morinaga S, Onodera S, Tomiyama I, Imada T, et al. The buried bumper syndrome: an early complication of percutaneous endoscopic gastrostomy. Hepato-gastroenterology. 2002;49(46):1183–4.

81. Sheers R, Chapman S. The buried bumper syndrome: a complication of percutaneous endoscopic gastrostomy. Gut. 1998;43(4):586.

82. Klein S, Heare BR, Soloway RD. The "buried bumper syndrome": a complication of percutaneous endoscopic gastrostomy. Am J Gastroenterol. 1990;85(4):448–51.

83. Anagnostopoulos GK, Kostopoulos P, Arvanitidis DM. Buried bumper syndrome with a fatal outcome, presenting early as gastrointestinal bleeding after percutaneous endoscopic gastrostomy placement. J Postgrad Med. 2003;49(4):325–7.

84. Larson DE, Burton DD, Schroeder KW, DiMagno EP. Percutaneous endoscopic gastrostomy. Indications, success, complications, and mortality in 314 consecutive patients. Gastroenterology. 1987;93(1):48–52.

85. Grant JP. Percutaneous endoscopic gastrostomy. Initial placement by single endoscopic technique and long-term follow-up. Ann Surg. 1993;217(2):168–74.

86. Safadi BY, Marks JM, Ponsky JL. Percutaneous endoscopic gastrostomy. Gastrointest Endosc Clin N Am. 1998;8(3):551–68.

87. Committee ASoP, Anderson MA, Ben-Menachem T, Gan SI, Appalaneni V, Banerjee S, et al. Management of antithrombotic agents for endoscopic procedures. Gastrointest Endosc. 2009;70 (6):1060–70.

88. Ahmad J, Thomson S, McFall B, Scoffield J, Taylor M. Colonic injury following percutaneous endoscopic-guided gastrostomy insertion. BMJ Case Rep. 2010;2010.

89. Guloglu R, Taviloglu K, Alimoglu O. Colon injury following percutaneous endoscopic gastrostomy tube insertion. J Laparoendosc Adv Surg Tech A. 2003;13(1):69–72.

90. Blum CA, Selander C, Ruddy JM, Leon S. The incidence and clinical significance of pneumoperitoneum after percutaneous endoscopic gastrostomy: a review of 722 cases. Am Surg. 2009;75(1):39–43.

91. Gottfried EB, Plumser AB, Clair MR. Pneumoperitoneum following percutaneous endoscopic gastrostomy. A prospective study. Gastrointest Endosc. 1986;32(6):397–9.

92. Foutch PG, Talbert GA, Waring JP, Sanowski RA. Percutaneous endoscopic gastrostomy in patients with prior abdominal surgery: virtues of the safe tract. Am J Gastroenterol. 1988;83(2):147–50.

93. Heuss LT, Froehlich F, Beglinger C. Changing patterns of sedation and monitoring practice during endoscopy: results of a nationwide survey in Switzerland. Endoscopy. 2005;37(2):161–6.

94. Fujiwara Y, Arakawa T, Fukuda T, Kimura S, Uchida T, Obata A, et al. Diagnosis of borderline adenomas of the stomach by endoscopic mucosal resection. Endoscopy. 1996;28(5):425–30.

95. Muehldorfer SM, Stolte M, Martus P, Hahn EG, Ell C, Multicenter Study Group Gastric P. Diagnostic accuracy of forceps biopsy versus polypectomy for gastric polyps: a prospective multicentre study. Gut. 2002;50(4):465–70.

96. Lanza FL, Graham DY, Nelson RS, Godines R, McKechnie JC. Endoscopic upper gastrointestinal polypectomy. Report of 73 polypectomies in 63 patients. Am J Gastroenterol. 1981;75 (5):345–8.

97. Hsieh YH, Lin HJ, Tseng GY, Perng CL, Li AF, Chang FY, et al. Is submucosal epinephrine injection necessary before polypectomy? A prospective, comparative study. Hepatogastroenterology. 2001;48(41):1379–82.

98. Muhldorfer SM, Kekos G, Hahn EG, Ell C. Complications of therapeutic gastrointestinal endoscopy. Endoscopy. 1992;24 (4):276–83.

99. Bardan E, Maor Y, Carter D, Lang A, Bar-Meir S, Avidan B. Endoscopic ultrasound (EUS) before gastric polyp resection: is it mandatory? J Clin Gastroenterol. 2007;41(4):371–4.

100. Committee AT, Hwang JH, Konda V, Abu Dayyeh BK, Chauhan SS, Enestvedt BK, et al. Endoscopic mucosal resection. Gastrointest Endosc. 2015;82(2):215–26.

101. Tomizawa Y, Iyer PG, Wong Kee Song LM, Buttar NS, Lutzke LS, Wang KK. Safety of endoscopic mucosal resection for Barrett's esophagus. Am J Gastroenterol. 2013;108(9):1440–7 (quiz 8).

102. Oka S, Tanaka S, Kaneko I, Mouri R, Hirata M, Kawamura T, et al. Advantage of endoscopic submucosal dissection compared with EMR for early gastric cancer. Gastrointest Endosc. 2006;64 (6):877–83.

103. Catalano F, Trecca A, Rodella L, Lombardo F, Tomezzoli A, Battista S, et al. The modern treatment of early gastric cancer: our experience in an Italian cohort. Surg Endosc. 2009;23(7):1581–6.

104. Nakamoto S, Sakai Y, Kasanuki J, Kondo F, Ooka Y, Kato K, et al. Indications for the use of endoscopic mucosal resection for early gastric cancer in Japan: a comparative study with endoscopic submucosal dissection. Endoscopy. 2009;41(9):746–50.

105. Okano A, Hajiro K, Takakuwa H, Nishio A, Matsushita M. Predictors of bleeding after endoscopic mucosal resection of gastric tumors. Gastrointest Endosc. 2003;57(6):687–90.

106. Konda VJ, Gonzalez Haba Ruiz M, Koons A, Hart J, Xiao SY, Siddiqui UD, et al. Complete endoscopic mucosal resection is effective and durable treatment for Barrett's-associated neoplasia. Clin Gastroenterol Hepatol. 2014;12(12):2002–10 (e1–2).

107. van Vilsteren FG, Pouw RE, Seewald S, Alvarez Herrero L, Sondermeijer CM, Visser M, et al. Stepwise radical endoscopic resection versus radiofrequency ablation for Barrett's oesophagus with high-grade dysplasia or early cancer: a multicentre randomised trial. Gut. 2011;60(6):765–73.

108. Park YM, Cho E, Kang HY, Kim JM. The effectiveness and safety of endoscopic submucosal dissection compared with endoscopic mucosal resection for early gastric cancer: a systematic review and metaanalysis. Surg Endosc. 2011;25(8):2666–77.

109. Fanning SB, Bourke MJ, Williams SJ, Chung A, Kariyawasam VC. Giant laterally spreading tumors of the duodenum: endoscopic resection outcomes, limitations, and caveats. Gastrointest Endosc. 2012;75(4):805–12.

110. Larghi A, Lightdale CJ, Memeo L, Bhagat G, Okpara N, Rotterdam H. EUS followed by EMR for staging of high-grade dysplasia and early cancer in Barrett's esophagus. Gastrointest Endosc. 2005;62(1):16–23.

111. Fujishiro M, Yahagi N, Kakushima N, Kodashima S, Muraki Y, Ono S, et al. Endoscopic submucosal dissection of esophageal squamous cell neoplasms. Clin Gastroenterol Hepatol. 2006;4 (6):688–94.

112. Peters FP, Kara MA, Rosmolen WD, ten Kate FJ, Krishnadath KK, van Lanschot JJ, et al. Stepwise radical endoscopic resection is effective for complete removal of Barrett's esophagus with early neoplasia: a prospective study. Am J Gastroenterol. 2006;101(7):1449–57.

113. Qumseya B, Panossian AM, Rizk C, Cangemi D, Wolfsen C, Raimondo M, et al. Predictors of esophageal stricture formation post endoscopic mucosal resection. Clin Endosc. 2014;47 (2):155–61.

114. Yoshida N, Naito Y, Kugai M, Inoue K, Wakabayashi N, Yagi N, et al. Efficient hemostatic method for endoscopic submucosal dissection of colorectal tumors. World J Gastroenterol. 2010;16 (33):4180–6.

115. Chung IK, Lee JH, Lee SH, Kim SJ, Cho JY, Cho WY, et al. Therapeutic outcomes in 1000 cases of endoscopic submucosal dissection for early gastric neoplasms: Korean ESD Study Group multicenter study. Gastrointest Endosc. 2009;69(7):1228–35.

116. Koh R, Hirasawa K, Yahara S, Oka H, Sugimori K, Morimoto M, et al. Antithrombotic drugs are risk factors for delayed postoperative bleeding after endoscopic submucosal dissection for gastric neoplasms. Gastrointest Endosc. 2013;78(3):476–83.

117. Yang Z, Wu Q, Liu Z, Wu K, Fan D. Proton pump inhibitors versus histamine-2-receptor antagonists for the management of iatrogenic gastric ulcer after endoscopic mucosal resection or endoscopic submucosal dissection: a meta-analysis of randomized trials. Digestion. 2011;84(4):315–20.

118. Lian J, Chen S, Zhang Y, Qiu F. A meta-analysis of endoscopic submucosal dissection and EMR for early gastric cancer. Gastrointest Endosc. 2012;76(4):763–70.

119. Jung JH, Choi KD, Ahn JY, Lee JH, Jung HY, Choi KS, et al. Endoscopic submucosal dissection for sessile, nonampullary duodenal adenomas. Endoscopy. 2013;45(2):133–5.

120. Guo HM, Zhang XQ, Chen M, Huang SL, Zou XP. Endoscopic submucosal dissection vs endoscopic mucosal resection for superficial esophageal cancer. World J Gastroenterol. 2014;20 (18):5540–7.

121. Nakajima T, Saito Y, Tanaka S, Iishi H, Kudo SE, Ikematsu H, et al. Current status of endoscopic resection strategy for large, early colorectal neoplasia in Japan. Surg Endosc. 2013;27 (9):3262–70.

122. Takahashi H, Arimura Y, Masao H, Okahara S, Tanuma T, Kodaira J, et al. Endoscopic submucosal dissection is superior to conventional endoscopic resection as a curative treatment for early squamous cell carcinoma of the esophagus (with video). Gastrointest Endosc. 2010;72(2):255–64 (e1–2).

123. Mizuta H, Nishimori I, Kuratani Y, Higashidani Y, Kohsaki T, Onishi S. Predictive factors for esophageal stenosis after endoscopic submucosal dissection for superficial esophageal cancer. Dis Esophagus. 2009;22(7):626–31.

124. Ono S, Fujishiro M, Niimi K, Goto O, Kodashima S, Yamamichi N, et al. Predictors of postoperative stricture after esophageal endoscopic submucosal dissection for superficial squamous cell neoplasms. Endoscopy. 2009;41(8):661–5.

125. Kim JS, Kim BW, Shin IS. Efficacy and safety of endoscopic submucosal dissection for superficial squamous esophageal neoplasia: a meta-analysis. Dig Dis Sci. 2014;59(8):1862–9.

126. Isomoto H, Yamaguchi N, Minami H, Nakao K. Management of complications associated with endoscopic submucosal dissection/endoscopic mucosal resection for esophageal cancer. Dig Endosc. 2013;25(Suppl 1):29–38.

127. Mori H, Rafiq K, Kobara H, Fujihara S, Nishiyama N, Oryuu M, et al. Steroid permeation into the artificial ulcer by combined steroid gel application and balloon dilatation: prevention of esophageal stricture. J Gastroenterol Hepatol. 2013;28(6):999–1003.

128. Wen J, Lu Z, Yang Y, Liu Q, Yang J, Wang S, et al. Preventing stricture formation by covered esophageal stent placement after endoscopic submucosal dissection for early esophageal cancer. Dig Dis Sci. 2014;59(3):658–63.

129. Dulai GS, Jensen DM, Cortina G, Fontana L, Ippoliti A. Randomized trial of argon plasma coagulation vs. multipolar electrocoagulation for ablation of Barrett's esophagus. Gastrointest Endosc. 2005;61(2):232–40.

130. Luman W, Lessels AM, Palmer KR. Failure of Nd–YAG photocoagulation therapy as treatment for Barrett's oesophagus —a pilot study. Eur J Gastroenterol Hepatol. 1996;8(7):627–30.

131. Michopoulos S, Tsibouris P, Bouzakis H, Sotiropoulou M, Kralios N. Complete regression of Barrett's esophagus with heat probe thermocoagulation: mid-term results. Gastrointest Endosc. 1999;50(2):165–72.

132. Sampliner RE, Faigel D, Fennerty MB, Lieberman D, Ippoliti A, Lewin K, et al. Effective and safe endoscopic reversal of nondysplastic Barrett's esophagus with thermal electrocoagulation combined with high-dose acid inhibition: a multicenter study. Gastrointest Endosc. 2001;53(6):554–8.

133. Prost B, Poncet G, Scoazec JY, Saurin JC. Unusual complications of argon plasma coagulation. Gastrointest Endosc. 2004;59 (7):929–32.

134. Roman S, Saurin JC, Dumortier J, Perreira A, Bernard G, Ponchon T. Tolerance and efficacy of argon plasma coagulation for controlling bleeding in patients with typical and atypical manifestations of watermelon stomach. Endoscopy. 2003;35 (12):1024–8.

135. Herrera S, Bordas JM, Llach J, Gines A, Pellise M, Fernandez-Esparrach G, et al. The beneficial effects of argon plasma coagulation in the management of different types of gastric vascular ectasia lesions in patients admitted for GI hemorrhage. Gastrointest Endosc. 2008;68(3):440–6.

136. Overholt BF, Wang KK, Burdick JS, Lightdale CJ, Kimmey M, Nava HR, et al. Five-year efficacy and safety of photodynamic therapy with Photofrin in Barrett's high-grade dysplasia. Gastrointest Endosc. 2007;66(3):460–8.

137. Petersen BT, Chuttani R, Croffie J, DiSario J, Liu J, Mishkin D, et al. Photodynamic therapy for gastrointestinal disease. Gastrointest Endosc. 2006;63(7):927–32.

138. Dunkin BJ, Martinez J, Bejarano PA, Smith CD, Chang K, Livingstone AS, et al. Thin-layer ablation of human esophageal epithelium using a bipolar radiofrequency balloon device. Surg Endosc. 2006;20(1):125–30.

139. Smith CD, Bejarano PA, Melvin WS, Patti MG, Muthusamy R, Dunkin BJ. Endoscopic ablation of intestinal metaplasia containing high-grade dysplasia in esophagectomy patients using a balloon-based ablation system. Surg Endosc. 2007;21(4):560–9.

140. Shaheen NJ, Sharma P, Overholt BF, Wolfsen HC, Sampliner RE, Wang KK, et al. Radiofrequency ablation in Barrett's esophagus with dysplasia. N Engl J Med. 2009;360(22):2277–88.

141. Pouw RE, Gondrie JJ, Van Vilsteren FG, Sondermeijer C, Rosmolen W, Curvers WL, et al. Complications following circumferential radiofrequency energy ablation of Barrett's esophagus containing early neoplasia. Gastrointestinal Endoscopy. 67(5):AB145.

142. Lyday WD, Corbett FS, Kuperman DA, Kalvaria I, Mavrelis PG, Shughoury AB, et al. Radiofrequency ablation of Barrett's esophagus: outcomes of 429 patients from a multicenter community practice registry. Endoscopy. 2010;42(4):272–8.

143. Vahbzadeh B, Rastogi A, Bansal A, Sharma P. Use of a plastic endoprosthesis to successfully treat esophageal perforation following radiofrequency ablation of Barrett's esophagus. Endoscopy. 2011;43(1):67–9.

144. Greenwald BD, Dumot JA, Abrams JA, Lightdale CJ, David DS, Nishioka NS, et al. Endoscopic spray cryotherapy for esophageal cancer: safety and efficacy. Gastrointest Endosc. 2010;71(4):686–93.

145. Greenwald BD, Dumot JA, Horwhat JD, Lightdale CJ, Abrams JA. Safety, tolerability, and efficacy of endoscopic low-pressure liquid nitrogen spray cryotherapy in the esophagus. Dis Esophagus. 2010;23(1):13–9.

146. Repici A, Hassan C, Sharma P, Conio M, Siersema P. Systematic review: the role of self-expanding plastic stents for benign oesophageal strictures. Aliment Pharmacol Ther. 2010;31(12):1268–75.

147. Bakken JC, Wong Kee Song LM, de Groen PC, Baron TH. Use of a fully covered self-expandable metal stent for the treatment of benign esophageal diseases. Gastrointest Endosc. 2010;72(4):712–20.

148. van Boeckel PG, Dua KS, Weusten BL, Schmits RJ, Surapaneni N, Timmer R, et al. Fully covered self-expandable metal stents (SEMS), partially covered SEMS and self-expandable plastic stents for the treatment of benign esophageal ruptures and anastomotic leaks. BMC Gastroenterol. 2012;12:19.

149. Dua KS, Latif SU, Yang JF, Fang TC, Khan A, Oh Y. Efficacy and safety of a new fully covered self-expandable non-foreshortening metal esophageal stent. Gastrointest Endosc. 2014;80(4):577–85.

150. Kozarek R, Baron T, Song HY. Self-expandable stents in the gastrointestinal tract. New York: Springer; 2012.

151. Knyrim K, Wagner HJ, Bethge N, Keymling M, Vakil N. A controlled trial of an expansile metal stent for palliation of esophageal obstruction due to inoperable cancer. N Engl J Med. 1993;329(18):1302–7.

152. Sandha GS, Marcon NE. Expandable metal stents for benign esophageal obstruction. Gastrointest Endosc Clin N Am. 1999;9(3):437–46.

153. Ackroyd R, Watson DI, Devitt PG, Jamieson GG. Expandable metallic stents should not be used in the treatment of benign esophageal strictures. J Gastroenterol Hepatol. 2001;16(4):484–7.

154. Hirdes MM, Vleggaar FP, Van der Linde K, Willems M, Totte ER, Siersema PD. Esophageal perforation due to removal of partially covered self-expanding metal stents placed for a benign perforation or leak. Endoscopy. 2011;43(2):156–9.

155. Hramiec JE, O'Shea MA, Quinlan RM. Expandable metallic esophageal stents in benign disease: a cause for concern. Surg Laparosc Endosc. 1998;8(1):40–3.

156. Shenfine J, McNamee P, Steen N, Bond J, Griffin SM. A randomized controlled clinical trial of palliative therapies for patients with inoperable esophageal cancer. Am J Gastroenterol. 2009;104(7):1674–85.

157. Jacobson BC, Hirota W, Baron TH, Leighton JA, Faigel DO. Standards of practice committee. American Society for gastrointestinal E. The role of endoscopy in the assessment and treatment of esophageal cancer. Gastrointest Endosc. 2003;57(7):817–22.

158. Kozarek RA, Ball TJ, Patterson DJ. Metallic self-expanding stent application in the upper gastrointestinal tract: caveats and concerns. Gastrointest Endosc. 1992;38(1):1–6.

159. Tierney W, Chuttani R, Croffie J, DiSario J, Liu J, Mishkin DS, et al. Enteral stents. Gastrointest Endosc. 2006;63(7):920–6.

160. Wenger U, Luo J, Lundell L, Lagergren J. A nationwide study of the use of self-expanding stents in patients with esophageal cancer in Sweden. Endoscopy. 2005;37(4):329–34.

161. Siersema PD, Tan TG, Sutorius FF, Dees J, van Blankenstein M. Massive hemorrhage caused by a perforating Gianturco-Z stent resulting in an aortoesophageal fistula. Endoscopy. 1997;29(5):416–20.

162. Homs MY, Wahab PJ, Kuipers EJ, Steyerberg EW, Grool TA, Haringsma J, et al. Esophageal stents with antireflux valve for tumors of the distal esophagus and gastric cardia: a randomized trial. Gastrointest Endosc. 2004;60(5):695–702.

163. Gaidos JK, Draganov PV. Treatment of malignant gastric outlet obstruction with endoscopically placed self-expandable metal stents. World J Gastroenterol. 2009;15(35):4365–71.

164. Tringali A, Didden P, Repici A, Spaander M, Bourke MJ, Williams SJ, et al. Endoscopic treatment of malignant gastric and duodenal strictures: a prospective, multicenter study. Gastrointest Endosc. 2014;79(1):66–75.

165. Maetani I, Ukita T, Tada T, Shigoka H, Omuta S, Endo T. Metallic stents for gastric outlet obstruction: reintervention rate is lower with uncovered versus covered stents, despite similar outcomes. Gastrointest Endosc. 2009;69(4):806–12.

166. Piesman M, Kozarek RA, Brandabur JJ, Pleskow DK, Chuttani R, Eysselein VE, et al. Improved oral intake after palliative duodenal stenting for malignant obstruction: a prospective multicenter clinical trial. Am J Gastroenterol. 2009;104(10):2404–11.

167. Baron TH. Minimizing endoscopic complications: endoluminal stents. Gastrointest Endosc Clin N Am. 2007;17(1):83–104 (vii).

168. El-Tawil AM. Trends on gastrointestinal bleeding and mortality: where are we standing? World J Gastroenterol. 2012;18(11):1154–8.

169. Hwang JH, Shergill AK, Acosta RD, Chandrasekhara V, Chathadi KV, Decker GA, et al. The role of endoscopy in the management of variceal hemorrhage. Gastrointest Endosc. 2014;80(2):221–7.

170. Garcia-Tsao G, Sanyal AJ, Grace ND, Carey W. Practice guidelines committee of the American Association for the study of liver D, practice parameters committee of the American College of G. Prevention and management of gastroesophageal varices and variceal hemorrhage in cirrhosis. Hepatology. 2007;46(3):922–38.

171. Chavez-Tapia NC, Barrientos-Gutierrez T, Tellez-Avila F, Soares-Weiser K, Mendez-Sanchez N, Gluud C, et al. Meta-analysis: antibiotic prophylaxis for cirrhotic patients with upper gastrointestinal bleeding—an updated Cochrane review. Aliment Pharmacol Ther. 2011;34(5):509–18.

172. Soares-Weiser K, Brezis M, Tur-Kaspa R, Leibovici L. Antibiotic prophylaxis for cirrhotic patients with gastrointestinal bleeding. Cochrane Database Syst Rev. 2002(2):CD002907.

173. Koch DG, Arguedas MR, Fallon MB. Risk of aspiration pneumonia in suspected variceal hemorrhage: the value of prophylactic endotracheal intubation prior to endoscopy. Dig Dis Sci. 2007;52(9):2225–8.

174. Laine L, Cook D. Endoscopic ligation compared with sclerotherapy for treatment of esophageal variceal bleeding. A meta-analysis. Ann Intern Med. 1995;123(4):280–7.

175. Schuman BM, Beckman JW, Tedesco FJ, Griffin JW Jr, Assad RT. Complications of endoscopic injection sclerotherapy: a review. Am J Gastroenterol. 1987;82(9):823–30.

176. Poza Cordon J, Froilan Torres C, Burgos Garcia A, Gea Rodriguez F, Suarez de Parga JM. Endoscopic management of esophageal varices. World J Gastrointest Endosc. 2012;4(7):312–22.

177. Young MF, Sanowski RA, Rasche R. Comparison and characterization of ulcerations induced by endoscopic ligation of esophageal varices versus endoscopic sclerotherapy. Gastrointest Endosc. 1993;39(2):119–22.

178. Sarin SK, Sachdev G, Nanda R, Batra SK, Anand BS. Comparison of the two time schedules for endoscopic sclerotherapy: a prospective randomised controlled study. Gut. 1986;27(6):710–3.

179. Westaby D, Melia WM, Macdougall BR, Hegarty JE, Williams R. Injection sclerotherapy for oesophageal varices: a prospective

randomised trial of different treatment schedules. Gut. 1984;25 (2):129–32.

180. Shephard H, Barkin JS. Omeprazole heals mucosal ulcers associated with endoscopic injection sclerotherapy. Gastrointest Endosc. 1993;39(3):474–5.

181. Dai C, Liu WX, Jiang M, Sun MJ. Endoscopic variceal ligation compared with endoscopic injection sclerotherapy for treatment of esophageal variceal hemorrhage: a meta-analysis. World J Gastroenterol. 2015;21(8):2534–41.

182. Avgerinos A, Armonis A, Stefanidis G, Mathou N, Vlachogiannakos J, Kougioumtzian A, et al. Sustained rise of portal pressure after sclerotherapy, but not band ligation, in acute variceal bleeding in cirrhosis. Hepatology. 2004;39(6):1623–30.

183. Piai G, Cipolletta L, Claar M, Marone G, Bianco MA, Forte G, et al. Prophylactic sclerotherapy of high-risk esophageal varices: results of a multicentric prospective controlled trial. Hepatology. 1988;8(6):1495–500.

184. Yuki M, Kazumori H, Yamamoto S, Shizuku T, Kinoshita Y. Prognosis following endoscopic injection sclerotherapy for esophageal varices in adults: 20-year follow-up study. Scand J Gastroenterol. 2008;43(10):1269–74.

185. Schmitz RJ, Sharma P, Badr AS, Qamar MT, Weston AP. Incidence and management of esophageal stricture formation, ulcer bleeding, perforation, and massive hematoma formation from sclerotherapy versus band ligation. Am J Gastroenterol. 2001;96 (2):437–41.

186. Koch H, Henning H, Grimm H, Soehendra N. Prophylactic sclerosing of esophageal varices–results of a prospective controlled study. Endoscopy. 1986;18(2):40–3.

187. Stiegmann GV, Goff JS, Michaletz-Onody PA, Korula J, Lieberman D, Saeed ZA, et al. Endoscopic sclerotherapy as compared with endoscopic ligation for bleeding esophageal varices. N Engl J Med. 1992;326(23):1527–32.

188. Sorensen T, Burcharth F, Pedersen ML, Findahl F. Oesophageal stricture and dysphagia after endoscopic sclerotherapy for bleeding varices. Gut. 1984;25(5):473–7.

189. Deboever G, Elegeert I, Defloor E. Portal and mesenteric venous thrombosis after endoscopic injection sclerotherapy. Am J Gastroenterol. 1989;84(10):1336–7.

190. Stoltenberg PH, Goodale RL, Silvis SE. Portal vein thrombosis following combined endoscopic variceal sclerosis and vasopressin therapy for bleeding varices. Am J Gastroenterol. 1987;82 (12):1297–300.

191. Terada T, Nakanuma Y, Yonejima M, Yokoyama H, Koike N. Portal, mesenteric, and splenic venous thrombosis after endoscopic injection sclerotherapy. J Clin Gastroenterol. 1990;12 (2):238–9.

192. Ibrarullah M, Wagholikar G, Srinivas M, Mishra A, Reddy DG, Prasadbabu TL. Acute mesenteric venous thrombosis complicating endoscopic variceal sclerotherapy with absolute alcohol. Indian J Gastroenterol. 2003;22(1):27–9.

193. Alexander S, Korman MG, Sievert W. Cyanoacrylate in the treatment of gastric varices complicated by multiple pulmonary emboli. Intern Med J. 2006;36(7):462–5.

194. Neumann H, Scheidbach H, Monkemuller K, Pech M, Malfertheiner P. Multiple cyanoacrylate (histoacryl) emboli after injection therapy of cardia varices. Gastrointest Endosc. 2009;70(5):1025–6 (discussion 6).

195. Jia Y, Dwivedi A, Elhanafi S, Ortiz A, Othman M, Zuckerman M. Low risk of bacteremia after endoscopic variceal therapy for esophageal varices: a systematic review and meta-analysis. Endosc Int Open. 2015;3(5):E409–17.

196. Shaheen NJ, Stuart E, Schmitz SM, Mitchell KL, Fried MW, Zacks S, et al. Pantoprazole reduces the size of postbanding ulcers after variceal band ligation: a randomized, controlled trial. Hepatology. 2005;41(3):588–94.

197. Vanbiervliet G, Giudicelli-Bornard S, Piche T, Berthier F, Gelsi E, Filippi J, et al. Predictive factors of bleeding related to post-banding ulcer following endoscopic variceal ligation in cirrhotic patients: a case-control study. Aliment Pharmacol Ther. 2010;32(2):225–32.

198. Tayama C, Iwao T, Oho K, Toyonaga A, Tanikawa K. Effect of large fundal varices on changes in gastric mucosal hemodynamics after endoscopic variceal ligation. Endoscopy. 1998;30(1):25–31.

199. de la Pena J, Rivero M, Sanchez E, Fabrega E, Crespo J, Pons-Romero F. Variceal ligation compared with endoscopic sclerotherapy for variceal hemorrhage: prospective randomized trial. Gastrointest Endosc. 1999;49(4 Pt 1):417–23.

200. Laine L, el-Newihi HM, Migikovsky B, Sloane R, Garcia F. Endoscopic ligation compared with sclerotherapy for the treatment of bleeding esophageal varices. Ann Intern Med. 1993;119 (1):1–7.

201. Hwang JH, Fisher DA, Ben-Menachem T, Chandrasekhara V, Chathadi K, Decker GA, et al. The role of endoscopy in the management of acute non-variceal upper GI bleeding. Gastrointest Endosc. 2012;75(6):1132–8.

202. Rehman A, Iscimen R, Yilmaz M, Khan H, Belsher J, Gomez JF, et al. Prophylactic endotracheal intubation in critically ill patients undergoing endoscopy for upper GI hemorrhage. Gastrointest Endosc. 2009;69(7):e55–9.

203. Lohse N, Lundstrom LH, Vestergaard TR, Risom M, Rosenstock SJ, Foss NB, et al. Anaesthesia care with and without tracheal intubation during emergency endoscopy for peptic ulcer bleeding: a population-based cohort study. Br J Anaesth. 2015;114(6):901–8.

204. Liou TC, Lin SC, Wang HY, Chang WH. Optimal injection volume of epinephrine for endoscopic treatment of peptic ulcer bleeding. World J Gastroenterol. 2006;12(19):3108–13.

205. Laine L, McQuaid KR. Endoscopic therapy for bleeding ulcers: an evidence-based approach based on meta-analyses of randomized controlled trials. Clin Gastroenterol Hepatol. 2009;7(1):33–47 (quiz 1–2).

206. Marmo R, Rotondano G, Piscopo R, Bianco MA, D'Angella R, Cipolletta L. Dual therapy versus monotherapy in the endoscopic treatment of high-risk bleeding ulcers: a meta-analysis of controlled trials. Am J Gastroenterol. 2007;102(2):279–89 (quiz 469).

207. Sung JJ, Tsoi KK, Lai LH, Wu JC, Lau JY. Endoscopic clipping versus injection and thermo-coagulation in the treatment of non-variceal upper gastrointestinal bleeding: a meta-analysis. Gut. 2007;56(10):1364–73.

Pediatric EGD

11

Keisha R. Mitchell and Douglas S. Fishman

Introduction/History

Pediatric endoscopy has been an exciting and dynamic procedural field since its inception in the 1970s. With advancement in techniques, equipment and sedation, it has become a common, safe and effective procedure for the diagnosis and therapy treatment of common pediatric gastrointestinal and hepatobiliary disorders. This chapter will focus on upper endoscopy in pediatric patients. Although the procedure is very similar to that of adult endoscopy, there are specific pediatric considerations needed to ensure success. These include but are not limited to: the size of the patient, variety of equipment, differences in upper gastrointestinal tract anatomy, procedural preparation and sedation needs. In addition, there are specific disease states that are more likely to present in the pediatric age range when compared to adults, and appreciating the indications for the procedure is essential.

Basil Hirschowitz pioneered the fiberoptic endoscope in 1957, and with subsequent advances, it has been widely used for medical diagnostics in the adult population [1]. It was not until nearly two decades after its introduction when the first reports were published about the use of the endoscope in the pediatric population [2–6]. Prior to the 1970s, diagnostic studies for children mainly involved contrast radiologic studies. Video endoscopes have now become the mainstay of pediatric gastrointestinal endoscopy worldwide.

Electronic supplementary material
Supplementary material is available in the online version of this chapter at 10.1007/978-3-319-49041-0_11. Videos can also be accessed at https://link.springer.com/chapter/10.1007/978-3-319-49041-0_11.

K.R. Mitchell · D.S. Fishman (✉)
Section of Gastroenterology, Hepatology and Nutrition, Texas Children's Hospital, Baylor College of Medicine, 6701 Fannin Street Suite 1010, Houston, TX 77030, USA
e-mail: dougfishman@gmail.com

K.R. Mitchell
e-mail: krmitch20@gmail.com

The numerous advancements in equipment, technology and pediatric-specific endoscopy suites have made this procedure both safe and reliable in the diagnosis, management and therapeutic treatment of pediatric upper gastrointestinal diseases. This chapter will discuss pediatric-specific entities regarding this procedure.

Equipment

Anatomic and Developmental Differences

The neonatal esophagus ranges from 8 to 10 cm in length and 5 mm in diameter [7]. The range in length of the older pediatric esophagus continues to be variable prompting research studies to develop mathematical equations to predict [8]. In addition to esophageal length, the anatomic connections differ than that in adults. There are sharper angulations in the pediatric antrum making it more difficulty to view the pylorus than in an adult patient. This requires more deflection with the gastroscope to place it into view, and retroflexion to visualize the cardia can be challenging [9]. Similarly, the small intestine of newborns is much narrowed (10–15 mm) compared to adults. The turns of the proximal duodenum are also more acute in a smaller circumferential area making certain therapies more difficult (e.g., bleeding control for duodenal ulcers).

Equipment Types

In general, there is a universal "standard adult"-sized gastroscope (forward-viewing endoscope) that can be used for most adults. [It should be noted there are different categories of endoscopes, but for the purpose of this discussion, we will only be discussing the gastroscope]. The insertion tube lengths range from 925 to 1100 mm, the endoscope diameter ranges from 4.9 to 12.8 mm and the instrument's working channel size ranges from 2.0 to 3.8 mm [9]. Given the differing age and

© Springer International Publishing AG 2017
D.G. Adler (ed.), *Upper Endoscopy for GI Fellows*,
DOI 10.1007/978-3-319-49041-0_11

Table 11.1 Endoscope size

Weight (kg)	EGD
<2.5	<6-mm gastroscope
2.5–10	<6-mm gastroscope preferred; standard adult gastroscope can be considered especially if therapeutic intervention required
>10	Standard adult gastroscope

Adapted from Barth et al. [9]

sizes of pediatric patients, there is not a "one size fits all" gastroscope that can be used in all pediatric patients.

The decision on the type of gastroscope to be used in patients depends on numerous factors including the size, height and weight of the patient and the nature of the intended procedure (i.e., diagnostic vs therapeutic). The major size restrictions are due to the smaller upper esophageal sphincter and the narrower pylorus. Typically, an "adult" gastroscope can be used for patients weighing in excess of 10–15 kg. However, smaller diameter endoscopes are recommended for patients under 10 kg [10] (Table 11.1). Most endoscopic manufacturers have created "ultrathin" or "neonatal" devices with smaller working channels and outer diameters (Table 11.2).

There is a caveat regarding selecting an endoscope solely on weight because the actual procedure type must be considered. This is due to certain drawbacks that are created when the size of gastroscope is decreased. There is a trade-off with smaller endoscope size that translates to a smaller working channel. Smaller gastroscopes with smaller channels may limit suction which would be vital during a procedure for upper GI bleeding to adequately and efficiently view the source for diagnosis and therapeutic intervention. Similarly, the water pump may not be attached to the smaller gastroscopes.

Indications

As in adults, there are numerous indications for endoscopy (EGD) in children. However, there remain some differences. These can be seen in Table 11.3 [10]. Many of the differences are related to the difference in developmental ages in children and caused by accidental events, i.e., foreign body and caustic ingestions. In some cases, the endoscopy then becomes not only diagnostic but therapeutic.

Adverse Events

Adverse events in pediatric upper endoscopy occur infrequently (0–4%). In a multicenter experience of 10,236 procedures from the PEDS-CORI network, the immediate complication rate was reported to be 2.3% [11]. The majority were related to hypoxia (66% of total) and were reversible. Bleeding was more commonly reported during therapeutic procedures (1.5%). Younger age, higher ASA class, female sex and use of IV sedation, and the presence of a fellow were all significantly associated with increased adverse event rates. Other reported events that have been reported during pediatric EGD include: abdominal distention, perforation and unintended medication effects.

Disease-Specific Considerations

Gastrointestinal Bleeding

Pediatric gastrointestinal (GI) bleeding is a relatively common problem which carries a substantial risk of morbidity and mortality. A small series from Montreal demonstrated a 1.6% rate of gastrointestinal bleeding in ICU patients, but only limited characterizations of endoscopic interventions or other management strategies have been described in non-variceal GI bleeding [12]. Upper GI tract bleeding has been described in numerous conditions, commonly due to erosions, ulcers or vascular malformations (Figs. 11.1, 11.2, 11.3 and 11.4). However, across pediatric age groups, the etiologies of GI bleeding may differ (Table 11.4). It is also important to note that it is not uncommon to have lower gastrointestinal bleeding in children due to an upper GI source.

Current management of pediatric gastrointestinal bleeding employs a variety of medical, transfusion and

Table 11.2 Neonatal and pediatric gastroscopes

Manufacturer	Model	Insertion tube length/diameter (mm)	Biopsy channel/diameter (mm)
Olympus	GIF-N180	1100/4.9	1/2.0
	GIF-XP180 N	1100/5.5	1/2.0
Fujinon	EG530 N	1100/5.9	1/2.0
	EG530NP	1100/4.9	1/2.0
Pentax	EG1690 K	1100/5.4	1/2.0
	EG1870 K	1050/6.0	1/2.0

Adapted from Barth et al. [9]

Table 11.3 Common indications for pediatric EGD

Diagnostic	Dysphagia
	Odynophagia
	Complicated or chronic GERD
	Hematemesis
	Persistent epigastric pain
	Weight loss, failure to thrive
	Chronic diarrhea/malabsorption
	GI bleeding
	Caustic ingestion
	Evaluation of celiac disease (abnormal serologies, family history)
	Eosinophilic esophagitis (food impaction, atopic history)
	Evaluation of Helicobacter pylori
Therapeutic	Foreign body removal
	Stricture dilation/stent placement
	Esophageal variceal ligation
	Upper GI bleeding control
	Polypectomy/tumor Removal

Adapted from Lightdale et al. [10]

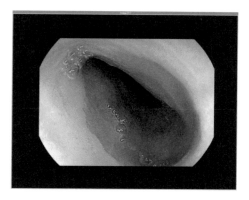

Fig. 11.2 A twelve-year-old with long segment Barrett's esophagus. (Courtesy of Dr. V. Enemuo)

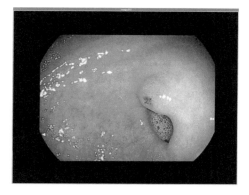

Fig. 11.3 A twelve-year-old with blue rubber bleb nevus syndrome

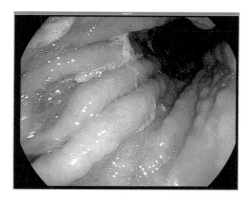

Fig. 11.1 A fourteen-year-old with Helicobacter gastritis. Diffuse nodularity is frequently seen in pediatric patients

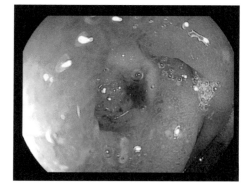

Fig. 11.4 A nine-year-old with Helicobacter gastritis and deep duodenal ulcer in the posterior bulb. (Courtesy of Dr. R. Himes)

endoscopic strategies. Red blood cell transfusion is also often necessary in the setting of acute blood loss caused by GI bleeding and should be available in the operating room. Additionally, fresh frozen plasma, platelets and other agents may be required. The major limitations in managing these cases are the size of the tools used for bleeding control. The majority of equipment including hemostatic clips and multipolar coagulation probes do not fit through the working channel. Also, the typical variceal band ligation cap (typically used in adults) is difficult to pass in children under 10 kg in size. Commonly used strategies for bleeding control in smaller patients may include an injection needle that can pass through a 2.0-mm channel or the argon plasma probe which can also pass through a smaller channel (Video 11.1). Alternatively, an attempt at using a larger caliber endoscope can be considered depending on the anticipated treatment. In our experience, we typically make a diagnostic assessment with the smallest appropriate endoscope and change endoscopes if needed for an intervention.

Table 11.4 Causes of upper gastrointestinal bleeding in pediatric patients

Age	Common	Rare
Birth to 1 year	Swallowed maternal blood Maternal breast inflammation Vitamin K deficiency Infectious esophagitis (Candida, HSV) Reflux esophagitis Gastritis or ulcer NSAID-induced gastritis or ulcer Duodenitis	Coagulation and bleeding diathesis Vascular malformations Duplication cysts Maternal NSAID use Pyloric stenosis Esophageal and gastric varices Foreign body Aortoesophageal fistula GVHD
Children and adolescents (1–18 years)	Esophagitis Esophageal and gastric varices H. pylori-induced ulcer NSAID-induced gastritis or ulcer Mallory–Weiss tear Inflammatory bowel disease Emetogenic gastritis	Vascular malformations Tumors (e.g., leiomyoma) Hematobilia GVHD

Celiac Disease

Celiac disease (CD) is an autoimmune condition involving the inability of the small intestine to properly respond to the breakdown and absorption of gluten. In celiac disease, the host's immune system is activated with the ingestion of gluten causing local inflammation, damage and destruction of the small intestine. Over time, this can lead to classic symptoms of celiac disease including failure to thrive, weight loss, diarrhea, abdominal pain and malnutrition.

This disease is particularly important to pediatric gastroenterologists because the classic symptoms typically begin during the childhood and adolescence. Studies performed in the USA and Europe estimate the prevalence to be 3–13/1000 or 1:300–1:80 of children between 2.5 and 15 years of age [13]. This understanding of the epidemiology of CD has greatly changed over the past few decades due to serologic tests in addition to advances in endoscopy. Until recently, it was not appreciated that a large majority of individuals can have a more chronic and insidious onset with milder symptoms than the classic, historical presentation thus making the diagnosis much more difficult [14].

Along with the changing epidemiology of CD, the diagnosis has also been a topic of numerous changes specific to endoscopy. Prior to the 1960s, the diagnosis of celiac disease was based solely on symptoms. In 1969, the European Society for the Pediatric Gastroenterology, Hepatology and Nutrition (ESPGHAN) developed the first diagnostic criteria for celiac disease. This included: (1) "structurally abnormal jejunal mucosa when taking a diet containing gluten," (2) "clear improvement of villous structure when taking a gluten-free diet," (3) "deterioration of the mucosa during challenge." With these criteria there was a minimum of three sets of biopsies required over a period of at least one year. The initial biopsy was performed to demonstrate damage, the second biopsy was performed after one year on a gluten-free diet to document healing and the third biopsy was performed after a few months of gluten re-introduction. Further revisions in 1990 stated that demonstrating the recurrence of histologic abnormalities after a gluten-free diet and gluten challenge was unnecessary as a part of the diagnostic criteria [15].

Histopathology remains the mainstay of the diagnosis for celiac disease. A clinical diagnosis alone was shown to be incorrect in >50% of cases [13]. In addition, celiac disease is a chronic condition involving a lifelong abstinence from gluten-containing products. Therefore, it is highly recommended that the diagnosis be confirmed with endoscopy and histologic evaluation before the treatment plan is initiated. Although symptoms may be "classic" there are other conditions that may manifest with similar symptoms. A recent report from ESPGHAN proposes a possibility of deferring biopsy if the serology is abnormal, and the patient has a specific HLA haplotype [16]. This was evaluated in a Canadian cohort that challenges this concept as an alternative diagnosis may be missed if strictly adhering to the proposed European guidelines [17]. Thus, the North American Society for Pediatric Gastroenterology, Hepatology and Nutrition (NASPGHAN) continues to recommend upper endoscopy with intestinal biopsy for confirmation of celiac disease.

Biopsy Technique

Celiac disease is patchy in nature with differences in severity at different locations in the small bowel [18]. For this reason, multiple duodenal biopsies need to be obtained in order to increase the probability of accurately confirming a diagnosis. Important locations to biopsy from include: the duodenal bulb, as well as distal segments of the duodenum, and duodenal–jejunal junction. At least six duodenal biopsies including at least two bulb biopsies should be performed to appropriately evaluate for celiac disease. This may be even more important in patients with early disease or milder symptoms, as their small intestinal architecture may not be evident endoscopically (Video 11.1).

Gross Pathology

Endoscopic features of CD can be varied. In a patient with mild disease, the mucosa may appear to be completely normal. However, in patients with severe disease, it is not uncommon to visualize diffuse disturbances in duodenal architecture. The most common macroscopic findings of duodenal villous atrophy include the absence of mucosal folds (Fig. 11.5a), scalloping (Fig. 11.5b) and submucosal blood vessels and a mosaic pattern of the mucosa [13]. Although these are most common, it is again important to note that affected patients may need subtotal to total villous atrophy for these to become visible endoscopically. In addition, the phrase "all that scallops is not celiac disease" has been coined to illustrate that celiac disease is only one of the disease states implicated with these gross abnormalities.

Histopathology

An experienced pediatric pathologist with specific experience with the evaluation of gastrointestinal mucosa should perform the evaluation of any obtained biopsy specimens; this increases the likelihood of an accurate diagnosis. The modified Marsh criteria (Table 11.5) are widely used for classifying histologic changes. It reveals four categories: pre-infiltrative (type 0), infiltrative (type 1), infiltrative-hyperplastic (type 2) and flat-destructive (type 3) and the atrophic-hypoplastic (type 4) lesion [19]. These criteria establish a grading severity for mucosal destruction and are not specific to celiac disease. However, with the appropriate clinical correlate, a diagnosis of celiac disease can be made.

Characteristically there are increases in intraepithelial lymphocytes (>30 lymphocytes/100 enterocytes), decrease in goblet cells, brush border abnormalities and villous flattening.

Eosinophilic Esophagitis

Eosinophilic esophagitis (EE) is a disorder isolated to the esophagus associated with eosinophilic infiltration in association with upper gastrointestinal symptoms. It is a relatively newly described disorder, and the incidence has increased over the past 20 years. As studied by Noel et al. [20] in the early 2000s, there was a fourfold increase in pediatric EE prevalence in the Midwest United States with a relative incidence of ~1/10,000 children per year. It is not uncommon for a patient to be initially (and incorrectly) diagnosed with gastroesophageal reflux (GERD) but then found not to respond to typical anti-reflux medications including proton pump inhibitors and H2 receptor antagonists [21].

EE can present in either childhood or adulthood; however, there are generally differences in the presentations [22]. Adults commonly present with intermittent dysphagia (29–100%) and food impaction (25–100%) [20]. Children may have nonspecific symptoms due to the inability to describe the sensation in the esophagus. Mostly commonly, the presenting symptoms are similar to GERD including heartburn or regurgitation. Other presenting symptoms in children that differ from adults include emesis, abdominal pain, failure to thrive, and diarrhea. Food impaction may occur more frequently as a presenting finding in adults, but this is not uncommon in the pediatric population. The pathologic process is unknown; however, it seems to be separate from GERD given that it does not lead to mucosal destruction or ulceration even in severe cases. Unlike GERD, which when progressive can lead to esophageal adenocarcinoma, there does not seem to be a link between EE and carcinoma.

Fig. 11.5 A four-year-old with celiac disease. Endoscopic findings include scalloping, nodularity, loss of folds and absence of a discrete villous appearance

(a)   **(b)**

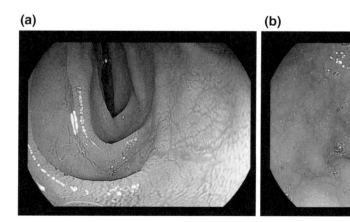

Table 11.5 Modified Marsh criteria

Marsh type	Intraepithelial lymphocytes/100 enterocytes	Crypts	Villi
0	<40	Normal	Normal
1	>40	Normal	Normal
2	>40	Increased	Normal
3a	>40	Increased	Mild atrophy
3b	>40	Increased	Marked atrophy
3c	>40	Increased	Absent

Adapted from Antonioli [19]

Biopsy Technique

In the past, it was common that in the absence of endoscopic findings of esophagitis only distal esophageal biopsies were obtained to evaluate EE (if at all). Newer recommendations advise the utility of biopsies in additional areas of the esophagus (mid and proximal) [22]. From these recent studies, it has been found that histopathologic abnormalities are common in biopsy specimens of even normal appearing mucosa. For this reason, it is also recommended that biopsies be taken in multiple levels of the esophagus even if it is grossly normal. In addition, biopsies should also be obtained from the stomach and duodenum to assess for other disease entities such as eosinophilic gastroenteritis and inflammatory bowel disease.

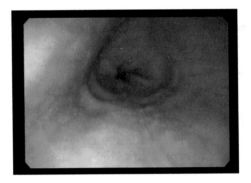

Fig. 11.6 A six-year-old with eosinophilic esophagitis. Furrowing and nodularity is prominent

Gross Pathology

Eosinophilic esophagitis, as with many other GI diseases, can have completely normal mucosa grossly. This does not exclude the diagnosis of EE. When there is more severe disease, there are common features seen on endoscopy. These include vertical lines, linear furrowing, white exudates, circular rings aka "felinization" or "trachealization," and strictures (Figs. 11.6 and 11.7). These are not pathognomonic of EE but can be helpful in diagnosis in the correct clinical context.

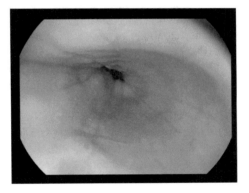

Fig. 11.7 A twelve-year-old female on tacrolimus with eosinophilic esophagitis. Furrowing and early trachealization is present

Histopathology

The key diagnostic criterion for diagnosing EE is based on the number of intraepithelial eosinophils. There has been much debate over the decades about the exact number of eosinophils that are sufficient to diagnosis EE. Recently, the criterion for diagnosis has been proposed as ≥ 15 intraepithelial eosinophils per high power field (HPF). Although some biopsy specimens may have <15 intraepithelial eosinophils per high power field (HPF), only 1 specimen is required to make the diagnosis [22]. For this reason, multiple

biopsy specimens are taken in order to increase the sensitivity. As above, the average number of biopsies suggested is 4–5 from different areas.

Inflammatory Bowel Disease

Inflammatory bowel disease (IBD) represents a class of autoimmune disorders affecting primarily the small intestine and the colon. This chiefly includes ulcerative colitis and

Crohn's disease, but there are other forms including inflammatory bowel disease-unspecified or indeterminate colitis which do not classically fit into either category. Distinguishing between ulcerative colitis and Crohn's disease is essential as it has therapeutic and prognostic implications. Ulcerative colitis involves continuous involvement starting in the rectum, whereas Crohn's disease has more patchy involvement. Although the prime involvement is in the lower tract, there can be some upper GI tract involvement, especially in Crohn's disease. In adults, there is strong link between inflammation within the terminal ileum, colon or perianal area and upper GI tract involvement in CD; therefore, routine upper endoscopy is not always recommended or warranted [23]. However, in the pediatric population, there is not as strong of an association between upper and lower tract disease especially in Crohn's disease and indeterminate colitis. Studies have shown than isolated upper GI tract abnormalities, specifically granulomas, may be present in 12–28% of patients newly diagnosed with IBD with completely normal colonoscopies [24]. This includes patients that have no symptoms of upper GI disease. This discrepancy between adult and pediatric IBD has prompted the recommendation that all pediatric patients with presumed IBD should undergo both upper endoscopy and colonoscopy as part of a full diagnostic evaluation.

Biopsy Technique

There is no current consensus on the number of upper gastrointestinal biopsies that should be taken in order to have the best sensitivity for making a diagnosis of Crohn's disease. However, it is recommended that multiple biopsies be taken from the upper and lower esophagus, stomach and duodenum. In one study, as many as 67% of patients had inflammation within the stomach, which is the most common area for abnormalities in the upper tract [25].

Polyposis Syndromes

Pediatric patients often undergo EGD for the management of polyposis. Specific recommendations and guidelines are in place for several disorders. Patients with Peutz–Jeghers syndrome, a hamartomatous polyposis syndrome, are recommended to have EGD with colonoscopy beginning at age 8 for evaluation and treatment of polyps and every three years if polyps are detected [26]. In our experience, patients may need an initial upper endoscopy prior to age 8 to decrease the risk of intussusception and bleeding. In patients with familial adenomatous polyposis (FAP), EGD is recommended when colonic adenomas are detected. This is appropriate for related syndromes as well such as Gardner

and Turcot syndrome [27, 28]. A side-viewing duodenoscope should be used to evaluate for ampullary adenomas in some polyposis syndromes, i.e., FAP, but the timing for the index examination is not well validated, but should be done by age eighteen. Patients with juvenile polyposis syndromes are recommended to have their first upper endoscopy at age 12 (and every 1–3 years thereafter) along with colonoscopy [27].

Therapeutic Interventions

Foreign Body Removal

Foreign body ingestion (FBI) is one of the major indications for pediatric endoscopies and can also be one of the most challenging. The majority of patients are <3 years of age [29]. There are many critical determining factors involving this procedure including object ingested, location of object, timing of the removal (emergent = <2 h, urgent = <24 h, elective = >24 h) versus watching waiting/observation, etc. (Video 11.1).

The presentation can range from patients who are completely asymptomatic to those severe symptoms including stridor, drooling and respiratory distress [30]. It is routinely stated that objects that are lodged within the esophagus require removal. 60–80% of FBIs are radiopaque making X-ray the first diagnostic step, but this clearly leaves a large number of patients with foreign bodies that are completely invisible on X-ray [29].

When foreign bodies are located in the stomach, this produces another difficult clinical scenario because the decision to intervene is solely based on the provider's clinical judgment to determine the likelihood of it moving past the duodenal bulb and only monitoring with serial X-rays. Other factors to consider are the reliability of a history given by family. If the family did not witness the exact object ingested, this again produces more clinical difficulty when deciding whether or not to endoscopically intervene.

Ingested Object

In contrast to adults, most FBIs in children are accidental and involve common household objects. The type of object ingested is of the utmost importance. Coins are the most common. Other objects include: magnets, button batteries, sharp objects and food [30].

- **Coins (and other blunt objects)**: Coins are very common ingested foreign bodies in children. Even if an ingested coin is thought to be lodged in the esophagus, it is important to perform both AP and lateral X-rays to rule

Fig. 11.8 AP and lateral views of a multi-coin ingestion in a 20-month-old (esophageal and gastric)

(a)   **(b)**

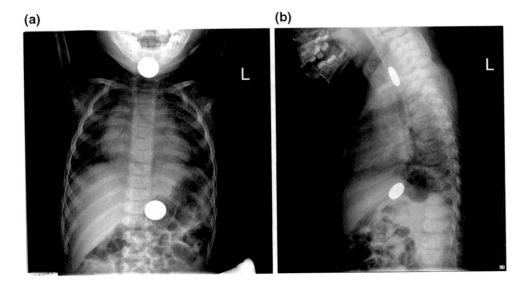

out tracheal impaction. In the AP position, the face of the coin is usually visualized if positioned in the esophagus whereas the side of the coin is usually front facing if lodged in the trachea [29]. This is only a general rule of thumb and there are exceptions.

The 3 sites in the esophagus that a coin can be impacted include the upper esophageal sphincter/thoracic inlet (60–70%), the mid-esophagus at the level of the aortic notch (10–20%) and the lower esophageal sphincter (20%). Coins at these locations should be removed within 12–24 h. Gastric coins are not routinely removed unless they remain present and do not pass spontaneously when observed by X-ray for 4–6 weeks. The family can also screen the stool for passage, although in practice this is often easier said than done [30] (Figs. 11.8 and 11.9).

- **Magnets**: The incidence of magnet ingestion has increased with the increasing incidence of incorporation of magnets into children's toys, the growing trend of adolescents with piercings (i.e., tongue or lip), and the increasing number of adult toys and desk objects that may contain many high-powered neodymium magnets. Magnets have the potential to cause the formation of enteroenteric fistulae between 2 or more magnets in bordering bowel loops; this can also lead to bowel perforation, necrosis and peritonitis.

Determining the number of magnets ingested is vital (Fig. 11.10). If only one magnet is ingested, then it may be treated like a standard ingested foreign body based on its shape and size and, in many cases, observation may be ideal. However, if there are 2 more magnets, if the magnets are adherent, or if there is uncertainty about the number of magnets, then removal is needed urgently. If the magnet can be reached endoscopically, then endoscopic removal should be performed as first-line therapy

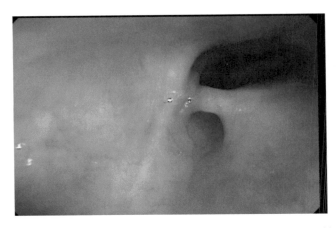

Fig. 11.9 Esophageal stricture after coin ingestion in a two-year-old with developmental delay. (Courtesy of Dr. C. Jensen)

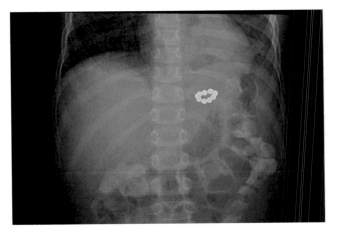

Fig. 11.10 Neodynium magnets in the gastric wall of a twelve-year-old child

[30]. However, if there is evidence of bowel entrapment or ischemia then a surgical consult should be performed concurrently. Many consensus papers have been written discouraging the production of toys with neodymium magnets, and since 2014 these have been banned in the USA, although many still exist and can be purchased on the secondary market.

- **Button Batteries**: Button batteries (BB) pose the highest risk to patients when they become lodged in the esophagus. An ingested button battery has become the leading cause for emergent endoscopic intervention in a patient with a swallowed foreign body. The mechanism of the injury is related to chemical or caustic injury to the mucosa via hydroxide radicals (alkaline) that cause an elevated pH. The main mechanism is not related to thermal burns as has been previously suggested. Animal models have shown a rise in pH from ingested button batteries can develop as early as 15 min after ingestion [29].

The most dangerous button batteries are lithium batteries as they have recently been manufactured in sizes with a larger diameter that makes them easier to lodge within the esophagus and to simultaneously have higher a conductance (Fig. 11.11). Severe complications that can develop following button battery ingestion include esophageal ulceration, perforation, development of tracheoesophageal fistula, aortoesophageal fistula and death (Fig. 11.12).

Ingested button batteries that have passed through the esophagus and are now in the stomach present a different challenge. There is no universal consensus on how to proceed in a patient with an intragastric button battery as some would argue to observe and others were perform endoscopic removal.

A clinical report by NASPGHAN recommends to "consider observation of patients with intragastric button batteries only if the following factors are present: <2 h duration since ingestion, battery <20 mm, absence of clinical symptoms and child 5 years of age or younger" [30]. However, in some studies esophageal damage had already occurred prior to the button battery settling in the stomach. Thus, there is a role in these patients to perform endoscopy, not only to remove the battery, but also to evaluate the integrity of the esophageal mucosa. Most agree that if a gastric battery has not passed after >48 h then it should be removed.

- **Sharp objects**: Sharp objects are not commonly ingested in the pediatric population. Adult gastroenterologists usually encounter them with patients that may have ingested the object intentionally (i.e., patients with psychiatric disease, prisoners, etc.). As a general rule, ingested sharp objects undergo endoscopic removal to reduce the risk of perforation and peritonitis. Most sharp objects can be removed with the sharp edge in the trailing

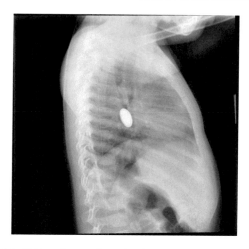

Fig. 11.11 Lithium battery ingestion in a three-year-old child. Note the two layers within the battery differentiating it from a coin. (Courtesy of Dr. M. Munden)

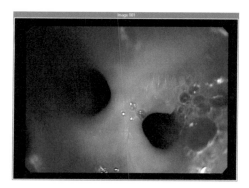

Fig. 11.12 Esophageal stricture after lithium battery ingestion in a two-year-old male

position as stated in the oft-repeated phrase "leading points perforate and trailing points don't." Sharp objects that children ingest include pens, pencils, pen caps and safety pins [29, 31].

- **Food Impaction**: Food impactions are far more common in adults than children. When they occur in children, food impactions are likely due to primary esophageal pathology such as eosinophilic esophagitis, strictures, etc. Food impactions should be treated endoscopically, both allowing for relief of obstruction and evaluation of the esophagus for underlying pathology [29]. Endoscopy in this setting can usually be performed electively unless the patient cannot control their secretions, in which case it should be performed urgently. The food bolus can either be removed in a retrograde manner or gently advanced into the stomach via the so-called push technique [30]. The push technique is not validated in children as there may be an undiagnosed stricture beyond the food bolus, although in many patients this is used as some boluses are not amenable to retrograde removal. As eosinophilic esophagitis may be the underlying cause, endoscopic biopsies are recommended at the time of foreign body or food impaction removal [22].

Caustic Ingestions

The accidental ingestion of inedible and caustic substance is another serious problem in the pediatric population with potential severe long-term complications. Patients are generally between the ages of 1 and 4 years old, when they first become mobile and are curious of their environments [32]. The type of injury and whether or not to intervene depends on a multitude of factors including, but not limited to, the substance ingested, the volume of the ingested substance, clinical symptoms and time course since ingestion.

Type of Substance Ingested

In most patients with caustic ingestions, injury to the esophagus occurs secondary to a chemical reaction. Ingested substances are generally classified as alkali or acidic. Alkali substances (aka bases) with pH of >11 or acids with a pH of <3 cause the most severe forms of injury. Commonly ingested products are listed in Table 11.6 [33].

Alkalis in liquid form are tasteless; therefore, they are can be swallowed with less difficulty and tend to cause more distal injuries. Injury is usually caused by liquefactive necrosis with diffusion of the caustic agent into and through the mucosa, sometimes affecting more distal layers of the esophageal wall. Acids, in general, have a poor taste, cause oral burning and are less well tolerated. Acids are much more difficult to swallow and may be regurgitated. Acids are less likely to cause distal injuries. Children are more likely to choke or aspirate when ingesting acids; this can lead to damage to the upper airway. The mechanism of injury with ingested acids is via coagulative necrosis which forms an

Table 11.6 Common caustic ingestion agents [32]

Type	Example
Alkali (bases)	Oven cleaners, liquid drain cleaners, disk batters, hair relaxers, household cleaners, dishwasher detergents
Acid	Toilet bowl cleaners, swimming pool cleaners, rust removers
Bleaches and others	Bleach, peroxide

Adapted from Lupa et al. [32]

Table 11.7 Zargar's mucosal injury classification [34]

Grade	Endoscopic visualization
0	Normal examination
1	Edema and hyperemia of the mucosa
2a	Friability, hemorrhages, erosions, blisters, whitish membranes, exudates and superficial ulcerations
2b	Grade 2a + deep discrete or circumferential ulcerations
3a	Small scattered areas of necrosis
3b	Extensive necrosis

eschar which generally prevents seepage of the offending agent into deeper tissue layers.

The degree of esophageal injury from caustic ingestions is measured by the endoscopic appearance. The Zargar grading system was described mainly in adults in 1991 (Table 11.7) [34].

The concept behind the grading system was to predict outcomes and future complications. Patients with a stage 2b or higher (circumferential) burn have a high likelihood of developing strictures. Therefore, it is recommended that these patients have nasogastric (NG) tubes placed with endoscopic visualization to prevent further erosive damage [32].

Clinical Manifestations and Therapy

Clinical presentations of patients with caustic injuries range from asymptomatic to complete airway occlusion requiring artificial airways and mechanical ventilation. Common symptoms include vomiting, cough, wheezing, shortness of breath, drooling and difficulty managing secretions. Patients who are completely asymptomatic can be observed in a controlled medical setting in order to monitor for late complications. Symptomatic patients should undergo endoscopy.

Late Complications

Esophageal strictures are the main complication of caustic ingestions. These can appear as early as three weeks after the index ingestion [33]. For this reason, all children with grade 2 burns or more should have a barium swallow within 2–3 weeks after injury to evaluate for any nascent strictures. Nearly all patients with grade 3 burns will develop strictures. The treatment of choice is balloon dilation to alleviate symptoms. This is generally a temporary solution as most patients will require repeat dilations and some progress to the point of stenting or, rarely, esophagectomy with colonic interposition.

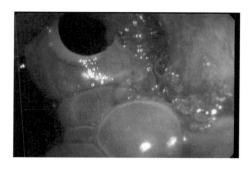

Fig. 11.13 Esophageal stricture and multiple blebs in a child with epidermolysis bullosa. (Courtesy of Dr. L. Karam)

Other Strictures Intervened upon by Upper Endoscopy

Congenital anomalies such as tracheoesophageal fistula are usually repaired surgically in infancy. These surgeries can commonly lead to esophageal strictures, which may present in a delayed manner. These strictures can typically by managed with endoscopic dilation; however, the use of self expanding stents has been reported as a treatment for these strictures and is often highly effective. Patients with moderate-to-severe forms of epidermolysis bullosa can also have significant esophageal strictures (Fig. 11.13). These patients may undergo numerous dilation procedures during the course of their life (Video 11.1).

Sedation for Pediatric Upper Endoscopy

There are three main types of sedation for GI procedures in pediatric patients: general anesthesia, deep sedation provided and moderate sedation (previously referred to as conscious sedation). The latter two are typically administered by a gastroenterologist or more commonly a practitioner trained in pediatric sedation; the former is administered by an anesthesiologist or a nurse anesthetist.

Unlike adults who may only undergo moderate sedation for common GI procedures, there are other considerations in pediatric endoscopy. In the early years of endoscopy, the gastroenterologist performing the procedure performed almost all sedation in parallel with the endoscopy. However, as patients who needed endoscopic procedures became smaller (premature infants) and endoscopic technology became more advanced and procedures more lengthy, the need for general anesthesia has become a more common route [26]. General anesthesia decreases in the amount of interruptions during the procedure and allows for continuous endoscopic therapy. In addition, the airway is completely protected, making accidental intubation of the airway with the endoscope difficult (although if this occurs there is usually no injury to airway structures). There are

significant costs to general anesthesia, especially when performed in an operating room. Many endoscopists will perform routine endoscopies outside of the operating room in a procedure suite via other means of sedation, greatly minimizing costs.

Pediatric Procedural Considerations

The procedural environment for pediatric patients undergoing endoscopy must have special modifications in order for a safe and relaxed experience for the patient and family. Unlike adults who will fully understand the reasoning for the specific procedure, children are generally apprehensive and not fully aware of the happenings of the day. For this reason, the procedural suite must be a comfortable place for both the patient and family. Nurses and technicians with pediatric training should endeavor to create a positive environment for children. Responsible staff should have PALS (Pediatric Advanced Life Support) or equivalent certification.

Pre-procedure

In the pre-procedure area, there must be adequate space for both the patient and the family. Parents or guardians should always be allowed to accompany the child until the last moment prior to the beginning of the procedure. This creates a sense of trust and also provides solidarity in that the child sees the parent/guardian in agreement with the medical team. Since patients will be fasting for many hours prior to the procedures, children are more apt than adults to suffer from dehydration, and therefore, intravenous fluid supplementation should be considered.

Reducing anxiety is also a high priority. There are various methods including involving pre-procedural tours of the procedure area, early introduction of child life experts and pre-procedural anxiolytics. Child life colleagues will have expertise in calming an anxious child with distraction techniques such as video games, demonstrations on dolls and deep breathing techniques.

Intra-procedure

As with all procedures, efficient and timely completion of the endoscopic task at hand should be the goal. Patient positioning is dependent on the mode of sedation; however, upper endoscopy can easily be performed in the supine or left lateral position. Care should be taken to have different scope sizes available in the event that equipment needs to be changed for the specific patient depending on needs dictated by size or endoscopic maneuver. Having differing sizes of equipment available in the room allows for shortened time lapses in the room. In addition, the appropriate media for biopsy specimens should always be available in the event that biopsies that were not previously planned should be taken. Care should be taken to limit insufflation and to frequently remove air from the stomach and bowel. Abdominal distention due to overinflation can lead to cardiovascular instability or challenges with ventilation. A recent modification in endoscopic practice has utilized CO_2 (carbon dioxide) gas for insufflation, which may decrease some of these effects.

Post-procedure

A pediatric patient should always awaken to a familiar face as this allows for less disorientation and anxiety. For this reason, families should be allowed into the recovery area as soon as possible after the completion of endoscopy. In addition, careful attention should be made to the proper positioning of the head and neck (especially in neonates and infants) as they have a tendency to obstruct the airway secondary to redundant posterior pharyngeal tissue. The recovery area should always be in direct view of staffing member (nurse or MD) who is able to visualize complications early in order to intervene quickly.

Quality Assessment in Pediatric Upper Endoscopy

Although there are no specific recommendations for the assessment of quality for pediatric upper endoscopy, some parallels can be drawn from both adult gastroenterology and that of pediatric colonoscopy. NASPGHAN training guidelines recommend at least 100 EGDs be performed as part of the fellowship training, along with at least 10 foreign body removals [35]. Complex endoscopic maneuvers such as endoscopic stent placement and hemostasis are less commonly performed, and trainees may have difficulty completing these in sufficient numbers prior to the completion of their training [36]. Trainees should also have a dedicated log for all endoscopic procedures. This will be needed at the time of completion of fellowship training as well as for future credentialing as an attending physician.

Conclusion

Performing EGD in pediatric patients requires an understanding of general endoscopy and an understanding of pediatric patients and disease states. A key difference

between pediatric and adult upper endoscopy is the need to use smaller equipment for smaller patients. Advances in endoscope and accessory technology will increase the ability to care for this unique population. Furthermore, improving safety and decreasing adverse rates is an ongoing task which can improve with a focus on quality assessment.

References

1. Hirschowitz BI, Curtiss LE, Peters CW, et al. Demonstration of a new gastroscopy, the "fiberscope". Gastroenterol. 1958;35:50–3.
2. Gleason WA Jr, Tedesco FJ, Keating JP, et al. Fiberoptic gastrointestinal endoscopy. J Pediatr. 1974;85(6):810–3.
3. Gans SL, Ament M, Christie DL, et al. Pediatric endoscopy with flexible fiberscopes. J Pediatr Surg. 1975;10(3):375–80.
4. Cadranel S, Rodesch P, Peeters JP, et al. Fiberendoscopy of the gastrointestinal tract in children. A series of 100 examinations. Am J Dis Child. 1977;131(1):41–5.
5. Graham DY, Klish WJ, Ferry GD, et al. Value of fiberoptic gastrointestinal endoscopy in infants and children. South Med J. 1978;71(5):558–60.
6. Kawai K, Murakami K, Misak F. Endoscopical observations on gastric ulcers in teenagers. Endoscopy. 1970;2:206–8.
7. Varadarajulu S, Baerjee S, Barth BA, et al. GI endoscopes. Gastrointest Endosc. 2011;74:1–6.
8. Day A, Marchant J, Bohane TD. Use of formulae to predict esophageal length in children undergoing PH probe studies. J Pediatr Gastroenterol Nutr. 2003;36:292–3.
9. Barth BA, Banerjee S, Bhat YM, et al. Equipment for pediatric endoscopy. Gastrointest Endosc. 2012;76(1):8–17.
10. Lightdale JL, Acosta R, Shergil AK, et al. Modifications in endoscopic practice for pediatric patients. Gastrointest Endosc. 2014;79:699–710.
11. Thakkar K, El-Serag H, Mattek N, et al. Complications of pediatric EGD: a 4-year experience in PEDS-CORI. Gastrointest Endosc. 2007;65:213–21.
12. Chaibou M, Tucci M, Dugas MA. Clinically significant upper gastrointestinal bleeding acquired in a pediatric intensive care unit: a prospective study. Pediatrics. 1998;102(4):933–8.
13. Hill I, Dirks MH, Liptak GS, et al. Guideline for the diagnosis and treatment of celiac disease in children: recommendations of the North American society for pediatric gastroenterology, hepatology and nutrition. J Pediatr Gastroenterol Nutr. 2005;40:1–19.
14. Lebenthal E, Shteyer E, Branski D. The Changing clinical presentation of celiac disease. Frontiers in celiac disease. Pediatr Adolesc Med. 2008;12:18–22.
15. Revised criteria for diagnosis of coeliac disease. Report of working group of European society of paediatric gastroenterology and nutrition. Arch Dis Child. 1990;65:909–11.
16. Husby S, et al. European Society for pediatric gastroenterology, hepatology, and nutrition guidelines for the diagnosis of coeliac disease. J Pediatr Gastroenterol Nutr. 2012;54(1):136–60.
17. Gidrewicz D, Potter K, Trevenen C, et al. Evaluation of the ESPGHAN celiac guidelines in a North American pediatric population. Am J Gastroenterol. 2015;110:760–7.
18. Shah VH, Rotterdam H, Kotler DP, Fasano A, Green PH. All that scallops is not celiac disease. Gastrointest Endosc. 2000;51(6):717–20.
19. Antonioli D. Celiac disease: a progress report. Mod Pathol. 2003;16(4):342–6.
20. Noel R, Putnam P, Rothenberg M. Eosinophilic Esophagitis. NEJM. 2004;351:940–1.

21. Ngo P, Furuta GT, Antonioli DA, et al. Eosinophils in the esophagus-peptic or allergic eosinophilic esophagitis? Case series of three patients with esophageal eosinophilia. Am J Gastroenterol. 2006;101(7):1666–70.

22. Furuta G, et al. Eosinophilic esophagitis in children and adults: a systematic review and consensus recommendations for diagnosis and treatment. Gastroenterology. 2007;133:1342–63.

23. Shergill AK, Lightdale JL, Bruining DH, et al. The role of endoscopy in inflammatory bowel disease. Gastroint Endosc. 2014;81:1101–25.

24. Bousvaros A, Antonioli DA, Colletti RB, et al. Differentiating ulcerative colitis from Crohn disease in children and young adults: report of a working group of the North American Society for Pediatric Gastroenterology, Hepatology, and Nutrition and the Crohn's and Colitis Foundation of America. J Pediatr Gastroenterol Nutr. 2007;44:653–74.

25. Castellaneta SP, et al. Diagnostic role of upper gastrointestinal endoscopy in pediatric inflammatory bowel disease. J Pediatr Gastrointest Nutr. 2004;39(3):257–61.

26. Beggs AD, Latchford AR, Vasen HFA, et al. Peutz-Jeghers syndrome: a systematic review and recommendations for management. Gut. 2010;59:975–86.

27. Syngal S, Brand RE, Church RE, et al. ACG clinical guideline: genetic testing and management of hereditary gastrointestinal cancer syndromes. Am J Gastroentero. 2015;110(2):223–63.

28. Munck A, Gargouri L, Alberti C, et al. Evaluation of guidelines for management of familial adenomatous polyposis in a multicenter pediatric cohort. J Pediatr Gastroenterol Nutr. 2011;53:296–302.

29. Kay M, Wyllie R. Foreign body ingestions in the pediatric population and techniques of endoscopic removal. Tech Gastrointest Endosc. 2013;15(1):9–17.

30. Kramer RE, Lerner DG, Lin T, et al. Management of ingested foreign bodies in children: a clinical report of the NASPGHAN endoscopy committee. J Pediatr Gastroenterol Nutr. 2015;60(4):562–74.

31. Jackson C, Jackson CL. Sharp objects. Disease of the air and food passages of foreign body origin. Philadelphia: Saunders; 1937.

32. Lupa M, Magne J, Guarisco J, Amedee R. Update on the diagnosis and treatment of caustic ingestion. Ochsner J. 2009;9(2):54–9.

33. Kay M, Wylie R. Caustic ingestions in pediatrics. Curr Opin Pediatr. 2009;21:651–4.

34. Zargar SA, Kochhar R, Mehta S, et al. The role of fiberoptic endoscopy in the management of corrosive ingestion and modified endoscopic classification of burns. Gastrointest Endosc. 1991;37:165.

35. Leichtner A, Gillis LA, Gupta S, et al. NASPGHAN guidelines for training in pediatric gastroenterology. J Pediatr Gastroenterol Nutr. 2013;56(Suppl. 1):S1–38.

36. Lerner DG, Li BU, Mamula P, et al. Challenges in meeting fellowship procedural guidelines in pediatric therapeutic endoscopy and liver biopsy. J Pediatr Gastroenterol Nutr. 2014;58 (1):27–33.

Evaluation and Management of Mucosal and Submucosal Lesions in the Foregut

12

Dino Beduya and Gulshan Parasher

Introduction

"Submucosal lesion" is a loosely applied term, often used to describe a bulge or prominence seen on endoscopy when the lesion has overlying normal mucosa encountered during gastrointestinal (GI) endoscopy. A more appropriate term would be "subepithelial lesion" (SEL) since submucosa is a distinct histologic layer in the gastrointestinal wall and such lesions can arise from any layer, although the term "submucosal lesion" remains in widespread use. The majority of these lesions are located within the gut wall (intramural), although these prominences may be extramural in 15–30% of cases, as a result of impressions made by surrounding structures [1]. In the foregut, these extramural structures include normal organs such as the liver, spleen, gall bladder, kidney, vertebra, and blood vessels (Fig. 12.1) [2]. Extramural pathologic conditions include pancreatic cysts and pseudocysts, splenic artery aneurysms, enlarged lymph nodes, mediastinal masses, duplication cysts of GI or bronchogenic origin, and lung cancer [2–4]. This chapter will focus on intramural subepithelial lesions in the foregut, including endoscopic diagnosis and management.

Electronic supplementary material
Supplementary material is available in the online version of this chapter at 10.1007/978-3-319-49041-0_12. Videos can also be accessed at https://link.springer.com/chapter/10.1007/978-3-319-49041-0_12.

D. Beduya · G. Parasher (✉)
Division of Gastroenterology and Hepatology, University of New Mexico School of Medicine, Albuquerque, USA
e-mail: gparasher@salud.unm.edu

D. Beduya
e-mail: dbeduya@salud.unm.edu

Incidence and Clinical Presentation

Subepithelial lesions are encountered in 0.3–3.5% of upper endoscopies [5, 6]. The majority of these lesions are in the stomach (51.6–75.5%), followed by esophagus (18.5–41.3%), and duodenum (6–7.1%) [5, 7]. Because a biopsy is not performed or warranted for most SELs, histologically confirmed diagnosis is not available in a majority of cases [1]. A presumptive diagnosis is made based on appearance on endoscopy, endoscopic ultrasound (EUS), and other imaging modalities [1, 2, 4, 8].

Among cases with a histologic diagnosis, 41.8–63.8% are confirmed to be gastrointestinal stromal tumors (GISTs), 21.9–34.3% are leiomyomas, 1.4–10.4% are lipomas, 2.9–8.7% are granular cell tumors, 7.5% are heterotopic pancreas, 3.0–5.5% are cysts, including duplication cysts, and 2.6% are carcinoid tumors [1, 4, 7, 8]. The proportion of the different types of foregut SELs vary based on location. For example, in a study which included only gastric SELs, 30.5% were GISTs, 30.1% were heterotopic pancreas, 15.5% were leiomyomas, 5.8% were lipomas, and 2.2% were schwannomas [9]. Other diagnoses include heterotopic liver, leiomyosarcoma, lymphoma, bronchial carcinoma, and metastasis (renal cell primary, ovarian primary). Of note, in the studies on SEL with histologic confirmation, reasons for tissue acquisition included hypoechogenicity on imaging, size >10 mm, increase in size by >25%, and worrisome endosonographic changes. This indicates that the above incidence rates for the different types of SELs cannot be applied to SELs as a whole.

The majority of small SELs do not increase in size or develop worrisome endosonographic features. In a retrospective study of gastric SELs ≤ 30 mm followed for up to 13 years (median 7 years), only 8.5% (84 of 989) showed a significant increase in size, developed ulceration, and/or had their appearance on EUS change over a median period of 24 months [10]. Twenty-five lesions underwent resection or enucleation; 19 of the 25 (76%) were found to be GISTs [10]. Of 65 hypoechoic foregut SELs (size 7–29 mm)

© Springer International Publishing AG 2017
D.G. Adler (ed.), *Upper Endoscopy for GI Fellows*,
DOI 10.1007/978-3-319-49041-0_12

139

Fig. 12.1 Splenic artery. Endoscopy shows a pulsatile prominence in the posterior gastric wall. Varying views on EUS shows a tubular, also round anechoic structure. Doppler examination shows pulsatile flow

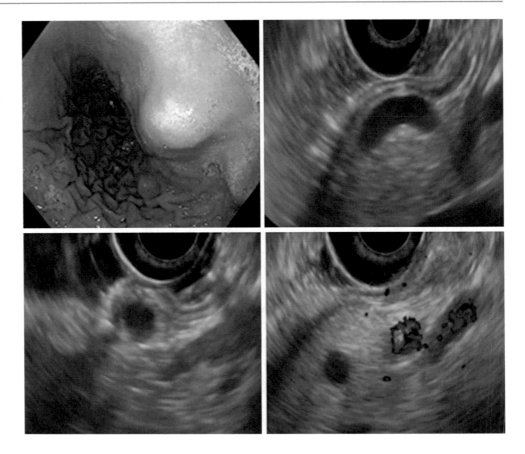

prospectively followed for up to 9 years (median 2.5 years), 16 (25%) increased in size. Nine had a tissue diagnosis, 6 of which were GISTs [7].

Most foregut SELs are asymptomatic and incidentally discovered during upper endoscopy or abdominal surgery for an unrelated indication. If present, symptoms are often related to the location and size of the lesion. Dysphagia is mostly reported in cases of esophageal SELs when the size of the lesion is >1 cm. Vomiting or other obstructive symptoms can be the presenting symptom for large gastric SELs near the pylorus (Fig. 12.2). Duodenal SELs can be complicated by jaundice and, rarely, pancreatitis [2, 4, 11]. Other presenting symptoms of foregut SELs include GI bleeding (overt, with hematemesis or melena, or occult resulting in anemia), abdominal pain, and chest discomfort.

Diagnosis

A diagnosis cannot be made for all SELs solely based on endoscopic visualization. However, upper endoscopy is 95% accurate in identifying a subepithelial lesion as solid, cystic, or vascular [12]. Also, for lipomas, indentation with a closed biopsy forceps during endoscopy (the "pillow sign") is

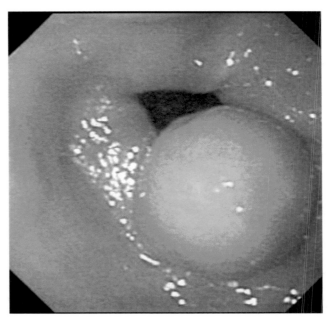

Fig. 12.2 Giant antral lipoma causing intermittent obstruction of the pylorus in a 61-year-old woman with intermittent vomiting. *Image courtesy* Douglas G. Adler MD

98.8% specific [1]. Upper endoscopy can be used to biopsy suspected lipomas in a tunneled manner—if this reveals adipose tissue this is termed the "naked fat" sign. Also upper endoscopy has a sensitivity of 87–98%, but a low specificity of 29–64% in determining whether the lesion is intramural or extramural [1, 2].

Endoscopic ultrasound (EUS) plays an important role in the diagnosis and management of SELs. It is superior to endoscopy in determining whether a lesion is intramural or extramural, with a sensitivity of 92% sensitive and specificity of 100% [2]. EUS helps narrow the differential diagnoses of an SEL based on the echogenicity and layer of origin (Table 12.1). EUS imaging alone is sufficient for diagnosing lipomas, simple cysts, and varices [13, 14]. However, a presumptive diagnosis by EUS without performing biopsy is correct in only 45.5–48% of cases [1, 15]. This is because several SELs (GIST, leiomyoma, schwannoma, heterotopic pancreas) have overlapping endosonographic features. EUS is also helpful in predicting risk of malignancy. Large size (≥3 cm) and irregular margins in hypoechoic SELs [16], as well as the presence of perilesional lymphadenopathy, correlate with malignancy or indeterminate malignant potential. EUS allows evaluation for candidacy for endoscopic resectability of an SEL. Findings which indicate that a tumor is generally not amenable to endoscopic resection include (1) extension to the muscularis propria, (2) the presence of lymphadenopathy, and (3) size >2 cm [17, 18].

EUS is frequently used to perform tissue acquisition, usually by EUS-guided fine-needle aspiration (FNA). Diagnostic rate for EUS-guided FNA or biopsy ranges from 34 to 91% [14]. In a recent meta-analysis which included 17 studies from 2004 to 2014, the overall diagnostic rate was found to be 59.9% in 978 cases. There was no difference in the diagnostic rate among fine-needle aspiration, needle biopsy, and trucut biopsy, as well as 19-gauge, 22-gauge, and 25-gauge needles. Only studies which used ability to perform immunohistochemical staining as a parameter for specimen adequacy were included [14]. Other techniques (mucosal incision or unroofing, resection, and dissection) are available which allow for acquisition of more tissue.

Endoscopic mucosal resection (EMR) is a technique which allows not only deeper sampling but also complete removal of a small, superficial lesion via endoscopy. EMR is essentially a variation of the technique of standard polypectomy as performed during colonoscopy and involves submucosal injection of a fluid, usually saline or saline diluted with epinephrine to create a submucosal cushion, followed by band ligation and removal of the lesion via electrocautery with a polypectomy snare (Fig. 12.3). A lesion is considered amenable to EMR if it is less than 2 cm, not invading the musclaris propria, and with no surrounding lymphadenopathy [17, 18]. Endoscopic submucosal dissection (ESD) is another technique that allows en bloc lesion removal, for lesions >2 cm. Margin-negative (curative) resection can be achieved and surgery avoided via ESD, allowing preservation of the native organ. Compared to EMR, ESD has a higher risk of bleeding and perforation a longer procedure duration and is limited to referral centers [19]. Endoscopic full thickness resection can also be performed for deeper lesions (involving the muscularis propria), but this procedure also limited to only a few tertiary centers [20, 21].

Other imaging modalities have been used to characterize SELs. These include computed topography (CT) scan, magnetic resonance imaging (MRI), and magnetic resonance

Table 12.1 EUS features of different SELs

	Echogenicity	Layer of origin	Homogeneity	Margin
Lipoma	Intensely hyperechoic	SM	Homogenous	Distinct
Heterotopic pancreas	Hypoechoic or mixed	Mainly SM, also MM and MP	Heterogenous	Mostly indistinct
Carcinoid	Isoechoic or slightly hypoechoic	Mainly SM, also MP	Homogenous	Distinct
Duplication cyst	Anechoic	Any	Homogenous	Distinct
GIST	Hypoechoic or mixed	Mainly MP, rarely MM, SM	Homogenous or heterogenous	Mostly distinct (irregular margins suggest intermediate or high risk of malignancy)
Leiomyoma	Hypoechoic	Mainly MP, also MM	Mostly homogenous	Distinct
Schwannoma	Hypoechoic	Mucosa, SM, MP, serosa	Homogenous	Distinct
Granular cell tumor	Hypoechoic	Mucosa, MM, SM, MP	Homogenous or mildly inhomogenous	Distinct

SM submucosa, *MM* muscularis mucosa, *MP* muscularis propria

Fig. 12.3 Endoscopic mucosal resection of a gastric carcinoid. Lesion is suctioned with a cap-fitted endoscope and band ligation is performed, followed by snare resection

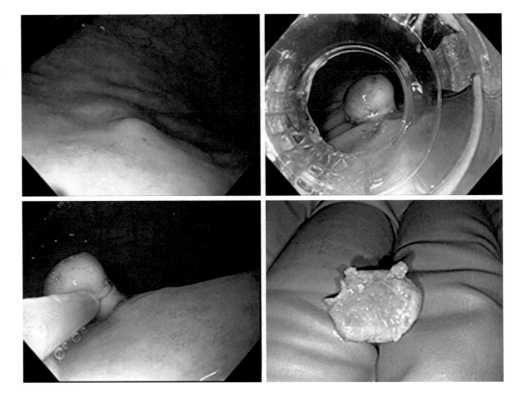

pancreatography (MRCP). Both CT and MRI take advantage of fat content and are able to specifically diagnosis lipomas [22, 23]. Overall accuracy of multidetector CT in detecting and classifying SELs is 85.3% and 78.8%, respectively [24]. While EUS is generally better than CT in detecting foregut SELs, rarely, CT can show a lesion not visualized on EUS if it is too far from the gut wall to be seen clearly [24].

Management

Management of foregut SELs depends on the presence of symptoms attributable to the lesion, as well as concern for a malignant or a potentially malignant condition. Symptomatic lesions should, in general, be treated by endoscopic or surgical resection or enucleation. For duplication cysts, marsupialization is also an option but is rarely required. For asymptomatic lesions, the decision of whether or not to biopsy can be individualized.

If a lesion appears yellow in hue and the "pillow sign" or the "naked fat" signs are positive, the lesion is likely a lipoma and further biopsy is not typically warranted. If a lesion appears vascular (such as a varix, which is often serpiginous and has a bluish hue) or cystic, endoscopic biopsies should not be performed until the target lesion is further evaluated by EUS. On EUS, a varix appears as a round or tubular anechoic structure, usually deep to the submucosa, and Doppler examination shows flow in the

structure [25]. If an SEL appears solid, forceps biopsy should be considered. Forceps biopsy is low yield [4, 5, 26] but is often sufficient for carcinoid tumors since these lesions tend to invade the mucosa [27]. If the biopsy of a solid-appearing lesion is non-diagnostic, EUS should be pursued. Alternatively, repeat endoscopy in 1 year can be considered if the lesion is <1 cm and the patient is not enthusiastic about further evaluation. If EUS shows concerning features such as a hypoechoic mass >3 cm in size, referral for surgery should be considered. For hypoechoic lesions less than <3 cm, deeper biopsy (endoscopic mucosal resection, EUS FNA or biopsy, mucosal dissection) may be performed [28].

Foregut SELs

Lipomas

Gastrointestinal lipomas are benign, slowly growing tumors [29]. They can occur in any part of the GI tract but are most commonly found in the colon (65–75%). Four to eight percent of GI lipomas are found in the stomach [23, 29]. Microscopically, they are made up of a fibrous capsule containing mature adipose tissue lobules and thin regular fibrovascular septa [22].

Lipomas are often asymptomatic and incidentally found during endoscopy. Rarely, large lipomas can present with intussusception, GI obstruction, acute, and chronic bleeding, manifesting with anemia.

Prior to the advent of CT and endoscopy, the diagnosis of a lipoma was usually made after surgical intervention [23, 30]. Gastrointestinal lipomas are seen as a fatty density with distinct margins on CT. On MRI, they are characterized by hyperintensity on T1-weighted images [23]. Endoscopy usually shows a yellow to red-orange smooth-surfaced mass. Indentation with a closed biopsy, the "pillow sign," is 98.8% specific. However, this sign is only 40% sensitive for lipomas [1]. In such cases, EUS can be used for further evaluation. On EUS, GI lipomas usually appear as a homogenous hyperechoic lesion with distinct margins (Fig. 12.4). In some cases, they can have a more atypical and heterogeneous appearance. Approximately 90–95% arise from the submucosal layer, the rest from the subserosa [31]. EUS features are characteristic, and no further diagnostic intervention is usually needed [12]. Biopsies are generally unnecessary and should be limited only to cases with atypical imaging [29].

GI lipomas have essentially no malignant potential. Surveillance and treatment are not indicated for incidental lipomas. For symptomatic lipomas, surgical or endoscopic resection can be performed. Removal by endoscopy is contraindicated if EUS shows layer of origin is the serosa or if there is infiltration of the muscularis propria [31].

Pancreatic Rests

A pancreatic rest AKA heterotopic pancreas is pancreatic tissue outside of its normal location. It can be seen anywhere in the GI tract but can be found outside it as well (pelvis, thorax, mesentery, spleen). These lesions are found in up to 2% of the population [32]. Pancreatic rests have been reported in 0.2% of surgical operations involving the upper GI tract and 0.6–13% of autopsies [33]. Heterotopic pancreas can be found in patients at any age but is most often discovered in the fifth and sixth decades of life, more commonly in males. In the GI tract, it is most frequently seen in the gastric antrum, along the greater curve, in the prepyloric space [33].

Pancreatic rests are often asymptomatic. The most common complaint in symptomatic patients is abdominal pain. Other symptoms include GI bleeding, gastric outlet obstruction, biliary obstruction, and weight loss [31, 32]. Pancreatitis, pseudocyst, and cystic neoplasms can arise in heterotopic pancreas rarely [32, 33].

The classic appearance of heterotopic pancreas on endoscopy is a smooth subepithelial lesion with central umbilication, which corresponds with the opening of a partial or complete ductal structure. This umbilication is found in approximately half of cases. Size ranges from 0.1 to 5 cm, usually 0.6–3 cm [34]. Heterotopic pancreas is usually found in the antrum, 2–6 cm from the pylorus, in the 3–7 o' clock position [35]. Compared with gastric mesenchymal tumors (GISTs, leiomyomas, schwannomas), size <3 cm and location in the middle or lower third of the stomach is 92% sensitive and 78% for heterotopic pancreas [36].

On EUS, a pancreatic rest frequently has a hypoechoic or mixed echogenicity [13, 26, 34, 37]. Margins are indistinct in 72–80% of cases, owing to the lobular structure of the acinous tissue at the margin [24, 26, 37]. The layer of origin is mainly the submucosa, although these lesions can also (less commonly) originate from the muscularis propria and muscularis mucosa [13, 37]. Anechoic areas within a lesion can be seen corresponding to ductal or cystic structures [26, 37].

Histologic diagnosis of heterotopic pancreas is often difficult using endoscopic biopsy forceps [26]. Up to 12.5% of heterotopic pancreas can be diagnosed by endoscopic biopsy alone [32], 36% with biopsy or snare [35]. EUS FNA of pancreatic rests is rarely indicated.

Management of pancreatic rests remains controversial. Malignant transformation has been reported but is exceptionally rare, and an invasive approach is generally not recommended in asymptomatic patients [37]. Tissue acquisition may not always be required, particularly for lesions

Fig. 12.4 Lipoma

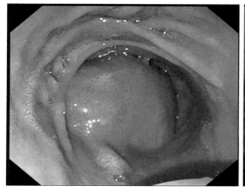
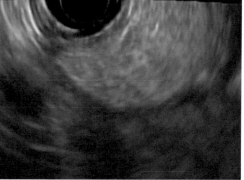

with a typical appearance on endoscopy or EUS [35]. It is proposed that a pancreatic rest should be removed when it is enlarging or the diagnosis is in doubt, besides lesions causing symptoms [34]. Endoscopic resection appears safe and effective in small-sized lesions (∼1 cm) [35].

Spindle Cell Lesions: GIST and Leiomyoma

GISTs are the most common soft tissue sarcoma of the GI tract. They can arise anywhere along the digestive tract, the stomach being the most common primary site (60%) followed by jejunum and ileum (30%). Duodenal GISTs account for 4–5% and rectal GISTs 4% [38, 39].

GISTs have an incidence of 14–20 per million. They are typically found in older adults (median age of 60–65 years). There is a slight male preponderance. Cases are extremely rare in patients younger than 21 years [40].

Close to a third of GISTs are asymptomatic and found incidentally during surgery, imaging, or endoscopy. Of those with symptoms, most present with ulcer-like symptoms or GI bleeding [40].

All GISTs are potentially malignant. Risk of metastases depends on tumor site, size, and mitotic index. For GISTs with malignant behavior, the most common sites of metastases are the liver and peritoneal cavity [40]. Lymph node metastases are extremely rare [39]. It can take up to several years before a primary GIST metastasizes [40].

Most gastrointestinal smooth muscle tumors referred to in the older literature as leiomyomas, leiomyosarcomas, and leiomyoblastomas would now be considered GISTs [38]. However, there remains a subset of GI smooth muscle tumors referred to as leiomyomas (or "true" leiomyomas), leiomyosarcomas, and leiomyoblastomas which are distinct from GISTs. Whereas all GISTs are considered to have malignant potential, leiomyomas are essentially invariably benign [41]. They are more common than GISTs in the esophagus [38]. They stain positive for desmin and negative for c-KIT (CD117) antigenic stain, in contrast to GISTs

which stain positive for c-KIT and negative for desmin [42, 43].

On EUS, GISTs and leiomyomas appear as hypoechoic, well-marginated tumors, mostly arising from the muscularis propria, but they can also originate from the muscularis mucosa (Fig. 12.5, Video 12.1) [9, 44]. Compared to leiomyomas, GISTs are sometimes more hyperechoic relative to the surrounding muscle echo. Marginal halo and hyperechogenic foci are also found more commonly in GISTs [41].

Biopsy of a primary GIST is needed before preoperative therapy at most institutions [39]. Needle aspiration or biopsy using EUS is preferred over the percutaneous route due to risk of intra-abdominal tumor dissemination, although percutaneous biopsy can be used to confirm metastasis [39]. Ninety-five percent of GISTs express the tyrosine kinase c-KIT (CD117). Immunohistochemical staining for CD 117 confirms the diagnosis. For c-KIT-negative GISTs, immunostaining for DOG1, a chloride channel protein, can be used [39]. Tissue obtained via needle aspiration or biopsy is not always adequate for immunostaining. Other techniques (such as incision or unroofing before biopsy) can be employed to increase tissue acquisition [45]. EUS core needle sampling is often superior to routine cytology with regard to obtaining adequate tissue for immunostaining.

CT with intravenous contrast is the initial imaging modality of choice for biopsy-proven GISTs. It allows for evaluation of extent of disease and the presence of metastases, thus conveying overall staging. A patient with a GIST can subsequently undergo surgery if there are no metastases and resection does not carry a significant risk of morbidity. If there is increased surgical morbidity (such as with pancreaticoduodenectomy for duodenal GISTs or esophagectomy for esophageal GISTs), preoperative imatinib or sunitinib scan be administered to allow for potential downstaging prior to surgery [39]. If there is response, resection should be considered. For progressive disease, options include radiofrequency ablation, embolization or chemoembolization, dose escalation of imatinib, and palliative radiotherapy

Fig. 12.5 Gastrointestinal stromal tumor

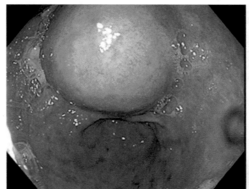
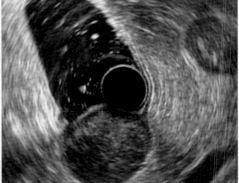

[39]. Endosonographic surveillance every 6–12 months is an option for gastric GISTs <2 cm without high-risk EUS features such as irregular border, cystic spaces, ulceration, echogenic foci, and heterogeneity, and many patients select observation, especially if they have other comorbidities that would make surgery high risk [39].

Carcinoid Tumors

Neuroendocrine aka carcinoid tumors are slow-growing tumors that arise from neuroendocrine cells and can occur anywhere in the body. The majority of these tumors (86%) are found in the GI tract [46]. Based on SEER registry data, the incidence of neuroendocrine tumors has increased from 1.09 per 100,000 in 1973 to 5.25 per 100,000 as of 2004, likely as a result of the explosive growth and use of endoscopy which identifies many of these lesions [46]. Gastric and duodenal carcinoids are most often diagnosed in the seventh decade of life [46, 47].

The most common site for digestive tract carcinoids is the rectum (29.8% of GI carcinoids), followed by jejunum and ileum (23.2%), stomach (10.4%), colon (6.9%), and duodenum (6.6%) [46]. This is a shift from earlier studies which showed the appendix as the most common site (42.7–49.4%) [47].

Most GI carcinoid tumors are asymptomatic. If present, symptoms include abdominal pain, vomiting, and GI bleeding [48]. Carcinoid syndrome (diarrhea, flushing, abdominal pain) is more common with extra-gastrointestinal primary (such as lung or bronchi) but can occur with GI carcinoids in the setting of liver metastases [49]. Primary GI carcinoids alone do not cause carcinoid syndrome as the biologically active metabolites are destroyed on first pass metabolism through the liver.

On endoscopy, carcinoid tumors can have varying appearances. In some cases, a carcinoid tumor appears as a smooth, round, subepithelial mass with yellowish hue, sometimes with a central depression. In other cases, the lesion can appear to be mucosal in nature. Most carcinoid lesions are firm when probed with a closed biopsy forceps. Most GI carcinoids are small (75% <1 cm) [48], but a tumor size of 23 cm has been reported [50]. EUS often shows a homogenous isoechoic or slightly hypoechoic mass, arising mostly from the submucosa layer (Fig. 12.6) [12]. It can also originate from the muscularis propria or even the mucosa [51]. Forceps biopsy is usually diagnostic [27].

Microscopically, carcinoid tumors show a typical pattern of small round or cuboidal cells with uniform dark nuclei, forming nests or islands and cords, in stroma made up of fibrous tissue and blood vessels [48]. Most stain positive for chromogranin A and synaptophysin [52].

Management of foregut carcinoids depends on several factors including tumor site, size, disease extent, and patient status (particularly surgical risk). Contrast-enhanced CT scans of the chest, abdomen and pelvis are recommended to evaluate for metastases [49]. For locoregional carcinoids in the duodenum, endoscopic resection is recommended if feasible, followed by surveillance endoscopy. EUS helps assess candidacy of a GI carcinoid for endoscopic resection. Extension into the muscularis propria, the presence of per-ilesional lymphadenopathy, and size >2 cm are findings that indicate a tumor is likely not amenable to resection via endoscopy [18].

In the management of gastric carcinoids, gastrin level needs to be measured to determine its type. For non-metastatic type 1 gastric carcinoids (associated with atrophic gastritis) with solitary or multiple tumors <2 cm, treatment options are endoscopic resection or observation. Endoscopy every 6–12 months for the first 3 years or annually thereafter should be performed, and if new lesions arise or tumor size increases, antrectomy should be considered [49]. For type 2 gastric carcinoid, which is associated with a true gastrinoma of the pancreas or the duodenum, the gastrin-producing tumor should be resected or enucleated.

Fig. 12.6 Carcinoid tumor

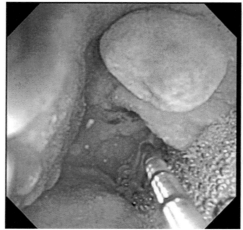
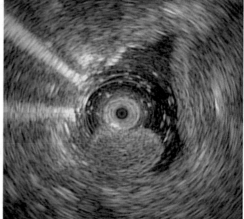

Proton pump inhibitors should be given to manage gastric hypersecretion and its attendant complications including diarrhea, peptic ulcer disease, reflux, and esophagitis. Type 3 gastric carcinoids are true sporadic lesions that arise in the setting of a normal serum gastrin level. These lesions are usually treated by primary gastric resection with lymphadenectomy as they tend to have a more aggressive nature. However, for a small (<2 cm) intraepithelial tumor, endoscopic or wedge resection may be considered [53]. Annual CT or MRI up to 10 years post-resection should be considered for type 3 gastric carcinoid [49].

Schwannoma

Schwannomas are rare mesenchymal tumors originating from nerve cell sheaths. They comprise 7.8% of mesenchymal tumors in the GI tract [54]. Most cases are found in individuals 30–50 years old (age range 10–90 years) [55–57]. GI tract schwannomas are more common among women, with varying female predominance [56].

The stomach is the most common site of GI tract schwannomas. Esophageal and small bowel schwannomas are rare [55, 56, 58]. Most gastric lesions are asymptomatic [56, 59]. Of those with symptoms, the most common complaint is abdominal pain. Gastric outlet obstruction can also occur with large lesions. Among patients with esophageal schwannoma, the predominant symptom is dysphagia [60]. A schwannoma in any site of the foregut can present with GI bleeding [55–58]. Reported lesion diameters range from 0.5 to 15.5 cm [56]. On endoscopy, a central depression or ulcer can be seen [54, 58].

EUS usually reveals a hypoechoic, well-defined lesion, similar to other mesenchymal tumors. The layer of origin for most GI schwannomas is the submucosa or the muscularis propria [54, 56], but they may also arise from the mucosa and serosa [55, 56].

Histologic analysis of schwannomas usually shows spindle cells with a lymphocytic peritumoral cuff [54, 56]. The hallmark for diagnosis is strong reactivity to S100 protein on immunohistochemistry [55]. Schwannomas also stain positive for neuron-specific enolase and Leu 7 antigen [55].

Reported cases of malignant foregut schwannomas are rare. Most investigators consider a mitotic index of 5 or more per 50 high power fields as the most reliable histologic factor that correlates with malignancy [61]. However, not all schwannomas with high rates of mitoses per high power field are malignant [56]. Clinically, malignancy should be suspected if there is an increase in size of the lesion over time or if symptoms are present [61]. Given that these cases are rare, the degree of size increase is considered significant

although the optimal timing of surveillance endoscopy is unclear. Surgical resection or enucleation is satisfactory in most patients with symptomatic schwannomas. Endoscopic removal (via snare, tunneling resection, excavation, or full thickness resection) has been reported for lesions up to 2.5 cm [21, 55]. A more extensive surgery (esophagectomy, partial gastrectomy) is preferred if there is evidence of non-metastatic malignancy [61].

Granular Cell Tumor

Granular cell tumors (GCTs) are tumors of neurogenic (Schwann cell) origin that can occur in different sites of the body. About 5–11% are found in the GI tract [62]. They are often diagnosed in the fifth decade of life. One-fourth to one-third of digestive tract GCTs occur in the esophagus [62, 63].

Most foregut GCTs are asymptomatic [62, 64]. Esophageal GCTs >1 cm can present with dysphagia [62]. GCTs appear as a firm white-gray to yellow nodule or plaque on endoscopy [64, 65]. They are usually solitary [62, 64, 66]. Size ranges from 0.1 to 10 cm [62, 66]. The majority (up to 75%) of GCTs are <1 cm in size [62, 64]. On EUS, they appear as a hypoechoic, homogenous, or mildly inhomogenous lesion, with smooth margins (Fig. 12.7) [12, 64, 67]. Most arise from the muscularis mucosa or submucosa. Rarely, the muscularis propria is involved [64, 66, 67].

Microscopically, a GCT consists of sheets of cells with a small, centrally located nucleus and a fine granular eosinophilic cytoplasm, hence the name [62]. Immunohistochemical staining is positive for S100 protein, neuron-specific enolase, laminin, and various myelin proteins [62]. Ninety-three to one hundred percent express CD56 [66]. Forceps biopsy can be diagnostic in 50–59% of foregut GCTs [66, 67]. Yield increases to 95% with snaring [67]. Most gastrointestinal GCTs are benign. Approximately 2–4% of GCTs are malignant. In general, distinction between benign and malignant GCTs cannot be made based on histology [62].

There is no universal agreement regarding the management of asymptomatic digestive tract GCTs. Symptomatic cases should be resected. Options for resection include EMR, ESD, submucosal tunneling endoscopic resection (STER), and surgery [63, 64]. In patients with esophageal GCTs without dysphagia, some authors do not recommend routine follow-up endoscopy; however, patients should be advised to contact their physicians should dysphagia develop [62]. Other authors recommend periodic follow-up with EGD and EUS. When the tumor is seen invading the deeper layers of the gut wall, surgical resection is warranted [67]. Optimal follow-up interval and duration are unclear.

Fig. 12.7 Granular cell tumor (hypoechoic spindle-shaped lesion between the *arrows*)

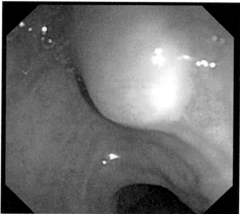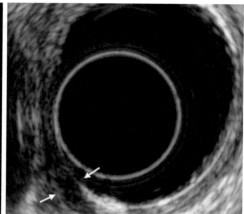

Duplication Cyst

Congenital cystic malformations are rare lesions of the GI tract. These are most commonly duplication cysts of gastrointestinal or bronchogenic origin. These cysts vary in their cyst lining and wall contents, suggesting different embryonic origins. Other differentials for cystic lesions in the GI tract include mesenteric cysts, pancreatic cysts, choledochal cysts, and splenic cysts [11, 68].

Proposed theories regarding the development of duplication cysts include errors of recanalization and fusion of longitudinal folds, adhesion of notochord and embryonic endoderm, and persistent embryological diverticula. No single theory may be satisfactory [69].

Symptomatic duplication cysts are found more commonly in children (majority in the first 3 months of life) and rarely in adults [69, 70]. Many adults with duplication cysts have these identified as incidental findings on endoscopy or imaging performed for other reasons. The reported age range for duplication cysts is from newborn to 83 years [11, 69, 71]. Female-to-male ratio is 1:1–3:1 [11, 68, 69].

Duplication cysts can occur anywhere in the digestive tract. Fifteen to forty-two percent are found in the esophagus, 2–12% in the duodenum, and 2–8% in the stomach [11, 69, 71, 72]. Most patients with esophageal and gastric duplication cysts are asymptomatic, although esophageal duplication cysts can cause dysphagia and/or chest pain [70, 73]. Duodenal duplication cysts present with non-specific complaints including abdominal pain, nausea, and vomiting [11, 74]. Up to 53% of duodenal duplication cysts are complicated with pancreatitis [11], possibly by intermittent blockage of the pancreatic duct by the cyst or cyst contents [11, 74]. Spontaneous cyst infection can also occur [11, 73].

Duplication cysts appear as a soft, round, or ovoid subepithelial lesion on endoscopy [68, 74]. The overlying mucosa is usually normal appearing. Size ranges from <1 to 13 cm. Most duodenal cysts are to 2–4 cm in diameter [11].

On EUS, a duplication cyst appears as a well-defined, homogenous, anechoic structure. Cyst wall layers can also be appreciated, often allowing them to be diagnosed just based on EUS alone [51, 68].

Duplication cysts can be demonstrated on CT and MRI. CT shows a well-circumscribed, walled lesion with a fluid or homogenous low density [69, 74]. On MRI, cysts appear hyperintense on T2-weighted images. The cyst content typically does not enhance, but wall enhancement can be seen when a cyst is infected [70, 73]. Gastric and duodenal duplication cysts sometimes communicate with the bile duct or pancreatic duct, and this can be demonstrated by an MRCP. Duplication cysts can be diagnosed prenatally with ultrasound.

Biopsy and aspiration of a duplication cyst should, in general, be avoided due to risk of infection and obliteration of the surgical fields [72]. In some cases, duplication cysts can mimic other solid lesions and undergo FNA. If this occurs, patients can be treated with prophylactic antibiotics to reduce the risk of cyst infection. For symptomatic cases, organ-sparing surgical resection is preferred [11, 68, 71]. Endoscopic treatment (submucosal dissection, marsupialization, incision, and snare) is also an option [11, 68, 75].

It should be noted that malignancy can arise from a duplication cyst in rare cases [76]. Management of asymptomatic duplication cysts is controversial [71]. Some authors recommend treatment to prevent complications [11]. Others recommend watchful waiting [71].

Conclusion

A variety of mucosal and submucosal lesions are commonly encountered on upper endoscopy. Some of these lesions are completely benign with no malignant potential, while others warrant more aggressive investigation and, ultimately, removal. While EUS is not mandatory in the evaluation of all of these lesions, EUS combined with standard upper endoscopy can often allow for more definitive characterization of many of these lesions.

References

1. Hwang JH, Saunders MD, Rulyak SJ, Shaw S, Nietsch H, Kimmey MB. A prospective study comparing endoscopy and EUS in the evaluation of GI subepithelial masses. Gastrointest Endosc. 2005;62(2):202–8.
2. Rösch T, Kapfer B, Will U, Baronius W, Strobel M, Lorenz R, et al. Accuracy of endoscopic ultrasonography in upper gastrointestinal submucosal lesions: a prospective multicenter study. Scand J Gastroenterol. 2002;37(7):856–62.
3. Oztas E, Oguz D, Kurt M, Etik DO, Cicek B, Kekilli M, et al. Endosonographic evaluation of patients with suspected extraluminal compression or subepithelial lesions during upper gastrointestinal endoscopy. Eur J Gastroenterol Hepatol. 2011;23(7): 586–92.
4. Ardengh JC, Vaiciunas S, Kemp R, Venco F, Lima-Filho ER, dos Santos JS. Upper endoscopy versus endosonography in differential diagnosis of gastrointestinal bulging. Arq Gastroenterol. 2011;48 (4):236–41.
5. Lim YJ, Son HJ, Lee J-S, Byun YH, Suh HJ, Rhee PL, et al. Clinical course of subepithelial lesions detected on upper gastrointestinal endoscopy. World J Gastroenterol. 2010;16 (4):439–44.
6. Imaoka H, Sawaki A, Mizuno N, Takahashi K, Nakamura T, Tajika M, et al. Incidence and Clinical Course of Submucosal Lesions of the Stomach. Gastrointest Endosc. 2005;61(5):AB167.
7. Kushnir VM, Keswani RN, Hollander TG, Kohlmeier C, Mullady DK, Azar RR, et al. Compliance with surveillance recommendations for foregut subepithelial tumors is poor: results of a prospective multicenter study. Gastrointest Endosc. 2015;81 (6):1378–84.
8. Brand B, Oesterhelweg L, Binmoeller KF, Sriram PVJ, Bohnacker S, Seewald S, et al. Impact of endoscopic ultrasound for evaluation of submucosal lesions in gastrointestinal tract. Dig Liver Dis. 2002;34(4):290–7.
9. Seo SW, Hong SJ, Han JP, Choi MH, Song J-Y, Kim HK, et al. Accuracy of a scoring system for the differential diagnosis of common gastric subepithelial tumors based on endoscopic ultrasonography. J Dig Dis. 2013;14(12):647–53.
10. Kim M-Y, Jung H-Y, Choi KD, Song HJ, Lee JH, Kim DH, et al. Natural history of asymptomatic small gastric subepithelial tumors. J Clin Gastroenterol. 2011;45(4):330–6.
11. Chen J-J, Lee H-C, Yeung C-Y, Chan W-T, Jiang C-B, Sheu J-C. Meta-analysis: the clinical features of the duodenal duplication cyst. J Pediatr Surg. 2010;45(8):1598–606.
12. Boyce GA, Sivak MV, Rösch T, Classen M, Fleischer DE, Boyce HW, et al. Evaluation of submucosal upper gastrointestinal tract lesions by endoscopic ultrasound. Gastrointest Endosc. 1991;37(4):449–54.
13. Yasuda K, Cho E, Nakajima M, Kawai K. Diagnosis of submucosal lesions of the upper gastrointestinal tract by endoscopic ultrasonography. Gastrointest Endosc. 1990;36(2 Suppl): S17–20.
14. Zhang X-C, Li Q-L, Yu Y-F, Yao L-Q, Xu M-D, Zhang Y-Q, et al. Diagnostic efficacy of endoscopic ultrasound-guided needle sampling for upper gastrointestinal subepithelial lesions: a meta-analysis. Surg Endosc. 2015.
15. Karaca C, Turner BG, Cizginer S, Forcione D, Brugge W. Accuracy of EUS in the evaluation of small gastric subepithelial lesions. Gastrointest Endosc. 2010;71(4):722–7.
16. Nickl N, Gress F, McClave S, Fockens P, Chak A, Savides T, et al. Hypoechoic Intramural Tumor Study: Final Report. Gastrointest Endosc. 2002;55(5):AB98.
17. ASGE Technology Committee, Kantsevoy SV, Adler DG, Conway JD, Diehl DL, Farraye FA, et al. Endoscopic mucosal resection and endoscopic submucosal dissection. Gastrointest Endosc. 2008;68(1):11–8.
18. Varas MJ, Gornals JB, Pons C, Espinós JC, Abad R, Lorente FJ, et al. Usefulness of endoscopic ultrasonography (EUS) for selecting carcinoid tumors as candidates to endoscopic resection. Rev Esp Enferm Dig. 2010;102(10):577–82.
19. Bhatt A, Abe S, Kumaravel A, Vargo J, Saito Y. Indications and Techniques for Endoscopic Submucosal Dissection. Am J Gastroenterol. 2015;110(6):784–91.
20. Huang LY, Cui J, Lin SJ, Zhang B, Wu CR. Endoscopic full-thickness resection for gastric submucosal tumors arising from the muscularis propria layer. World J Gastroenterol. 2014;20 (38):13981–6.
21. Li B, Liang T, Wei L, Ma M, Huang Y, Xu H, et al. Endoscopic interventional treatment for gastric schwannoma: a single-center experience. Int J Clin Exp Pathol. 2014;7(10):6616–25.
22. Taylor AJ, Stewart ET, Dodds WJ. Gastrointestinal lipomas: a radiologic and pathologic review. AJR Am J Roentgenol. 1990;155(6):1205–10.
23. Regge D, Lo Bello G, Martincich L, Bianchi G, Cuomo G, Suriani R, et al. A case of bleeding gastric lipoma: US, CT and MR findings. Eur Radiol. 1999;9(2):256–8.
24. Okten RS, Kacar S, Kucukay F, Sasmaz N, Cumhur T. Gastric subepithelial masses: evaluation of multidetector CT (multiplanar reconstruction and virtual gastroscopy) versus endoscopic ultrasonography. Abdom Imaging. 2012;37(4):519–30.
25. Hwang JH, Rulyak SD, Kimmey MB. American Gastroenterological Association Institute. American Gastroenterological Association Institute technical review on the management of gastric subepithelial masses. Gastroenterology. 2006;130(7): 2217–28.
26. Matsushita M, Hajiro K, Okazaki K, Takakuwa H. Gastric aberrant pancreas: EUS analysis in comparison with the histology. Gastrointest Endosc. 1999;49(4 Pt 1):493–7.
27. Karita M, Tada M. Endoscopic and histologic diagnosis of submucosal tumors of the gastrointestinal tract using combined strip biopsy and bite biopsy. Gastrointest Endosc. 1994;40(6): 749–53.
28. Eckardt AJ, Wassef W. Diagnosis of subepithelial tumors in the GI tract. Endoscopy, EUS, and histology: bronze, silver, and gold standard? Gastrointest Endosc. 2005;62(2):209–12.
29. Alberti D, Grazioli L, Orizio P, Matricardi L, Dughi S, Gheza L, et al. Asymptomatic giant gastric lipoma: what to do? Am J Gastroenterol. 1999;94(12):3634–7.
30. Lemer J. Haemorrhage from a polypoid lipoma of duodenum. Proc R Soc Med. 1971;64(4):395.
31. Nakamura S, Iida M, Suekane H, Matsui T, Yao T, Fujishima M. Endoscopic removal of gastric lipoma: diagnostic value of endoscopic ultrasonography. Am J Gastroenterol. 1991;86 (5):619–21.
32. Lai EC, Tompkins RK. Heterotopic pancreas. Review of a 26 year experience. Am J Surg. 1986;151(6):697–700.
33. Trifan A, Târcoveanu E, Danciu M, Huţanaşu C, Cojocariu C, Stanciu C. Gastric heterotopic pancreas: an unusual case and review of the literature. J Gastrointestin Liver Dis. 2012;21 (2):209–12.

34. Faigel DO, Gopal D, Weeks DA, Corless C. Cap-assisted endoscopic submucosal resection of a pancreatic rest. Gastrointest Endosc. 2001;54(6):782–4.

35. Bain AJ, Owens DJ, Tang RS, Peterson MR, Savides TJ. Pancreatic rest resection using band ligation snare polypectomy. Dig Dis Sci. 2011;56(6):1884–8.

36. Otani Y, Yoshida M, Saikawa Y, Wada N, Kubota T, Kumai K, et al. Discrimination between gastric ectopic pancreas and mesenchymal tumours, including GIST—from 12 years' surgical experience in one institute. Aliment Pharmacol Ther. 2006;2 (1):292–6.

37. Kim J-H, Lim JS, Lee YC, Hyung WJ, Lee JH, Kim M-J, et al. Endosonographic features of gastric ectopic pancreases distinguishable from mesenchymal tumors. J Gastroenterol Hepatol. 2008;23(8 Pt 2):e301–7.

38. Miettinen M, Lasota J. Gastrointestinal stromal tumors–definition, clinical, histological, immunohistochemical, and molecular genetic features and differential diagnosis. Virchows Arch Int J Pathol. 2001;438(1):1–12.

39. National Comprehensive Cancer Network. Soft Tissue Sarcoma (Version 1.2015) [Internet] [cited 6 Nov 2015]. Available from http://www.nccn.org/professionals/physician_gls/pdf/sarcoma.pdf.

40. Miettinen M, Lasota J. Gastrointestinal stromal tumors. Gastroenterol Clin North Am. 2013;42(2):399–415.

41. Kim GH, Park DY, Kim S, Kim DH, Kim DH, Choi CW, et al. Is it possible to differentiate gastric GISTs from gastric leiomyomas by EUS? World J Gastroenterol. 2009;15(27):3376–81.

42. Kuhlgatz J, Sander B, Golas MM, Gunawan B, Schulze T, Schulten H-J, et al. Differential diagnosis of gastrointestinal leiomyoma versus gastrointestinal stromal tumor. Int J Colorectal Dis. 2006;21(1):84–8.

43. Stelow EB, Murad FM, Debol SM, Stanley MW, Bardales RH, Lai R, et al. A limited immunocytochemical panel for the distinction of subepithelial gastrointestinal mesenchymal neoplasms sampled by endoscopic ultrasound-guided fine-needle aspiration. Am J Clin Pathol. 2008;129(2):219–25.

44. Kim MN, Kang SJ, Kim SG, Im JP, Kim JS, Jung HC, et al. Prediction of risk of malignancy of gastrointestinal stromal tumors by endoscopic ultrasonography. Gut Liver. 2013;7(6):642–7.

45. de la Serna-Higuera C, Pérez-Miranda M, Díez-Redondo P, Gil-Simón P, Herranz T, Pérez-Martín E, et al. EUS-guided single-incision needle-knife biopsy: description and results of a new method for tissue sampling of subepithelial GI tumors (with video). Gastrointest Endosc. 2011;74(3):672–6.

46. Yao JC, Hassan M, Phan A, Dagohoy C, Leary C, Mares JE, et al. One hundred years after "carcinoid": epidemiology of and prognostic factors for neuroendocrine tumors in 35,825 cases in the United States. J Clin Oncol. 2008;26(18):3063–72.

47. Godwin JD. Carcinoid tumors. An analysis of 2837 cases. Cancer. 1975;36(2):560–9.

48. Crowder BL, Judd ES, Dockerty MB. Gastrointestinal carcinoids and the carcinoid syndrome: clinical characteristics and therapy. CA Cancer J Clin. 1968;18(4):212–8.

49. National Comprehensive Cancer Network. Neuroendocrine tumors (Version 1.2015) [Internet] [cited 9 Nov 2015]. Available from http://www.nccn.org/professionals/physician_gls/pdf/neuroendocrine.pdf.

50. Thomas RM, Baybick JH, Elsayed AM, Sobin LH. Gastric carcinoids. An immunohistochemical and clinicopathologic study of 104 patients. Cancer. 1994;73(8):2053–8.

51. Yasuda K, Nakajima M, Yoshida S, Kiyota K, Kawai K. The diagnosis of submucosal tumors of the stomach by endoscopic ultrasonography. Gastrointest Endosc. 1989;35(1):10–5.

52. Oberg K. Neuroendocrine gastrointestinal tumours. Ann Oncol. 1996;7(5):453–63.

53. Saund MS, Al Natour RH, Sharma AM, Huang Q, Boosalis VA, Gold JS. Tumor size and depth predict rate of lymph node metastasis and utilization of lymph node sampling in surgically managed gastric carcinoids. Ann Surg Oncol. 2011;18(10):2826–32.

54. Daimaru Y, Kido H, Hashimoto H, Enjoji M. Benign schwannoma of the gastrointestinal tract: a clinicopathologic and immunohistochemical study. Hum Pathol. 1988;19(3):257–64.

55. Naus PJ, Tio FO, Gross GW. Esophageal schwannoma: first report of successful management by endoscopic removal. Gastrointest Endosc. 2001;54(4):520–2.

56. Voltaggio L, Murray R, Lasota J, Miettinen M. Gastric schwannoma: a clinicopathologic study of 51 cases and critical review of the literature. Hum Pathol. 2012;43(5):650–9.

57. Takemura M, Yoshida K, Takii M, Sakurai K, Kanazawa A. Gastric malignant schwannoma presenting with upper gastrointestinal bleeding: a case report. J Med Case Rep. 2012;6:37.

58. Seno K, Itoh M, Endoh K, Joh T, Yokoyama Y, Takeuchi T, et al. Schwannoma of the duodenum causing melena. Intern Med Tokyo Jpn. 1994;33(10):621–3.

59. Hong HS, Ha HK, Won HJ, Byun JH, Shin YM, Kim AY, et al. Gastric schwannomas: radiological features with endoscopic and pathological correlation. Clin Radiol. 2008;63(5):536–42.

60. Vinhais SN, Cabrera RA, Nobre-Leitão C, Cunha TM. Schwannoma of the esophagus: computed tomography and endosonographic findings of a special type of schwannoma. Acta Radiol. 2004;45(7):718–20.

61. Wang S, Zheng J, Ruan Z, Huang H, Yang Z, Zheng J. Long-term survival in a rare case of malignant esophageal schwannoma cured by surgical excision. Ann Thorac Surg. 2011;92(1):357–8.

62. Voskuil JH, van Dijk MM, Wagenaar SS, van Vliet AC, Timmer R, van Hees PA. Occurrence of esophageal granular cell tumors in The Netherlands between 1988 and 1994. Dig Dis Sci. 2001;46 (8):1610–4.

63. Chen W, Zheng X, Jin L, Pan X, Ye M. Novel diagnosis and treatment of esophageal granular cell tumor: report of 14 cases and review of the literature. Ann Thorac Surg. 2014;97(1):296–302.

64. Nie L, Xu G, Wu H, Huang Q, Sun Q, Fan X. Granular cell tumor of the esophagus: a clinicopathological study of 31 cases. Int J Clin Exp Pathol. 2014;7(7):4000–7.

65. Lack EE, Worsham GF, Callihan MD, Crawford BE, Klappenbach S, Rowden G, et al. Granular cell tumor: a clinicopathologic study of 110 patients. J Surg Oncol. 1980;13(4):301–16.

66. An S, Jang J, Min K, Kim M-S, Park H, Park YS, et al. Granular cell tumor of the gastrointestinal tract: histologic and immunohistochemical analysis of 98 cases. Hum Pathol. 2015;46(6):813–9.

67. Palazzo L, Landi B, Cellier C, Roseau G, Chaussade S, Couturier D, et al. Endosonographic features of esophageal granular cell tumors. Endoscopy. 1997;29(9):850–3.

68. Eom JS, Kim GH, Song GA, Baek DH, Ryu KD, Lee KN, et al. Gastric duplication cyst removed by endoscopic submucosal dissection. Korean J Gastroenterol. 2011;58(6):346–9.

69. Kim DH, Kim JS, Nam ES, Shin HS. Foregut duplication cyst of the stomach. Pathol Int. 2000;50(2):142–5.

70. Scatizzi M, Calistri M, Feroci F, Girardi LR, Moraldi L, Rubio CA, et al. Gastric duplication cyst in an adult: case report. Vivo. 2005;19(6):975–8.

71. Geng Y-H, Wang C-X, Li J-T, Chen Q-Y, Li X-Z, Pan H. Gastric foregut cystic developmental malformation: case series and literature review. World J Gastroenterol. 2015;21(2):432–8.

72. Soares R, Gasparaitis A, Waxman I, Chennat J, Patti M. Esophageal duplication cyst. Dis Esophagus. 2011;24(3):E21–2.

73. Agarwal A, Singla S, Bansal M, Ozdemir A. Infected esophageal duplication cyst masquerading as pericarditis. Intern Med Tokyo Jpn. 2012;51(6):689–90.

74. Carbognin G, Guarise A, Biasiutti C, Pagnotta N, Procacci C. Duodenal duplication cyst identified with MRCP. Eur Radiol. 2000;10(8):1277–9.

75. Lee YC, Kim YB, Kim JK, Shin SJ, Hwang JC, Lim SG, et al. Endoscopic treatment of a large gastric duplication cyst with hook-knife and snare (with video). Gastrointest Endosc. 2011;73 (5):1039–40.

76. Kuraoka K, Nakayama H, Kagawa T, Ichikawa T, Yasui W. Adenocarcinoma arising from a gastric duplication cyst with invasion to the stomach: a case report with literature review. J Clin Pathol. 2004;57(4):428–31.

Thiruvengadam Muniraj and Linda S. Lee

Introduction

Enteroscopy is defined as direct endoscopic examination of the small intestine, extending into the jejunum and/or the ileum with use of a fiberoptic endoscope [1]. While capsule endoscopy is often used to evaluate the small intestine, enteroscopy is needed for interventions. Due to the long length ($\sim$450 cm) and tortuous nature of the small intestine without significant anchoring points, deep enteroscopy has remained more challenging than routine endoscopy which includes esophagogastroduodenoscopy (EGD) and colonoscopy. Recent innovations in endoscopy and introduction of newer device-assisted deep enteroscopic techniques have made examination of entire small intestine possible. Such devices include double-balloon enteroscopy (DBE), single-balloon enteroscopy (SBE), spiral enteroscopy (SE), and the most recent through-the-scope balloon-assisted enteroscopy.

History of Enteroscopy

About 30 years ago, the modalities available to examine the small bowel were imaging techniques including small bowel follow-through and small bowel enteroclysis, and if any lesion was identified, the patient was taken to surgery for intraoperative enteroscopy. Intraoperative enteroscopes (IOE) with rigid sigmoidoscope passed through operative laparotomy were initially used in the 1950s [2]. Then in the 1970s, flexible endoscopes were available for intraoperative enteroscopy with or without enterotomy. IOE had a high diagnostic yield, but was accompanied by high surgical morbidity [2, 3].

Sonde enteroscopy was first proposed as a non-operative way to examine the small intestine [4, 5]. The sonde enteroscope (Olympus SIF-SW) (Fig. 13.1) was introduced in 1986 and claimed as a better tool than small bowel imaging available at that time in management of small bowel diseases [6, 7]. It is a thin floppy scope with a balloon tip which is generally passed transnasally and advances by exploiting intestinal peristalsis [5, 8]. Endoscopic examination of the small bowel is performed during withdrawal of the scope. It has no biopsy or therapeutic channel and, therefore, is solely a diagnostic tool. Due to prolonged procedure time, poor tolerance by the patient, limited visualization due to lack of tip deflection, uncontrolled nature of withdrawal, and lack of biopsy/therapeutic capabilities, sonde enteroscopy never became very popular and is obsolete now. However, by proving that better evaluation of small bowel was possible than conventional imaging, it led to innovations with future enteroscopic devices [9–11].

In the 1990s, **push enteroscopy (PE)** was introduced as an alternative using a specifically designed enteroscope with or without an overtube, or a colonoscope without an overtube [13]. PE is limited to examining the proximal 100–150 cm of the small intestine, compared with the overriding advantage of sonde enteroscopy which was capable of examining the entire small intestine [14]. The combination of push and sonde enteroscopy has been proven valuable in the evaluation of obscure gastrointestinal bleeding [15]. The diagnostic yield of push enteroscopy ranges from as low as 3% to as high as 70%, with the majority of findings being vascular lesions [16–18]. The main disadvantages of PE are looping of the enteroscope, patient discomfort, and the inability to examine the distal small bowel.

Electronic supplementary material
Supplementary material is available in the online version of this chapter at 10.1007/978-3-319-49041-0_13. Videos can also be accessed at https://link.springer.com/chapter/10.1007/978-3-319-49041-0_13.

T. Muniraj
Section of Digestive Diseases, Yale University School of Medicine, New Haven, CT 06520, USA
e-mail: thiruvengadam.muniraj@yale.edu

L.S. Lee (✉)
Division of Gastroenterology, Hepatology and Endoscopy, Brigham and Women's Hospital, Harvard Medical School, Boston, MA 02115, USA
e-mail: lslee@partners.org

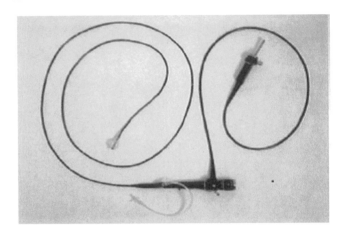

Fig. 13.1 Sonde enteroscope [12]

The landscape changed dramatically in 2001 with the introduction of wireless video capsule endoscopy (VCE) [19, 20] which revolutionized small bowel endoscopic imaging making sonde enteroscopy a rarely used procedure and PE often limited to patients with proximal small bowel lesions seen on VCE.

Currently, three different VCEs (PillCam, Covidien Inc., Dublin, Ireland; Endocapsule EC-10, Olympus America Inc., Center Valley, PA, USA; and MiroCam Intromedic Co Ltd, Seoul, Korea) are commercially available. Once swallowed, their battery last for 8–10 h and all three can take approximately 2 pictures every second. We have over a decade of experience using VCE, and the diagnostic yield is around 60% [21–23]. If an abnormality is detected with VCE, deep enteroscopy is then performed. As VCE was widely adopted, identification of small bowel lesions led to innovations in enteroscopes with the development of DBE in 2001 [24], SBE in 2007 [25], SE in 2008[26], and most recently through-the-scope single-balloon enteroscopy (TTS-SBE) in 2013[27].

Indications for Deep Enteroscopy

Deep enteroscopy has both diagnostic and therapeutic applications. The most common indication for deep enteroscopy is evaluation of obscure gastrointestinal (GI) bleeding [28]. Other indications include evaluation of imaging abnormalities, anemia, small bowel Crohn's disease, strictures, ulcers, polyps, masses, foreign bodies, lymphoma, other infiltrative diseases, and jejunal feeding tube placement (Table 13.1). While any procedure performed with a gastroscope or colonoscope can be accomplished with an enteroscope, due to looping and difficulty in advancing tools out of the biopsy channel, it may be challenging to perform

more complex therapeutics such as endoscopic mucosal resection and endoscopic submucosal dissection.

Double-Balloon Enteroscopy (DBE)

DBE is a novel enteroscopy technique first reported in Japan by Hironori Yamamoto in 2001 [24], and commercially developed by Fujinon Corporation (Tokyo, Japan). This is also known as '**push-and-pull enteroscopy**' [55], which uses a novel method whereby an endoscope and a soft flexible overtube, each of which has an inflatable balloon attached to its distal end, are employed together and an external pump system aids in inflating the balloons; both balloons can be inflated and deflated separately [56]. There is a standard 200-cm-long DBE scope (Fujinon EN-450P5) with 8.5 mm outer diameter and 2.2 mm channel size (Fig. 13.2) and also a couple of therapeutic DBE scopes (Fujinon EN-450T5 and Fujinon EN-450T5/W), which accommodate both endoscopic retrograde cholangiopancreatography (ERCP) and colonoscopy accessories with 2.8 and 3.2 mm working channels. The slim Fujinon EN-450P5 aids smooth antegrade insertion enabling visualization for diagnostic purposes, whereas the Fujinon EN-450T5 and Fujinon EN-450T5/W scopes allow the use of almost all therapeutic accessories including the argon plasma coagulation (APC) probe, hemoclip, and diathermic coagulator. A shorter 152-cm-long therapeutic DBE scope with 2.8 mm working channel (Fujinon EC-450BI5) is primarily used for cases of incomplete colonoscopy and for ERCP in patients with surgically altered anatomy (Table 13.2).

Once the DBE with the overtube is inserted in the usual fashion into the small bowel, the endoscope is advanced through the overtube with the inflated balloon on the overtube acting as an anchor maintaining a stable position (Fig. 13.3). Once the enteroscope has been advanced as far as possible, the enteroscope balloon is inflated, the overtube balloon deflated, and the overtube advanced along the enteroscope. Then the overtube balloon is inflated followed by reduction of loops by pulling back on both the overtube and the enteroscope. The enteroscope balloon is deflated to allow further advancement of the enteroscope. The process is repeated until the entire small bowel is visualized or the farthest extent is reached at which point tattoo should be applied (see Video 13.1). Either the enteroscope balloon or the overtube balloon or both are kept inflated at all times to maintain anchorage in the small intestine, enabling the steady insertion of the enteroscope (Fig. 13.3). DBE is used in the retrograde approach as well as with intubation of the ileum. The depth of insertion is greater with the antegrade than with the retrograde approach (360 $\pm$ 178 cm versus 182 $\pm$ 165 cm from the pylorus, $p < 0.0001$) [58].

Table 13.1 Common indications for deep enteroscopy

1. Obscure GI bleeding—evaluation and control [29]
2. Evaluation of abnormal lesions noted in imaging (VCE, CT, CTE, MRE)—small bowel tumors/polyps [30–34]
3. Work-up of iron-deficiency anemia [35, 36]
4. Placement of jejunal feeding tube [37, 38]
5. Evaluation of symptoms in patients with altered GI anatomy—e.g., Roux-en-Y gastric bypass and Billroth-II [39–41]
6. Evaluation of NSAID-related small bowel injury [42]
7. Evaluation of Crohn's disease [43]
8. Evaluation of malabsorption and celiac disease [44, 45]
9. Stricture balloon dilation [46, 47]
10. ERCP in altered anatomy [48–52]
11. Polyp surveillance in patients with familial adenomatous polyposis (FAP) [53]
12. Foreign body retrieval [54]

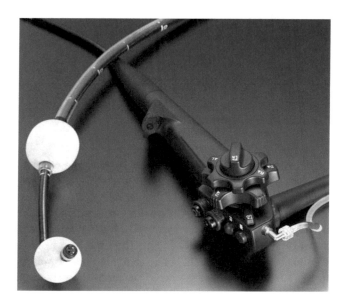

Fig. 13.2 Double-balloon enteroscope (*Courtesy* Fujinon Corporation)

Table 13.2 Double-balloon endoscope specifications

	EN-450P5	EN-450T5	EN-450T5/W	EC-450BI5
Field of view	120°	140°		
Distal end diameter (mm)	8.5	9.4		
Bending capcity				
Up/down	180°			
Left/right	160°			
Forceps channel diameter (mm)	2.2	2.8		
Working length (mm)	2000			1520
Total length (mm)	2300			1820

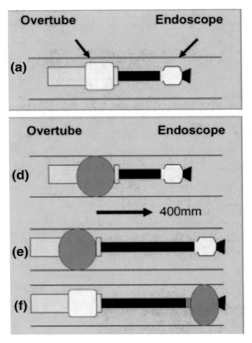

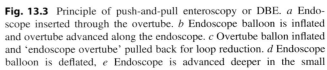

Fig. 13.3 Principle of push-and-pull enteroscopy or DBE. *a* Endoscope inserted through the overtube. *b* Endoscope balloon is inflated and overtube advanced along the endoscope. *c* Overtube ballon inflated and 'endoscope overtube' pulled back for loop reduction. *d* Endoscope balloon is deflated, *e* Endoscope is advanced deeper in the small intestine. *f* Endoscope balloon is inflated and overtube advanced along the endoscope. *g* Overtube balloon is inflated, and after a pull back of 'endoscope overtube' to straighten the scope, endoscope balloon is deflated and endoscope advanced further [57] (Reproduced with permission)

DBE is superior to PE with a higher success rate for deep small bowel intubation and an increased diagnostic yield [59]. The diagnostic yield using DBE is between 40 and 80% leading to a subsequent change in management in 57–84% of patients [58–61]. On a review from 66 studies, Xin et al. noted an overall rate of positive findings of 68% with the highest diagnostic yield (86%) occurring for the indication of small bowel obstruction. Inflammatory lesions were most commonly identified in overall 33% of cases followed by vascular lesions in 29% and neoplasms in 23% [62]. For the indication of small bowel GI bleeding, vascular lesions were most frequent in 40% followed by inflammatory lesions in 30% and neoplastic lesions in 22%.

Although the detection rate for obscure GI bleeding with VCE is superior to DBE, these procedures are complementary. An initial diagnostic imaging employing VCE might be followed by therapeutic and interventional DBE [63]. The time index, defined as lesion location as a percentage of the mouth–cecum time [64], from VCE helps in choosing the best insertion route (antegrade vs. retrograde) for DBE [65], and also VCE-directed DBE increases the diagnostic yield in obscure GI bleeding [66]. It has been suggested that the retrograde DBE approach should be the initial approach when the lesion is at a location greater than 75% of the timeline of the capsule study (i.e., time index >0.75) [64].

The success rate of total enteroscopy ranges widely from 20 to 44% with 98% of the successful cases requiring both an antegrade and a retrograde approach [62, 67] Given such low-to-average success rates of total enteroscopy with DBE, endoscopists should remember to set expectations not only to patients, but also to themselves to avoid disappointment and to avoid unduly prolonging the procedure.

The complication rates with DBE range from 2 to 9% [62, 67] and apart from the usual expected complications, which include perforation, bleeding, and aspiration pneumonia, pancreatitis is seen in some cases (0.5%) [68, 69]. The cause for pancreatitis in DBE (when ERCP is not performed) is thought to be prolonged inflation of the balloon near the ampulla. Of note, perforation is significantly higher (3%) in patients with post-surgical anatomy, especially with the retrograde approach (10%) [68].

Relative Contraindications for DBE

As with any other endoscopic procedure, DBE should not be performed whenever a small bowel perforation or high-grade intestinal obstruction is suspected or the risks of the procedure outweigh the potential benefits. DBE involves forceful distention and traction, and therefore, conditions with pre-existing weakened intestinal wall, such as recently created intestinal anastomosis, severely ulcerated small intestine, and small bowel lymphoma undergoing active chemotherapy is susceptible to perforation with DBE [70].

Learning Curve for DBE

As with other procedures, technical skill in performing DBE improves with experience. While some studies show no learning curve for antegrade DBE [71], others demonstrate a significant decline in overall procedural time and fluoroscopy time after the initial 10 DBE cases [58]. The average time taken for adequate insertion is long and reported as 102 ± 38 min [58]. The improvement in procedure duration was observed only for anterograde cases, and not with retrograde examinations. About 30 retrograde cases are required for stable overtube intubation into the ileum [71]. More than 150 DBE procedures are necessary for increased rate of total enteroscopy and helpful DBEs that provide definitive explanation of symptoms or imaging abnormality, therapy, or guide management [72].

Single-Balloon Enteroscopy (SBE)

The SBE system was first introduced in 2007 by Olympus Corporation [25, 56]. SBE uses an enteroscope with a 2.8 mm working channel and an overtube which is equipped with a silicone balloon at its tip that can be inflated and deflated (Fig. 13.4) [25]. There is no balloon attached to the enteroscope. The basic insertion technique is similar for both SBE and DBE. However, in SBE the scope tip is deflected to anchor onto the small intestine, rather than using a second

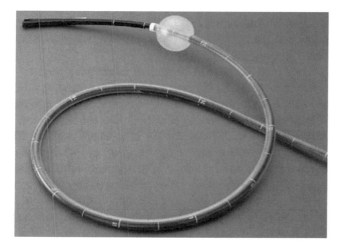

Fig. 13.4 Single-balloon enteroscope (*Courtesy* Olympus America Inc. Center Valley, PA, USA)

balloon. The overtube is advanced to the distal portion of the scope at which point the overtube balloon is inflated. The enteroscope tip is subsequently returned to luminal view and advanced as far as possible. At this point, the enteroscope scope is deflected for anchoring, the overtube balloon is deflated, and the overtube advanced over the enteroscope. The overtube balloon is inflated, the tip of the enteroscope is straightened, and both the overtube and enteroscope are reduced. This pleats the small intestine onto the overtube, and the enteroscope can be advanced again. This sequential technique of advancement and withdrawal is repeated until the scope can no longer be advanced or the target lesion is reached (Fig. 13.5) (see Video 13.1). When compared to DBE, SBE is technically easier to perform and appears to provide similar diagnostic and therapeutic yield [73, 74]. With SBE, a mean distance of 203.8 ± 87.6 cm from the pylorus with the antegrade approach and 72.1 ± 41.1 cm from the ICV with the retrograde approach can be achieved [74]. Both SBE and DBE are useful in performing ERCP in patients with surgically altered anatomy [40, 75, 76].

Spiral Overtube-Assisted Endoscopy (SE)

Spiral enteroscopy, which was originally designed as a urinary catheter in 2006, is a newer technique for deep small bowel intubation that uses a special single-use overtube [Discovery Small Bowel (DSB)] with soft spiral coils to pleat small bowel and facilitate antegrade small bowel enteroscopy. The DSB is 118 cm long with 16 mm outer diameter and 9.8 mm inner diameter, which accommodates an enteroscope or pediatric colonoscope [78]. The proximal end of the overtube has two handles for rotation, a locking device, and a port for lubrication. Using the DSB overtube over enteroscopes was first reported in 2008, [26] and DSB was also FDA approved in 2008 as an overtube (Endo-Ease Discovery SB, Spirus Medical, Stoughton, MA) that facilitates endoluminal advancement through the small intestine (Fig. 13.6). The overtube is lubricated and locked onto the enteroscope with the distal end of the overtube ending 25 cm proximal to the tip of the scope. If general anesthesia is used, the endotracheal balloon should be deflated as the DSB is advanced into the esophagus. Once the enteroscope is distal to the ligament of Treitz, the overtube is unlocked and the scope advanced forward. The overtube is then advanced to the tip of the scope, locked in place, and clockwise rotation of the Discovery SB is performed, similar to the mechanism used with a corkscrew. This pleats the small bowel onto the overtube. Then the overtube is unlocked, the enteroscope advanced forward, and the handles rotated counterclockwise to release the mucosa from the overtube. The Discovery SB overtube should be fixed to the enteroscope for spiral

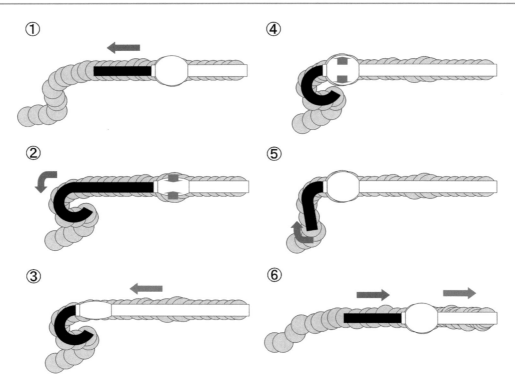

Fig. 13.5 Principles of insertion in SBE [1]. Insert enteroscope as deep as possible [2]. Angulate the enteroscope to anchor it on the intestinal wall and deflate the balloon [3]. Advance the overtube along the enteroscope [4]. Inflate the balloon to fix the tube to the intestinal wall [5]. Release the angulation [6]. Withdraw the overtube and enteroscope to shorten the intestine. From Kawamura et al. [77], with the permission from Elsevier

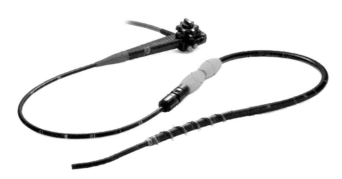

Fig. 13.6 Spiral enteroscopy–endo-ease discovery SB system (*Courtesy* of Spirus Medical)

advancement or unlocked when conventional manipulation of the endoscope is needed.

The maximum depth of insertion beyond the ligament of Treitz (approximately 250 cm) for SE is comparable with DBE and SBE [79–81]. While the procedure time of about 60 min does not significantly differ between SBE and DBE, the mean procedure time is significantly less with SE (41 min) than with DBE or SBE [74, 82]. Recent prospective studies concluded that the only advantage of SE is that it involves significantly shorter examination times, but that SE was no better than DBE with regard to the depth of insertion or the rate of complete enteroscopies achieved [81, 83]. Complication rates with SE are similar to that of DE [84].

Spiral enteroscopy can be performed in post-gastric surgery patients and used for ERCP in surgically altered anatomy. Spiral-assisted ERCP (SE-ERCP) in patients with Roux-en-Y anatomy is comparable with SBE-assisted ERCP in terms of successful cannulation (40 and 48%, respectively) and therapy (89 and 100%, respectively), procedure time, and complications [85].

Spiral enteroscopy can be used in a retrograde approach to visualize the ileum. A newer modification of the overtube, Endo-Ease Vista Retrograde (Spirus Medical, Stoughton, MA), was demonstrated to have high success rate in intubation of the terminal ileum [86]. In a recent study of 22 patients who underwent retrograde spiral enteroscopy, the terminal ileum was intubated in all patients with median depth of insertion from the ileocecal valve of 100 cm (range 50–150 cm) [86]. Similar to DBE and SBE, prior VCE results seem helpful in determining the route of SE and increasing the diagnostic yield for spiral enteroscopy [87].

Through-the-Scope Single-Balloon Enteroscopy

In 2013, a novel through-the-scope (TTS) single-balloon enteroscope system (NaviAid™ AB Advancing Balloon, Pentax Medical, Tokyo, Japan) was introduced. Through-the-scope balloon-assisted enteroscopy (TTS-BAE) is a novel technique that utilizes a standard endoscope with a 3.7 mm working channel without the need for an overtube. The TTS balloon system includes a single-use latex-free balloon catheter designed for anchoring in the small bowel and a balloon inflation/deflation system. Once the ligament of Treitz or the terminal ileum is reached, the balloon is advanced in front of the endoscope until resistance is felt. The balloon is then inflated and the endoscope is advanced forward while applying traction on the balloon [88]. Once the balloon is reached by the endoscope, it is deflated and this push-and-pull technique is repeated to advance through the small bowel. The catheter may be removed and reinserted to allow for therapeutic intervention while maintaining the endoscope position [89] (Figs. 13.7 and 13.8).

Procedure time to point of maximal insertion is much shorter (~ 15.5 min) than the other forms of deep enteroscopy (~ 45–60 min) with comparable diagnostic yield (45%) and depth of insertion (~ 158 cm from the pylorus or 110 cm proximal to the ileocecal valve) [27, 89, 90]. No complications have been reported to date in the few studies of TTS-BAE [89, 90]. It may be particularly useful in assisting ERCP and metallic stent deployment in patients with strictures.

Comparison Among Different Enteroscopic Methods

The two most commonly used enteroscopic methods in current practice are double-balloon enteroscopy and single-balloon enteroscopy. Both of these not only have excellent depth of insertion, but also stabilize the intestine for good endoscopic control during interventions. There are numerous head-to-head studies comparing these two; however, many of these studies are not well done and difficult to compare. Most studies show that DBE can be advanced a bit further than SBE, but this is still debatable (Table 13.3) [73, 74, 81, 83, 91]. Procedure duration is shorter for SE than for DBE and SBE. Although the rate of successful complete enteroscopy appears superior for DBE compared with SE and SBE, this result does not necessarily translate to an increase in diagnostic or therapeutic yield.

A retrospective study of 250 patients compared the antegrade to retrograde approach. There were 182 antegrade procedures (91 SBE, 52 DBE, and 39 SE) and 68 retrograde approaches (23 SBE, 37 DBE, and 8 SE). The antegrade approach provided higher diagnostic and therapeutic yield than the retrograde route in patients with suspected small bowel disease [94].

Overall, the studies suggest that DBE, SBE, and SE have comparable diagnostic and therapeutic yields. Therefore, the endoscopist should choose the method based on availability and his/her experience after considering the basic characteristics of these techniques (Table 13.4).

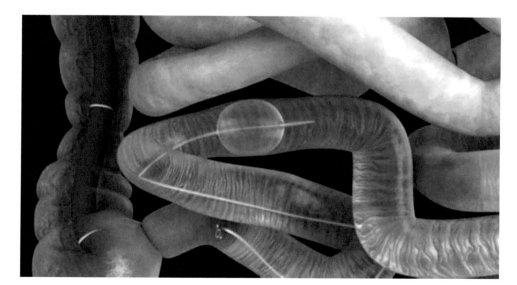

Fig. 13.7 TTS-BAE—once the endoscope has passed the ligament of Treitz, the through-the-scope balloon catheter is inserted through the biopsy channel, advanced ahead of the endoscope until resistance is encountered, and the balloon is inflated. From Ali et al. [89]. With the permission from Elsevier

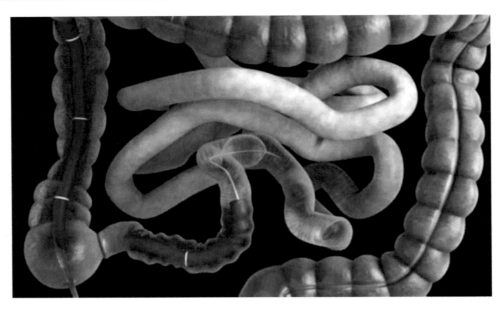

Fig. 13.8 TTS-BAE—once the balloon is inflated, anchoring the bowel, the endoscope is advanced by pushing it forward while pulling the catheter back until the balloon is reached. The balloon is then deflated and the previous push-and-pull technique is repeated. From Ali et al. [89]. With permission from Elsevier

Table 13.3 Comparison of outcomes among different enteroscopic methods

Study	Design	N	Procedure time, min	Depth of insertion, cm from pylorus	Diagnostic yield %	Therapeutic yield %
DBE vs SBE						
Efthymiou et al. [74]	RCT	66 vs. 53	60 vs. 60	234 vs. 204	53 vs. 57	26 vs. 32
Domagk et al. [73]	RCT	65 vs. 65	105 vs. 96	253 vs. 258	43 vs. 37	9 vs. 5
May et al. [82]	RCT	50 vs. 50	67 vs. 54[a]	–	52 vs. 42	72 vs. 48
DBE vs SE						
Rahmi et al. [80]	P	191 vs. 50	60 vs. 55	200 vs. 220	–	–
Messer et al. [83]	RCT	13 vs. 13	60 vs. 43[a]	346 vs. 268[a]	46 vs. 69	92
May et al. [81]	RCT	10 vs.10	65 vs. 43[a]	310 vs. 250[a]	–	–
Frieling et al. [92]	P	17 vs. 18	42 vs. 47	260 vs. 250	47.1 vs. 33.4	–
SBE vs SE						
Khashab et al. [93]	R	52 vs. 53	53 vs.47	222 vs. 301[a]	59.6 vs. 43.4	33 vs. 15

DBE double-balloon enteroscopy; *SBE* single-balloon enteroscopy; *SE* spiral enteroscopy; *RCT* randomized controlled trial; *P* prospective study; *R* retrospective study
[a]Statistically significant $p < 0.05$

Conclusion

Enteroscopic techniques have evolved significantly over the past two decades. Deep enteroscopy should be used as a complement to VCE. The time index of identified lesions on VCE should be utilized to select the appropriate approach for enteroscopy. All the currently available enteroscopic modalities have their own advantages and limitations. Although there are fine differences among the different enteroscopic modalities, the yield (both diagnostic and therapeutic) is quite comparable. Therefore, the selection of the enteroscopic technique should be based on the availability and technical experience of the endoscopist. Though deep enteroscopy is a well-tolerated procedure, care should

Table 13.4 Comparison of characteristics among enteroscopic techniques

Characteristic	DBE	Spiral	SBE	TTS balloon
Depth of insertion	Deepest	Deeper	Deep	Unclear
Procedure time	Long	Relatively faster	Relatively faster	Fastest
Therapeutic capability	Full	Full	Full	Full
On demand option	No	No	No	Yes
Other features		Need two providers		Uses standard endoscope/colonoscope with 3.7-mm channel

Table 13.5 General tips for successful deep enteroscopy

1. Set expectations: Both the patient and physician should remember that there is a chance of being unsuccessful almost half of the time

2. Time: These procedures can take a long time; therefore, the first important principle is that one should not schedule deep enteroscopies for half-hour slots and should plan with enough time

3. VCE: Review VCE or at least the report, as this will provide a very useful road map to where the likely target lesion is located. For example, if the lesion is identified within the proximal two-thirds of the small bowel, an antegrade method is chosen

4. Anesthesia is recommended for sedation as these are prolonged procedures

5. CO_2 is preferable as air can get trapped in distal small bowel loops, creating a mass-like effect and limiting flexibility of the small bowel

6. Stabilize the enteroscope before beginning any therapy as the small bowel is more mobile

7. Fluoroscopy: If available, fluoroscopy may help identify and reduce loops

8. Consider using a cap at the tip of the enteroscope for improved visualization with less use of insufflation

9. Tattoo the farthest extent reached

10. An excellent bowel preparation is important for the retrograde approach

be taken to remember some of the practical points as given in Table 13.5 to ensure a successful procedure without complications.

References

1. Leighton JA. The role of endoscopic imaging of the small bowel in clinical practice. Am J Gastroenterol. 2011;106(1):27–36; quiz 7.
2. Strodel WE, Eckhauser FE, Knol JA, Nostrant TT, Dent TL. Intraoperative fiberoptic endoscopy. Am Surg. 1984;50(6):340–4.
3. Kopacova M, Bures J, Rejchrt S, Siroky M, Bedrna J, Ferko A, et al. Intraoperative enteroscopy–personal experience from 1995 to 2002. Casopis lekaru ceskych. 2003;142(5):303–6.
4. Lewis BS. The history of enteroscopy. Gastrointest Endosc Clin N Am. 1999;9(1):1–11.
5. Tada M, Akasaka Y, Misaki F, Kwaie K. Clinical evaluation of a sonde-type small intestinal fiberscope. Endoscopy. 1977;9(1):33–8.
6. Waye JD. Small-intestinal endoscopy. Endoscopy. 2001;33(1):24–30.
7. Gostout CJ. Sonde enteroscopy. Technique, depth of insertion, and yield of lesions. Gastrointest Endosc Clin N Am. 1996;6(4):777–92.
8. Tada M, Shimizu S, Kawai K. A new transnasal sonde type fiberscope (SSIF type VII) as a pan-enteroscope. Endoscopy. 1986;18(4):121–4.
9. Waye JD. Small-bowel endoscopy. Endoscopy. 2003;35(1):15–21.
10. Lewis BS, Kornbluth A, Waye JD. Small bowel tumours: yield of enteroscopy. Gut. 1991;32(7):763–5.
11. Morris AJ, Wasson LA, MacKenzie JF. Small bowel enteroscopy in undiagnosed gastrointestinal blood loss. Gut. 1992;33(7):887–9.
12. MacKenzie JF. Atlas of enteroscopy. Springer: Berlin; 1998.
13. Shimizu S, Tada M, Kawai K. Development of a new insertion technique in push-type enteroscopy. Am J Gastroenterol. 1987;82(9):844–7.
14. Yamamoto H, Kita H. Enteroscopy. J Gastroenterol. 2005;40(6):555–62.
15. Berner JS, Mauer K, Lewis BS. Push and sonde enteroscopy for the diagnosis of obscure gastrointestinal bleeding. Am J Gastroenterol. 1994;89(12):2139–42.
16. Raju GS, Gerson L, Das A, Lewis B. American Gastroenterological Association (AGA) Institute technical review on obscure gastrointestinal bleeding. Gastroenterology. 2007;133(5):1697–717.
17. Zaman A, Katon RM. Push enteroscopy for obscure gastrointestinal bleeding yields a high incidence of proximal lesions within reach of a standard endoscope. Gastrointest Endosc. 1998;47(5):372–6.
18. Chak A, Cooper GS, Canto MI, Pollack BJ, Sivak MV Jr. Enteroscopy for the initial evaluation of iron deficiency. Gastrointest Endosc. 1998;47(2):144–8.
19. Appleyard M, Glukhovsky A, Swain P. Wireless-capsule diagnostic endoscopy for recurrent small-bowel bleeding. New England J Med. 2001;344(3):232–3.
20. Iddan G, Meron G, Glukhovsky A, Swain P. Wireless capsule endoscopy. Nature. 2000;405(6785):417.
21. Scapa E, Jacob H, Lewkowicz S, Migdal M, Gat D, Gluckhovski A, et al. Initial experience of wireless-capsule endoscopy for evaluating occult gastrointestinal bleeding and suspected small bowel pathology. Am J Gastroenterol. 2002;97(11):2776–9.

22. Liao Z, Xu C, Li ZS. Completion rate and diagnostic yield of small-bowel capsule endoscopy: 1 vs. 2 frames per second. Endoscopy. 2010;42(5):360–4.

23. Liao Z, Gao R, Xu C, Li ZS. Indications and detection, completion, and retention rates of small-bowel capsule endoscopy: a systematic review. Gastrointest Endosc. 2010;71(2):280–6.

24. Yamamoto H, Sekine Y, Sato Y, Higashizawa T, Miyata T, Iino S, et al. Total enteroscopy with a nonsurgical steerable double-balloon method. Gastrointest Endosc. 2001;53(2):216–20.

25. Tsujikawa T, Saitoh Y, Andoh A, Imaeda H, Hata K, Minematsu H, et al. Novel single-balloon enteroscopy for diagnosis and treatment of the small intestine: preliminary experiences. Endoscopy. 2008;40(1):11–5.

26. Akerman PA, Agrawal D, Cantero D, Pangtay J. Spiral enteroscopy with the new DSB overtube: a novel technique for deep peroral small-bowel intubation. Endoscopy. 2008;40(12):974–8.

27. Kumbhari V, Saxena P, Khashab MA. A new through-the-scope balloon-assisted deep enteroscopy platform. Gastrointest Endosc. 2014;79(4):694.

28. DiSario JA, Petersen BT, Tierney WM, Adler DG, Chand B, Conway JD, et al. Enteroscopes. Gastrointest Endosc. 2007;66 (5):872–80.

29. Westerhof J, Weersma RK, Koornstra JJ. Investigating obscure gastrointestinal bleeding: capsule endoscopy or double balloon enteroscopy? Neth J Med. 2009;67(7):260–5.

30. Yoshida N, Wakabayashi N, Nomura K, Konishi H, Yamamoto H, Mitsufuji S, et al. Ileal mucosa-associated lymphoid tissue lymphoma showing several ulcer scars detected using double-balloon endoscopy. Endoscopy. 2004;36(11):1022–4.

31. Iwamoto M, Yamamoto H, Kita H, Sunada K, Hayashi Y, Sato H, et al. Double-balloon endoscopy for ileal GI stromal tumor. Gastrointest Endoscopy. 2005;62(3):440–1; discussion 1.

32. Kunihiro K, Manabe N, Hata J, Kamino D, Nakao M, Mitsuoka Y, et al. Gastrointestinal stromal tumor in jejunum: diagnosis using contrast-enhanced ultrasonography and double-balloon enteroscopy. Dig Dis Sci. 2006;51(7):1236–40.

33. Ross A, Mehdizadeh S, Tokar J, Leighton JA, Kamal A, Chen A, et al. Double balloon enteroscopy detects small bowel mass lesions missed by capsule endoscopy. Dig Dis Sci. 2008;53(8):2140–3.

34. Yamagami H, Oshitani N, Hosomi S, Suekane T, Kamata N, Sogawa M, et al. Usefulness of double-balloon endoscopy in the diagnosis of malignant small-bowel tumors. Clin Gastroenterol Hepatol Official Clin Pract J Am Gastroenterol Assoc. 2008;6 (11):1202–5.

35. Tomba C, Sidhu R, Sanders DS, Mooney PD, Branchi F, Locatelli M, et al. Celiac disease and double-balloon enteroscopy: what can we achieve?: The experience of 2 European tertiary referral centers. J Clin Gastroenterol. 2015.

36. Gerson LB, Fidler JL, Cave DR, Leighton JA. ACG clinical guideline: diagnosis and management of small bowel bleeding. Am J Gastroenterol. 2015;110(9):1265–87; quiz 88.

37. Shetzline MA, Suhocki PV, Workman MJ. Direct percutaneous endoscopic jejunostomy with small bowel enteroscopy and fluoroscopy. Gastrointest Endosc. 2001;53(6):633–8.

38. Aktas H, Mensink PB, Kuipers EJ, van Buuren H. Single-balloon enteroscopy-assisted direct percutaneous endoscopic jejunostomy. Endoscopy. 2012;44(2):210–2.

39. Paduani GF, Saflatle-Ribeiro AV, Franco MC, Maluf-Filho F. Double-balloon enteroscopy-assisted endoscopic retrograde cholangiography for the treatment of a strictured Roux-en-Y hepaticojejunal anastomosis. Endoscopy. 2015;47 Suppl 1 UCTN: E381-2.

40. Itokawa F, Itoi T, Ishii K, Sofuni A, Moriyasu F. Single- and double-balloon enteroscopy-assisted endoscopic retrograde cholangiopancreatography in patients with Roux-en-Y plus hepaticojejunostomy anastomosis and Whipple resection. Dig Endosc Official J Jpn Gastroenterol Endosc Soc. 2014;26(Suppl 2):136–43.

41. Kurzynske FC, Romagnuolo J, Brock AS. Success of single-balloon enteroscopy in patients with surgically altered anatomy. Gastrointest Endosc. 2015;82(2):319–24.

42. Ishihara M, Ohmiya N, Nakamura M, Funasaka K, Miyahara R, Ohno E, et al. Risk factors of symptomatic NSAID-induced small intestinal injury and diaphragm disease. Aliment Pharmacol Ther. 2014;40(5):538–47.

43. Oshitani N, Yukawa T, Yamagami H, Inagawa M, Kamata N, Watanabe K, et al. Evaluation of deep small bowel involvement by double-balloon enteroscopy in Crohn's disease. Am J Gastroenterol. 2006;101(7):1484–9.

44. Fry LC, Bellutti M, Neumann H, Malfertheiner P, Monkemuller K. Utility of double-balloon enteroscopy for the evaluation of malabsorption. Dig Dis (Basel, Switzerland). 2008;26(2):134–9.

45. Hadithi M, Al-toma A, Oudejans J, van Bodegraven AA, Mulder CJ, Jacobs M. The value of double-balloon enteroscopy in patients with refractory celiac disease. Am J Gastroenterol. 2007;102(5):987–96.

46. Kroner PT, Brahmbhatt BS, Bartel MJ, Stark ME, Lukens FJ. Yield of double-balloon enteroscopy in the diagnosis and treatment of small bowel strictures. Dig Liver Dis Official J Ital Soc Gastroenterol Ital Assoc Study Liver. 2015.

47. Fukumoto A, Tanaka S, Yamamoto H, Yao T, Matsui T, Iida M, et al. Diagnosis and treatment of small-bowel stricture by double balloon endoscopy. Gastrointest Endosc. 2007;66(3 Suppl):S108–12.

48. Chu YC, Su SJ, Yang CC, Yeh YH, Chen CH, Yueh SK. ERCP plus papillotomy by use of double-balloon enteroscopy after Billroth II gastrectomy. Gastrointest Endosc. 2007;66(6):1234–6.

49. Kato H, Tsutsumi K, Harada R, Okada H, Yamamoto K. Short double-balloon enteroscopy is feasible and effective for endoscopic retrograde cholangiopancreatography in patients with surgically altered gastrointestinal anatomy. Dig Endosc Official J Jpn Gastroenterol Endosc Soc. 2014;26(Suppl 2):130–5.

50. Cheng CL, Liu NJ, Tang JH, Yu MC, Tsui YN, Hsu FY, et al. Double-balloon enteroscopy for ERCP in patients with Billroth II anatomy: results of a large series of papillary large-balloon dilation for biliary stone removal. Endosc Int Open. 2015;3(3):E216–22.

51. Ishii K, Itoi T, Tonozuka R, Itokawa F, Sofuni A, Tsuchiya T, et al. Balloon enteroscopy-assisted ERCP in patients with Roux-en-Y gastrectomy and intact papillae (with videos). Gastrointest Endosc. 2016;83(2):377-86.e6.

52. Itoi T, Ishii K, Sofuni A, Itokawa F, Tsuchiya T, Kurihara T, et al. Long- and short-type double-balloon enteroscopy-assisted therapeutic ERCP for intact papilla in patients with a Roux-en-Y anastomosis. Surg Endosc. 2011;25(3):713–21.

53. Matsumoto T, Esaki M, Yanaru-Fujisawa R, Moriyama T, Yada S, Nakamura S, et al. Small-intestinal involvement in familial adenomatous polyposis: evaluation by double-balloon endoscopy and intraoperative enteroscopy. Gastrointest Endosc. 2008;68 (5):911–9.

54. May A, Nachbar L, Ell C. Extraction of entrapped capsules from the small bowel by means of push-and-pull enteroscopy with the double-balloon technique. Endoscopy. 2005;37(6):591–3.

55. May A, Nachbar L, Ell C. Push-and-pull enteroscopy using a single-balloon technique for difficult colonoscopy. Endoscopy. 2006;38(4):395–8.

56. Hartmann D, Eickhoff A, Tamm R, Riemann JF. Balloon-assisted enteroscopy using a single-balloon technique. Endoscopy. 2007;39 (Suppl 1):E276.

57. May A. Current status of double balloon enteroscopy with focus on the Wiesbaden results. Gastrointest Endosc. 2007;66(3 Suppl): S12–4.

58. Mehdizadeh S, Ross A, Gerson L, Leighton J, Chen A, Schembre D, et al. What is the learning curve associated with double-balloon enteroscopy? Technical details and early experience in 6 U.S. tertiary care centers. Gastrointest Endosc. 2006;64 (5):740–50.

59. May A, Nachbar L, Schneider M, Ell C. Prospective comparison of push enteroscopy and push-and-pull enteroscopy in patients with suspected small-bowel bleeding. Am J Gastroenterol. 2006;101 (9):2016–24.

60. May A, Nachbar L, Ell C. Double-balloon enteroscopy (push-and-pull enteroscopy) of the small bowel: feasibility and diagnostic and therapeutic yield in patients with suspected small bowel disease. Gastrointest Endosc. 2005;62(1):62–70.

61. Di Caro S, May A, Heine DG, Fini L, Landi B, Petruzziello L, et al. The European experience with double-balloon enteroscopy: indications, methodology, safety, and clinical impact. Gastrointest Endosc. 2005;62(4):545–50.

62. Xin L, Liao Z, Jiang YP, Li ZS. Indications, detectability, positive findings, total enteroscopy, and complications of diagnostic double-balloon endoscopy: a systematic review of data over the first decade of use. Gastrointest Endosc. 2011;74(3):563–70.

63. Hadithi M, Heine GD, Jacobs MA, van Bodegraven AA, Mulder CJ. A prospective study comparing video capsule endoscopy with double-balloon enteroscopy in patients with obscure gastrointestinal bleeding. Am J Gastroenterol. 2006;101 (1):52–7.

64. Gay G, Delvaux M, Fassler I. Outcome of capsule endoscopy in determining indication and route for push-and-pull enteroscopy. Endoscopy. 2006;38(1):49–58.

65. Li X, Chen H, Dai J, Gao Y, Ge Z. Predictive role of capsule endoscopy on the insertion route of double-balloon enteroscopy. Endoscopy. 2009;41(9):762–6.

66. Li X, Dai J, Lu H, Gao Y, Chen H, Ge Z. A prospective study on evaluating the diagnostic yield of video capsule endoscopy followed by directed double-balloon enteroscopy in patients with obscure gastrointestinal bleeding. Dig Dis Sci. 2010;55(6): 1704–10.

67. Moschler O, May A, Muller MK, Ell C. Complications in and performance of double-balloon enteroscopy (DBE): results from a large prospective DBE database in Germany. Endoscopy. 2011;43 (6):484–9.

68. Gerson LB, Tokar J, Chiorean M, Lo S, Decker GA, Cave D, et al. Complications associated with double balloon enteroscopy at nine US centers. Clin Gastroenterol Hepatol Official Clin Pract J Am Gastroenterol Assoc. 2009;7(11):1177–82, 82.e1-3.

69. Moschler O, May AD, Muller MK, Ell C. Complications in double-balloon-enteroscopy: results of the German DBE register. Z Gastroenterol. 2008;46(3):266–70.

70. Yamamoto H, Kita H, Sunada K, Hayashi Y, Sato H, Yano T, et al. Clinical outcomes of double-balloon endoscopy for the diagnosis and treatment of small-intestinal diseases. Clin Gastroenterol hepatol Official Clin Pract J Am Gastroenterol Assoc. 2004;2(11):1010–6.

71. Tee HP, How SH, Kaffes AJ. Learning curve for double-balloon enteroscopy: findings from an analysis of 282 procedures. World J Gastrointest Endosc. 2012;4(8):368–72.

72. Gross SA, Stark ME. Initial experience with double-balloon enteroscopy at a U.S. center. Gastrointest Endosc. 2008;67 (6):890–7.

73. Domagk D, Mensink P, Aktas H, Lenz P, Meister T, Luegering A, et al. Single- vs. double-balloon enteroscopy in small-bowel diagnostics: a randomized multicenter trial. Endoscopy. 2011;43 (6):472–6.

74. Efthymiou M, Desmond PV, Brown G, La Nauze R, Kaffes A, Chua TJ, et al. SINGLE-01: a randomized, controlled trial comparing the efficacy and depth of insertion of single- and double-balloon enteroscopy by using a novel method to determine insertion depth. Gastrointest Endosc. 2012;76(5):972–80.

75. Tomizawa Y, Sullivan CT, Gelrud A. Single balloon enteroscopy (SBE) assisted therapeutic endoscopic retrograde cholangiopancreatography (ERCP) in patients with roux-en-y anastomosis. Dig Dis Sci. 2014;59(2):465–70.

76. Badamas JO. PI. ERCP in post-surgical patients In: Lee LS, editor. ERCP and EUS: a case-based approach. New York: Springer; 2015. p. 515–30.

77. Kawamura T, Yasuda K, Tanaka K, Uno K, Ueda M, Sanada K, et al. Clinical evaluation of a newly developed single-balloon enteroscope. Gastrointest Endosc. 2008;68(6):1112–6.

78. Akerman PA, Agrawal D, Chen W, Cantero D, Avila J, Pangtay J. Spiral enteroscopy: a novel method of enteroscopy by using the endo-ease discovery SB overtube and a pediatric colonoscope. Gastrointest Endosc. 2009;69(2):327–32.

79. Buscaglia JM, Dunbar KB, Okolo PI 3rd, Judah J, Akerman PA, Cantero D, et al. The spiral enteroscopy training initiative: results of a prospective study evaluating the discovery SB overtube device during small bowel enteroscopy (with video). Endoscopy. 2009;41 (3):194–9.

80. Rahmi G, Samaha E, Vahedi K, Ponchon T, Fumex F, Filoche B, et al. Multicenter comparison of double-balloon enteroscopy and spiral enteroscopy. J Gastroenterol Hepatol. 2013;28(6):992–8.

81. May A, Manner H, Aschmoneit I, Ell C. Prospective, cross-over, single-center trial comparing oral double-balloon enteroscopy and oral spiral enteroscopy in patients with suspected small-bowel vascular malformations. Endoscopy. 2011;43(6):477–83.

82. May A, Farber M, Aschmoneit I, Pohl J, Manner H, Lotterer E, et al. Prospective multicenter trial comparing push-and-pull enteroscopy with the single- and double-balloon techniques in patients with small-bowel disorders. Am J Gastroenterol. 2010;105 (3):575–81.

83. Messer I, May A, Manner H, Ell C. Prospective, randomized, single-center trial comparing double-balloon enteroscopy and spiral enteroscopy in patients with suspected small-bowel disorders. Gastrointest Endosc. 2013;77(2):241–9.

84. Morgan D, Upchurch B, Draganov P, Binmoeller KF, Haluszka O, Jonnalagadda S, et al. Spiral enteroscopy: prospective U.S. multicenter study in patients with small-bowel disorders. Gastrointest Endosc. 2010;72(5):992–8.

85. Lennon AM, Kapoor S, Khashab M, Corless E, Amateau S, Dunbar K, et al. Spiral assisted ERCP is equivalent to single balloon assisted ERCP in patients with Roux-en-Y anatomy. Dig Dis Sci. 2012;57(5):1391–8.

86. Nagula S, Gaidos J, Draganov PV, Bucobo JC, Cho B, Hernandez Y, et al. Retrograde spiral enteroscopy: feasibility, success, and safety in a series of 22 patients. Gastrointest Endosc. 2011;74 (3):699–702.

87. Mandaliya R, Korenblit J, O'Hare B, Shnitser A, Kedika R, Matro R, et al. Spiral enteroscopy utilizing capsule location index for achieving high diagnostic and therapeutic yield. Diagn Ther Endosc. 2015;2015:793516.

88. Kumbhari V, Storm AC, Okolo PI 3rd, Saxena P, Kalloo AN, Khashab MA. Efficient retrograde enteroscopy using a novel through-the-scope balloon. Surg Endosc. 2014;28(9):2745–6.

89. Ali R, Wild D, Shieh F, Diehl DL, Fischer M, Tamura W, et al. Deep enteroscopy with a conventional colonoscope: initial multicenter study by using a through-the-scope balloon catheter system. Gastrointest Endosc. 2015;82(5):855–60.

90. Kumbhari V, Storm AC, Khashab MA, Canto MI, Saxena P, Akshintala VS, et al. Deep enteroscopy with standard endoscopes using a novel through-the-scope balloon. Endoscopy. 2014;46 (8):685–9.

91. Takano N, Yamada A, Watabe H, Togo G, Yamaji Y, Yoshida H, et al. Single-balloon versus double-balloon endoscopy for achieving total enteroscopy: a randomized, controlled trial. Gastrointest Endosc. 2011;73(4):734–9.

92. Frieling T, Heise J, Sassenrath W, Hulsdonk A, Kreysel C. Prospective comparison between double-balloon enteroscopy and spiral enteroscopy. Endoscopy. 2010;42(11):885–8.

93. Khashab MA, Lennon AM, Dunbar KB, Singh VK, Chandrasekhara V, Giday S, et al. A comparative evaluation of single-balloon enteroscopy and spiral enteroscopy for patients with mid-gut disorders. Gastrointest Endosc. 2010;72(4):766–72.

94. Sanaka MR, Navaneethan U, Kosuru B, Yerneni H, Lopez R, Vargo JJ. Antegrade is more effective than retrograde enteroscopy for evaluation and management of suspected small-bowel disease. Clin Gastroenterol Hepatol Official Clin Pract J Am Gastroenterol Assoc. 2012;10(8):910–6.

Quality in Upper Endoscopy

Imran Sheikh and Jeffrey Tokar

Introduction

Upper endoscopy (EGD) is a diagnostic and therapeutic tool that is used widely in the management of esophageal, gastric, and small bowel disorders. In 2009, nearly seven million upper endoscopies were performed in the USA at an estimated cost over $12 billion [1]. Quality was defined by the Institute of Medicine in 1990 as "the degree to which health services for individuals and populations increase the likelihood of desired health outcomes and are consistent with current professional knowledge" [2]. Current trends in healthcare delivery indicate that "value" of medical services, including endoscopic services, will be a major driver of reimbursement in upcoming years. A formula that is frequently used to calculate or estimate value between two or more providers of similar service is quality divided by cost. Using this equation, it becomes clear that the value of a service offered by a provider (or group of providers with shared resources and aligned goals) can be increased by increasing the quality (numerator) related to how they deliver a service, decreasing the costs (denominator) associated with their provision of the service, or doing both. Quality has been receiving increasing attention by healthcare institutions, payors, and regulatory agencies.

The quality of health care can be measured by comparing the performance of an individual or a group of individuals to a benchmark. The parameter that is used for comparison (e.g., how often a provider instructs patients with peptic ulcers to take proton pump inhibitors) is termed a quality indicator and can be reported as a ratio between the incidence of correct performance and the opportunity for correct performance, as in the following equation: [3–5].

$$\text{Quality indicator} = \frac{\text{incidence of correct performance}}{\text{opportunity for correct performance}} \times 100\%.$$

This chapter discusses quality indicators (QIs) that have been identified by the various GI societies in the USA (the ASGE, ACG, and the AGA) as they pertain to the practice of upper endoscopy in 2016. In addition, in 2015, a joint task force known as the ASGE/ACG Task Force on Quality in Endoscopy published a series of articles discussing quality in endoscopy [3, 6–9]. These documents are perhaps the most systematic and concise reviews of a complex topic. It is imperative for trainees in gastrointestinal endoscopy, regardless of medical specialty, to familiarize themselves with the content of these documents.

For organizational purposes, the ASGE/ACG Task force divides the list of "quality indicators in endoscopy" into three distinct time periods: pre-procedure, intra-procedure, and post-procedure [3]. The ensuing discussion focuses on quality measures regarding diagnostic and therapeutic upper endoscopy as it relates to a practicing general gastroenterologist and the gastroenterology fellow in training.

Pre-procedure Quality Indicators (QIs)

The "pre-procedure" time period includes the points of contact pertaining to the upper endoscopy that occur between the patient and the endoscopy team prior to the delivery of sedation. In chronological order, this often begins with the initial consultation between the patient and his or her endoscopist, during which time an appropriate indication for upper endoscopy is identified and the upper endoscopy is suggested. A discussion and documentation of informed consent must occur during the pre-procedure period.

Electronic supplementary material
Supplementary material is available in the online version of this chapter at 10.1007/978-3-319-49041-0_14. Videos can also be accessed at https://link.springer.com/chapter/10.1007/978-3-319-49041-0_14.

I. Sheikh · J. Tokar (✉)
Department of Gastroenterology, Fox Chase Cancer Center, 333 Cottman Ave, Philadelphia, PA 19111, USA
e-mail: jeffrey.tokar@fccc.edu

I. Sheikh
e-mail: imran.sheikh@fccc.edu

Depending on the practice setting and framework within which the physician practices, this may be performed in detail at the time of the initial evaluation, on the day of the procedure, or a combination of both. In the modern practice of gastroenterology, many upper endoscopic examinations are performed in an "open-access" manner, with the endoscopist meeting the patient on the day of the procedure.

It is imperative that the upper endoscopy be performed by an appropriately trained and credentialed individual and that the following items are documented in the patient chart: a directed/focused history and physical, assessment of the patient's procedure-related risks, discussion of the timing of the upper endoscopy (which often *immediately* follows the history in the open-access setting), sedation plan, and pre-procedure preparation (including management of medications such as anticoagulants and antibiotics). Finally, immediately prior to the upper endoscopy, the performance of a "time-out" should be performed and documented [3, 6].

QI: Appropriate Indication

Generally speaking, medical and surgical procedures are indicated when diagnostic information is obtainable and/or the therapeutic potential of the procedure will improve the patient's outcome. Conversely, medical and surgical procedures are not indicated when the risks associated with them outweigh any perceived benefit [6]. For gastrointestinal endoscopy, the ASGE Standards of Practice Committee initially published a list of appropriate indication for endoscopic procedures in 2000 [10] and updated this list in 2012 [11]. Practicing endoscopists should familiarize themselves with this and future updated versions of this ASGE document. Of particular note, upper GI endoscopy is generally not indicated for routine surveillance of healed benign disease (excluding premalignant conditions) and is generally contraindicated when adequate patient cooperation or consent cannot be obtained or when a perforated viscus is known or suspected *unless the purpose of the endoscopy is to close the perforation itself* [12].

The ASGE/ACG Task force suggests that providers achieve this quality indicator (i.e., frequency with which upper endoscopy is performed for an appropriate indication) using a "performance target" over 80% and recommends that appropriate indication(s) are documented for each procedure, justifying the use of any nonstandard indication(s) in the medical record as well [6]. Studies have demonstrated that significantly more clinically relevant findings are obtained when GI endoscopy is performed for appropriate indications. This applies to both colonoscopy [13] and EGD [14]. As such, an important quality improvement goal of every

endoscopist should be minimization or elimination of procedures without appropriate indications.

QI: Appropriately Trained and Credentialed Endoscopist

Multiple training and credentialing guidelines have been published by the ASGE regarding the basic levels of competency and credentialing required to perform endoscopy. These emphasize the importance of using objective measures of an endoscopist's performance, in particular comparing performance to validated benchmarks (whenever possible). Ideally, competency for all endoscopists, regardless of subspecialty (e.g., GI and surgery), should be measured with comparable validated benchmarks, thereby establishing and documenting an endoscopist's ability to perform, at a minimum, the therapeutic interventions specific to a given endoscopic procedure. A high-quality upper endoscopy is one which is performed by an endoscopist who has met objective measures for competency whereby the desired objectives have been met and the potential for adverse events are minimized [6, 15–17].

QI: Informed Consent

The initial ASGE guidelines on informed consent for GI endoscopy were published in 1988 [18] and have since been updated, calling for a performance target (i.e., frequency with which informed consent is obtained and documented) exceeding 98% [6, 19]. According to these guidelines, the burden of legally obtaining adequate informed consent from the patient lies with the endoscopist prior to performing the endoscopic procedure [19]. If the patient is unable to consent due to incompetence or incapacitation, then their legal guardian or surrogate must consent on their behalf.

In the USA, the process of obtaining informed consent legally requires that the physician discloses information to the patient, enabling the patient to understand the procedure, evaluate the risks, benefits, and alternatives, and authorize a specific intervention [20]. Two standards of disclosure exist, and endoscopists are required to learn the applicable standard in the state they practice in.

The "physician-based" standard requires that the endoscopist discloses to the patient the amount of information that a reasonable, similarly situated endoscopist would. On the other hand, the "reasonable patient" standard requires the endoscopist to provide information that a reasonable layperson would consider material and significant when consenting to a proposed intervention [19].

It is prudent for an endoscopist to consult with the legal team within the confines of their practice setting when determining the informed consent standard they should use, the informed consent documentation they should complete, and the appropriateness of any audiovisual aides they may wish to use to facilitate the informed consent process.

In general terms, information regarding the indication, risks, benefits, alternatives, limitations, and personnel that will be involved in the endoscopic procedure should be disclosed. Patients should be aware of what occurs before, during, and after the procedure. Medications that are likely to be administered should be discussed with the patient. If an anesthesiology team will be present to deliver the sedation or anesthesia, a separate consent should be obtained by the anesthesia provider. It is not possible to anticipate and disclose every conceivable risk or complication of an invasive procedure; efforts should, therefore, focus on substantial risks that would influence a reasonable person's willingness to consent for a procedure. Reasonable alternatives to the endoscopy should be discussed, including those that may be more invasive or carry a riskier adverse event profile. Patients should also be counseled if no alternative exists and of the potential outcomes of declining endoscopy [19].

While informed consent is almost always necessary, there are four recognized exceptions to obtaining informed consent for surgical procedures. The clinical situations in which these are evoked are generally rare, especially as they relate to the performance of upper endoscopy. The first exception is when the patient has a life-threatening emergency with inadequate time available to obtain consent. Another exception is the invocation of therapeutic privilege: when the physician determines that providing the patient information would harm the patient. The third exception is when the patient, while knowledgeable and understanding of their right to informed consent, waives that right in writing. The final exception is the presence of a legal mandate in the form of a court order or statute where the patient's and/or public's welfare may overshadow the informed consent process [19].

QI: Documentation of Directed History and Physical Examination

The ASGE/ACG Task force and the American Society of Anesthesiologists (ASA) recommend that a pre-procedure assessment be documented prior to endoscopic procedures [6]. This documentation typically includes pertinent clinical history, medications, allergies, adverse reactions to prior anesthetics or sedatives, history of substance use or abuse, time of last oral intake, and a directed physical examination. Various organizations that accredit hospital endoscopy centers and ambulatory surgical centers, as well as third-party payors, may stipulate that this information be documented independent of the endoscopic procedure report. Endoscopists should familiarize themselves with local and institutional requirements and protocols for the documentation of the pre-procedure history and physical examination. The task force recommends a performance target over 98% for successful completion of the required documentation [6].

QI: Risk Assessment

Before sedation is administered, an assessment of potential adverse events associated with sedation should be performed and documented in the chart, based on the information gathered during focused history and physical examination discussed in the previous section [6]. Patients should be risk-stratified based on their individual ASA and Mallampati scores [6, 21], and the information obtained should be considered in the decision-making process regarding the endoscopic procedure. The Mallampati score assesses the upper airway using a visual scale in which an increasing score correlates with increasing difficulty encountered during endotracheal intubation. The ASA score takes into account a patient's comorbidities and ranks them on a scale from 1 to 6 (Table 14.1). The use of the ASA scoring system has been shown to predict adverse events related to sedation in endoscopy [22]. The ASGE/ACG Task force recommends a performance target over 98% for the documentation of risk assessment prior to endoscopy [6].

QI: Formulation and Documentation of a Sedation Plan

The ASGE/ACG Task force recommends a performance target over 98% for the formulation of a sedation plan prior to endoscopy. In the USA, upper endoscopy is typically performed with moderate sedation (also known as conscious sedation), deep sedation, or under general anesthesia. Rarely, upper endoscopy can be performed without sedation, often with the use of transnasal ultrathin endoscopes.

Moderate sedation is often delivered by an endoscopy nurse under the supervision and direction of the endoscopist. Moderate sedation involves administration of certain drugs to induce depression of consciousness to a degree in which patients are able to respond purposefully to verbal commands with or without light tactile stimulation. In moderate sedation, the patient is able to independently maintain a patent airway as well as maintain cardiovascular function [6].

Table 14.1 ASA physical status classification system

ASA class[a]	Definition
I	A normal healthy patient
II	A patient with mild systemic disease
III	A patient with severe systemic disease
IV	A patient with severe systemic disease that is a constant threat to life
V	A moribund patient who is not expected to survive without the operation
VI	A declared brain-dead patient whose organs are being removed for donor purposes

[a]The addition of "E" denotes emergency surgery whereby a delay in treatment would lead to a significant increase in the threat to life or body part

Deep sedation and general anesthesia are typically administered by the anesthesia team that works in conjunction with the endoscopy team. Deep sedation is a drug-induced depression of consciousness to a degree in which patients cannot be easily aroused but can respond purposefully after repeated or painful stimulation. In deep sedation, a patient's ability to independently maintain their ventilator function may become impaired and they may require assistance maintaining a patent and protected airway. Cardiovascular function, on the other hand, is usually maintained under deep sedation. General anesthesia is a drug-induced loss of consciousness during which patients cannot be aroused, even by painful stimulation. Under general anesthesia, a patient's ability to independently maintain their ventilatory function is frequently impaired and they frequently require ventilator support. Furthermore, cardiovascular function may be impaired during general anesthesia [6].

QI: Management of Pre-procedure Medications

Multiple medications that patients may be receiving prior to the day of upper endoscopy are of particular relevance and decisions regarding whether to continue or temporarily discontinue them must be considered on a case-by-case basis, guided by on the patient's history, indication for the upper endoscopy, and timing of the proposed procedure. A few examples of important medication-related pre-endoscopy decisions that occur frequently in clinical practice include whether to hold or continue any of the broad array of currently available antithrombotic therapies that many patients are receiving, when to administer prophylactic antibiotic therapy (e.g., endoscopy for PEG tube placement or endoscopy in the cirrhotic patient with acute upper GI bleeding), the use of vasoactive drugs prior to EGD for patients with suspected variceal bleeding, and the use of proton pump inhibitor (PPI) therapy when peptic ulcer bleeding is suspected.

QI: Antithrombotic Medications

Antithrombotic therapy includes antiplatelet agents as well as anticoagulant agents that are used to reduce the risk of thromboembolic events in patients with various cardiac, hematologic, neurologic, and vascular conditions such as embolic cerebrovascular accident, atrial fibrillation, venous thromboembolic disease, acute coronary syndrome, hypercoagulable conditions, and the presence of various indwelling endoprostheses. There has been significant development of novel pharmacotherapeutics over the last decade, and endoscopists should familiarize themselves with the recent ASGE Standards of Practice Committee guidelines which include recommendations for the management of these medications in the peri-procedural period [23].

Generally, diagnostic upper endoscopy is considered low risk for causing procedure-related bleeding, and the cessation of antithrombotic therapy is not routinely warranted. Some therapeutic upper endoscopic procedures, however, are considered high risk for procedure-related bleeding and may require cessation of certain antithrombotic medications. Patients at high risk for thromboembolic adverse events include those with atrial fibrillation associated with other specific cardiac conditions or a history of thromboembolism, mechanical mitral valve, coronary artery stents placed within one year in the setting of acute coronary syndrome, or non-stented percutaneous coronary intervention after myocardial infarction. Such patients may require consultation with their cardiologist, initiation of bridge therapy, or deferment of endoscopic evaluation until a management plan is established [6]. Of note, in many cases, endoscopy can be performed while maintaining antithrombotic or antiplatelet medication usage.

Most diagnostic upper endoscopic procedures can be performed safely without discontinuing aspirin prior to the procedure, and most patients can and should continue to take aspirin following their upper endoscopy. Patients who undergo certain endoscopic therapies, however, may require temporary cessation of antithrombotic therapy. Reinitiation of antithrombotic therapy in this group of patients should be individualized based on the type of endoscopic therapy they received and their individual risk of thromboembolism. The ASGE/ACG Task force recommends that antithrombotic medication use by the patient be recorded and that a plan regarding peri-procedural management of antithrombotic medications is both documented and communicated to the patient and the healthcare team [6].

QI: Prophylactic Antibiotic Therapy Prior to PEG Tube Placement

Prophylactic antibiotics are indicated prior to upper endoscopy with PEG tube placement [24], and their use should be discussed with the patient in the informed consent and documented in the medical record [19]. Antibacterial agents that cover cutaneous sources of bacterial infection, such as cefazolin, should be administered to patients undergoing PEG tube placement 30 min prior to the procedure (unless a contraindication to the use of cephalosporins exists or there is a high level of suspicion for cephalosporin-resistant organisms based on the patients prior to bacteriologic history and/or regional antimicrobial resistance patters) [24–26]. The ASGE/ACG Task force recommends a performance target over 98% for the administration of prophylactic antibiotic therapy prior to PEG tube placement [3].

QI: Prophylactic Antibiotic Therapy in a Cirrhotic Patient with Acute Upper GI Bleeding

Prophylactic antibiotics are indicated in patients with cirrhosis and acute upper GI bleeding. Oral fluoroquinolones or intravenous ceftriaxone should be administered independent of performing an upper endoscopy with the latter group of antibiotics reserved for patients with advanced cirrhosis, inability to take oral medications or in areas with high fluoroquinolone resistance [27–29]. The ASGE/ACG Task force has identified the frequency with which appropriate prophylactic antibiotics are given in this setting to be a "priority" quality indicator and recommends a performance target over 98% (priority indicators were selected from among all of the indicators discussed because of their clinical relevance and importance, evidence that significant variability exists in how frequently (or infrequently) the indicator is performed in clinical practice, and the feasibility of measuring the indicator) [3].

QI: Use of Vasoactive Drugs Prior to Upper Endoscopy for Patients with Suspected Variceal Bleeding

The use of vasoactive medications and their analogues (such as terlipressin and octreotide) has been associated with a significant improvement in hemostasis as well as with decreased mortality in patients presenting with variceal upper GI bleeding. At the present time, however, terlipressin is not approved for use in the USA [28]. Octreotide is often administered with an initial IV bolus of 50 mcg followed by a continuous infusion of 50 mcg per hour for a total of 3–5 days. The ASGE/ACG Task force recommends a performance target over 98% for the administration of vasoactive drugs prior to upper endoscopy for patients with suspected variceal bleeding [3].

QI: Use of Proton Pump Inhibitor (PPI) Therapy When Peptic Ulcer Bleeding Is Suspected

PPI therapy, if started when a patient presents with bleeding, has been found to reduce the proportion of high-risk stigmata seen at index endoscopy and the need for endoscopic therapy [30]. The ASGE/ACG Task force has identified the frequency with which PPI therapy is used for suspected peptic ulcer bleeding as a priority quality indicator, with a goal performance target over 98% [3].

QI: Team Pause (aka Time-Out)

A team pause, commonly referred to as a "time-out," should be performed prior to the administration of sedation and before insertion of the endoscope in all cases and should be performed even in patients undergoing unsedated endoscopy. During this pause, the endoscopy team reviews and records pertinent patient identifiers (e.g., name, date of birth, and medical record number), confirms the type of procedure to be performed and that all required equipment is available, and discusses whether pre-procedure medications are required and if they have been administered (e.g., prophylactic antibiotics). The purpose of the pause is to verify that the correct patient is undergoing the correct procedure. In the USA, the performance of a team pause is now mandated nationally by the Centers for Medicare & Medicaid Services as well as several other accrediting organizations. The pause provides an opportunity for the team to reassess, if necessary, pertinent aspects of the patient's history, including medication allergies, laboratory test, or radiologic data that may affect the safe and successful performance or safety of the endoscopic procedure. It may also provide an opportunity for the endoscopist to inform team members of planned interventions, the administration of certain pre-procedure medications, and confirmation of patient transportation from the endoscopy center after awakening from anesthesia. The ASGE/ACG Task force recommends a performance target over 98% for the frequency with which a team pause is conducted and documented [6].

Intra-procedure Quality Indicators

As defined by the ASGE/ACG Task Force on Quality in Endoscopy, the intra-procedure time period extends from the administration of sedation, or the insertion of the upper endoscope when no sedatives are used, up until the removal of the endoscope. This time period includes all the technical aspects of the procedure including any diagnostic and therapeutic maneuvers performed by the endoscopist as well as patient monitoring. Issues within this time period include patient monitoring, documentation of a comprehensive examination, and specific indicators related to the endoscopic management of Barrett's esophagus, peptic ulcer disease, upper GI bleeding, and celiac disease [3, 6].

QI: Patient Monitoring During Endoscopy

Monitoring of pulse oximetry, heart rate, respiratory rate, and blood pressure provides a means to detect potentially deleterious changes in a patient's cardiopulmonary status during sedation. Such recommendations have been set forth by ASA Task Force on Sedation and Analgesia by Non-Anesthesiologists and the ASGE Standards of Practice Committee [31, 32]. Such measures should be recorded at least every 5 min. With the advent of monitored anesthesia care in endoscopy, the use of deep sedation in upper endoscopy has increased, and while capnography monitoring has been linked with reduced hypoxemia in patients undergoing endoscopy with deep sedation, data supporting the routine use of capnography monitoring in patients undergoing moderate sedation are still limited [33]. The ASGE/ACG Task force recommends a performance target over 98% for the frequency with which patient monitoring during sedation is performed and documented.

QI: Documentation of a Comprehensive Endoscopic Examination

A complete upper endoscopy includes a comprehensive examination of the esophagus, stomach, and duodenum (see Video 14.1) with appropriate photodocumentation, especially when any clinically significant abnormality is encountered. At any point, if adequate visualization of any portion of the upper GI tract is impaired due to mucous, debris, blood, or other material, efforts to clear view are required to achieve a high-quality examination. If excessive food or luminal contents are found, the examination may need to be aborted.

Examination of the esophagus begins at the level of the upper esophageal sphincter. In light of the increased incidence of gastric cardia cancers in recent years, documentation during upper endoscopy should include a careful and "up-close" retroflexed inspection of the gastroesophageal junction (see Figs. 14.1 and 14.2) and cardia [34]. With the exception of gastric outlet obstruction, the upper endoscopy should proceed to the second portion of the duodenum and procedure documentation should confirm the extent of the examination (see Fig. 14.3). Other areas that may warrant photodocumentation include the pylorus (see Fig. 14.4) and the duodenal bulb (see Fig. 14.5). The ASGE/ACG Task force recommends a performance target for achieving a complete examination of the esophagus, stomach, and duodenum, including retroflexion in the stomach in over 98% of cases.

QI: Specific Indicators Related to the Endoscopic Management of Barrett's Esophagus

Specific quality indicators related to the endoscopic management of Barrett's esophagus (BE) include the frequency with which BE is appropriately measured and the frequency with which biopsy specimens are obtained in cases of suspected BE. In patients found to have salmon-colored mucosa suspicious of BE during upper endoscopy, it is imperative that the changes within the esophagus be characterized. This characterization includes a detailed examination of suspicious areas exhibiting nodularity, ulceration, depression, and changes in vascularity, along with the objective measurements of the extent that the salmon-colored mucosa extends into the tubular esophagus. A validated tool that can be used to measure the extent of BE is the Prague classification,

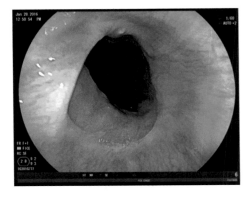

Fig. 14.1 Forward viewing examination of the gastroesophageal junction

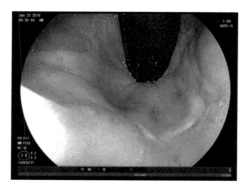

Fig. 14.2 Retroflexed view of the gastroesophageal junction and cardia

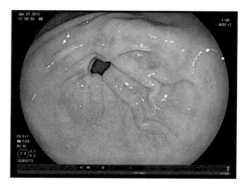

Fig. 14.4 Photodocumentation of the pylorus

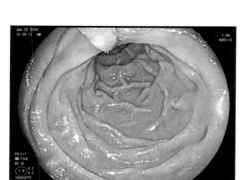

Fig. 14.3 Photodocumentation of the second portion of the duodenum showing the extent of examination

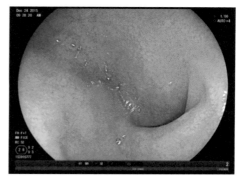

Fig. 14.5 Photodocumentation of the duodenal bulb

which describes both the circumferential and maximal extent of the BE.

The Prague classification defines the distance from the top of the gastric folds to the most proximal extent of the BE (including tongues of BE) as the maximal (M) extent of the BE. The distance from the top of the gastric folds to the most proximal extent of the *circumferential* involvement of the BE is the circumferential (C) measurement [35]. Thus, for example, a patient with Prague C3M4 has circumferential salmon-colored mucosa extending 3 cm above the top of the gastric fold (TGF) and the top of the most proximal tongue of salmon-colored mucosa extends 4 cm above the TGF. A diagnosis of BE requires documentation of salmon-colored columnar epithelium extending into the tubular esophagus and histologic confirmation of specialized (Barrett's) intestinal metaplasia.

Care should be taken to avoid labeling patients in whom biopsies from an "irregular Z-line" or gastroesophageal junction show intestinal metaplasia as having Barrett's esophagus. Some of these patients have gastric intestinal metaplasia or "junctional" metaplasia, rather than BE. Intestinal metaplasia of the Z-line, without dysplasia, is not known to carry sufficient cancer risk, and the ASGE/ACG

Task Force on Quality in Endoscopy advocates against routine surveillance unless actual Barrett's esophagus is demonstrated via careful documentation of landmarks [3, 36].

While the optimal frequency with which biopsy specimens should be obtained in cases of suspected BE has not been fully defined, four-quadrant biopsies every one to two centimeters throughout the length of the BE segment are currently recommended [3, 37]. The most recent ACG guidelines suggest that in patients with suspected BE, at least eight random biopsies be obtained to maximize the yield on histology. For patients with a short segment of BE (under three centimeters), in whom eight biopsies are unattainable, at least four biopsies per centimeter of circumferential BE, and one biopsy per centimeter in tongues of BE, should be taken [38]. In a recent study, the average time an endoscopist spends inspecting BE (the Barrett's inspection time, or BIT) correlates directly with the detection of concerning lesions. Patients who underwent endoscopies with longer BITs were significantly more likely to have endoscopically suspicious lesions than patients in whom BITs were shorter, and were more likely to receive a diagnosis of high-grade dysplasia or BE carcinoma. If confirmed by subsequent studies, BIT could conceivably be incorporated into future guidelines on quality examination for patients with BE [39].

Fig. 14.6 Proximal extent of BE as seen using white light (**a**) and electronic chromoendoscopy (**b**)

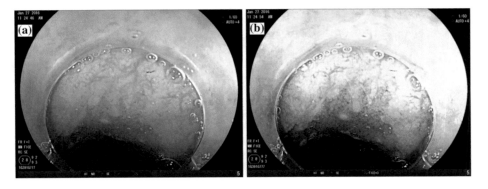

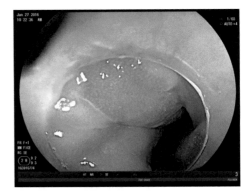

Fig. 14.7 A transparent cap can be fitted to the endoscope to aid visualization of Barrett's esophagus

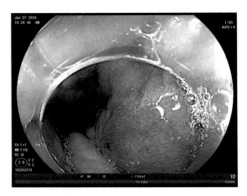

Fig. 14.8 Subtle nodular area detected in patient with Barrett's esophagus using electronic chromoendoscopy and a transparent cap. Endoscopic mucosal resection specimen of this area demonstrated high-grade dysplasia

The use of electronic chromoendoscopy can also aid in the diagnosis and surveillance of BE (see Fig. 14.6) [38]. The use of a transparent cap on the tip of the endoscope can facilitate inspection of BE segments (see Figs. 14.7 and 14.8), particularly in patients with significant tortuosity, angulation, or esophageal motility. Still, the use of a transparent cap is not widely practiced at this time.

QI: Specific Indicators Related to the Endoscopic Management of Peptic Ulcer Disease

The specific quality indicators related to the endoscopic management of peptic ulcer disease can be divided into the management of non-bleeding gastric ulcers and the management of gastric ulcers associated with bleeding. In patients with non-bleeding gastric ulcers, obtaining adequate and appropriate biopsy specimens from gastric tissue is paramount for the histological evaluation of underlying malignancy. While the optimal number and type of biopsy specimens has not been defined, it is worth noting that while single biopsy specimens may not detect malignancy in up to 30% of patients with gastric cancer, four or more biopsy specimens can detect over 95% of patients with gastric cancer [3, 40].

In upper endoscopy revealing peptic ulcer disease, at least one of the following ulcer stigmata should be noted: active bleeding, a non-bleeding visible vessel (pigmented protuberance), an adherent clot, the presence of a flat spot, or an ulcer with a clean base. These stigmata provide prognostic information on rebleeding rates and need for subsequent intervention. They help determine management strategies including the need for endoscopic therapy and the level of patient monitoring required after the endoscopic procedure (e.g., ICU, hospital ward and outpatient management). Endoscopic hemostasis should be performed in patients with spurting ulcers, oozing ulcers, and with non-bleeding visible vessels. The ASGE/ACG Task force identifies the frequency with which, barring any contraindications, endoscopic therapy is delivered for ulcers with active bleeding or with non-bleeding visible vessels as a priority quality indicator with a goal performance target over 98% [3]. In patients with ulcers and an overlying adherent clot, attempts to dislodge the clot may allow identification of underlying stigmata of hemorrhage that can be treated. If attempts at dislodgement are unsuccessful, the lesions can still be considered for endoscopic therapy.

Patients with bleeding peptic ulcer disease treated endoscopically should generally not be treated with epinephrine injection as monotherapy. When epinephrine injection is used, combination with a second treatment modality (thermal or mechanical therapy) provides superior results. Commonly used second modalities include heater probe thermal coagulation, multipolar coagulation, argon plasma coagulation, and endoscopic clipping. The effect of such treatments should be clearly documented in the endoscopy report [3, 41].

QI: Specific Indicators Related to the Endoscopic Management of Upper GI Bleeding

In the evaluation of any patient with upper GI bleeding, one of the first tasks the endoscopist is faced with is to locate and define the location of the bleeding lesion. Localization is often possible after a careful examination, but in cases with residual blood or continued bleeding impairing visualization, the cause of bleeding may not be identified. In these instances, a promotility agent (e.g., intravenous erythromycin) or attempts to reposition the patient may be helpful. Once the bleeding site is located, it's precise location and a description of the lesion should be detailed in the endoscopy report, such that a subsequent endoscopist (or interventional radiologist or surgeon) can locate the site if necessary [3, 42].

A second intra-procedural quality indicator regarding the endoscopic management of upper GI bleeding that was defined by the ASGE/ACG Task force is the frequency with which achievement of primary hemostasis of upper GI bleeding lesions is obtained [3]. The third intra-procedural, upper GI bleeding-related quality indicator provided by the task force states that variceal ligation should be the first endoscopic modality applied to patients with bleeding from esophageal varices. The use of octreotide has been discussed above and is a vital adjunct therapy in patients with acute variceal bleeding. Definitive therapy, however, is generally delivered endoscopically; variceal band ligation is preferred over sclerotherapy because of its greater safety and efficacy profile [43]. The task force recommends a performance target over 98% for the frequency with which variceal ligation is used as the first endoscopic treatment modality for esophageal varices [3].

QI: Specific Indicators Related to Endoscopy in Patients with Suspected Celiac Disease

In patients with suspected celiac disease, duodenal biopsies are instrumental in ascertaining the diagnosis and can be used to guide response to therapy in those with known celiac disease.

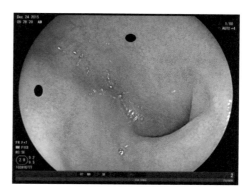

Fig. 14.9 Endoscopic view of the duodenal bulb. Black oval markers correspond to the 9 o'clock and 12 o'clock positions where bulbar biopsies can be obtained in the evaluation of celiac disease

Because of the potentially patchy nature of the disease, patients undergoing upper endoscopy with suspicion of celiac disease should have multiple biopsy specimens obtained from the duodenum. The AGA currently recommends at least one or two biopsies be obtained from the duodenal bulb (see Fig. 14.9) and at least four biopsies of the more distal duodenum [3, 44].

Post-procedure Quality Indicators

The ASGE/ACG Task force defines the post-procedure period as the interval between when the endoscope is removed from the patient to subsequent follow-up and includes activities such as communication with the patient and referring physician, providing the patient instructions, procedure documentation, recognition and documentation of adverse events, and pathology follow-up. Post-procedure quality indicators defined by the task force which are specific to upper endoscopy involve initiation of appropriate medications based on findings at upper endoscopy, making plans for subsequent testing based on findings at upper endoscopy or the patient's course after upper endoscopy, and the documentation of adverse events following upper endoscopy [3].

Various medications may need to be initiated based on findings at upper endoscopy. The task force currently recommends performance targets exceeding 98% for recommending PPI therapy in patients who undergo dilation for peptic esophageal strictures. They also recognize the frequency with which plans to test for Helicobacter pylori infection for patients diagnosed with gastric or duodenal ulcers are documented as a priority quality indicator with a goal performance target over 98% [3].

Finally, while endoscopic therapy delivered during the index upper endoscopy is often adequate, there are instances whereby rebleeding occurs. Selective repeat upper endoscopy for recurrent bleeding is effective and is supported by the quality in upper endoscopy task force. However, routine repeat or "second-look" endoscopy is not advocated [3, 45].

Conclusion

We are currently living in the era of quality in medicine, and endoscopy is no exception. Quality indicators for upper endoscopy have been carefully crafted and exist to provide a guide for best practices. Fellows and practicing endoscopists should be familiar with the quality indicators for upper GI endoscopy and incorporate them into their daily practice.

References

1. Peery AF, Dellon ES, Lund J, et al. Burden of gastrointestinal disease in the United States: 2012 update. Gastroenterology. 2012;143(1179–87):e1–3.
2. Lohr KN, editor. Medicare: a strategy for quality assurance. Washington, DC: National Academy Press; 1990.
3. Park WG, Shaheen NJ, Cohen J, et al. Quality indicators for EGD. Gastrointest Endosc. 2015;81:17–30.
4. Chassin MR, Galvin RW. The urgent need to improve health care quality. Institute of Medicine National Roundtable on Health Care Quality. JAMA. 1998;280:1000–5.
5. Petersen BT. Quality assurance for endoscopists. Best Pract Res Clin Gastroenterol. 2011;25:349–60.
6. Rizk MK, Sawhney MS, Cohen J, et al. Quality indicators common to all GI endoscopic procedures. Gastrointest Endosc. 2015;81:3–16.
7. Rex DK, Schoenfeld PS, Cohen J, et al. Quality indicators for colonoscopy. Gastrointest Endosc. 2015;81:31–53.
8. Adler DG, Lieb II JG, Cohen J, et al. Quality indicators for ERCP. Gastrointest Endosc. 2015; 81:54–66.
9. Wani S, Wallace MB, Cohen J, et al. Quality indicators for EUS. Gastrointest Endosc. 2015;81:67–80.
10. ASGE Standards of Practice Committee. Appropriate use of gastrointestinal endoscopy. American Society for Gastrointestinal Endoscopy. Gastrointest Endosc. 2000;52:831–7.
11. ASGE Standards of Practice Committee; Early DS, Ben-Menachem T, Decker GA, et al. Appropriate use of GI endoscopy. Gastrointest Endosc. 2012;75:1127–31.
12. Early DS, Ben-Menachem T, Decker GA, Evans JA, Fanelli RD, Fisher DA, et al. ASGE. Standards of practice committee. Appropriate use of GI endoscopy. Gastrointest Endosc. 2012;75:1127–31.
13. Morini S, Hassan C, Meucci G, et al. Diagnostic yield of open access colonoscopy according to appropriateness. Gastrointest Endosc. 2001;54:175–9.
14. Froehlich F, Repond C, Mullhaupt B, et al. Is the diagnostic yield of upper GI endoscopy improved by the use of explicit panel-based appropriateness criteria? Gastrointest Endosc. 2000;52:333–41.
15. Eisen GM, Baron TH, Dominitz JA, et al. Methods of granting hospital privileges to perform gastrointestinal endoscopy. Gastrointest Endosc. 2002;55:780–3.
16. Wexner SD, Litwin D, Cohen J, et al. Principles of privileging and credentialing for endoscopy and colonoscopy. Gastrointest Endosc. 2002;55:145–8.
17. ASGE Standards of Practice Committee. ASGE quality indicators for clinical application. Methods of privileging for new technology in gastrointestinal endoscopy. American Society for Gastrointestinal Endoscopy. Gastrointest Endosc. 1999;50:899–900.
18. American Society for Gastrointestinal Endoscopy. Guideline: informed consent for gastrointestinal endoscopy. Gastrointest Endosc. 1988;34(Suppl):26S–7S.
19. Standards of Practice Committee; Zuckerman MJ, Shen B, Harrison ME III, et al. Informed consent for GI endoscopy. Gastrointest Endosc. 2007;66:213–8.
20. Pape T. Legal and ethical considerations of informed consent. AORN J. 1997;65:1122–7.
21. Practice guidelines for sedation and analgesia by non-anesthesiologists. Anesthesiology. 2002;96:1004–17.
22. Enestvedt BK, Eisen GM, Holub J, et al. Is the American Society of Anesthesiologists classification useful in risk stratification for endoscopic procedures? Gastrointest Endosc. 2013;77:464–71.
23. Acosta RD, Abraham NS, Chandrasekhara V, et al. The management of antithrombotic agents for patients undergoing GI endoscopy. Gastrointest Endosc;83:3–16.
24. Lipp A, Lusardi G. Systemic antimicrobial prophylaxis for percutaneous endoscopic gastrostomy. Cochrane Database Syst Rev. 2006:CD005571.
25. Jain NK, Larson DE, Schroeder KW, et al. Antibiotic prophylaxis for percutaneous endoscopic gastrostomy: a prospective, randomized, double-blind clinical trial. Ann Intern Med. 1987;107:824–8.
26. Thomas S, Cantrill S, Waghorn DJ, et al. The role of screening and antibiotic prophylaxis in the prevention of percutaneous gastrostomy site infection caused by methicillin-resistant *Staphylococcus aureus*. Aliment Pharmacol Ther. 2007;25:593–7.
27. Chavez-Tapia NC, Barrientos-Gutierrez T, Tellez-Avila FI, et al. Antibiotic prophylaxis for cirrhotic patients with upper gastrointestinal bleeding. Cochrane Database Syst Rev. 2010:CD002907.
28. Garcia-Tsao G, Sanyal AJ, Grace ND, et al. Prevention and management of gastroesophageal varices and variceal hemorrhage in cirrhosis. Hepatology. 2007;46:922–38.
29. Fernandez J, Ruiz del Arbol L, Gomez C, et al. Norfloxacin vs ceftriaxone in the prophylaxis of infections in patients with advanced cirrhosis and hemorrhage. Gastroenterology. 2006;131:1049–56; quiz 1285.
30. Sreedharan A, Martin J, Leontiadis GI, et al. Proton pump inhibitor treatment initiated prior to endoscopic diagnosis in upper gastrointestinal bleeding. Cochrane Database Syst Rev. 2010: CD005415.
31. American Society of Anesthesiologists Task Force on Sedation, Analgesia by Non-Anesthesiologists. Practice guidelines for sedation and analgesia by non-anesthesiologists. Anesthesiology. 2002;96:1004–17.
32. Standards of Practice Committee; Lichtenstein DR, Jagannath S, Baron TH, et al. Sedation and anesthesia in GI endoscopy. Gastrointest Endosc. 2008;68:205–16.
33. ASGE Ensuring Safety in the Gastrointestinal Endoscopy Unit Task Force; Calderwood AH, Chapman FJ, Cohen J, et al. Quality indicators for safety in the gastrointestinal endoscopy unit. Gastrointest Endosc. 2014;79:363–72.
34. Jeon J, Luebeck EG, Moolgavkar SH. Age effects and temporal trends in adenocarcinoma of the esophagus and gastric cardia (United States). Cancer Causes Control. 2006;17:971–81.
35. Sharma P, Dent J, Armstrong D, et al. The development and validation of an endoscopic grading system for Barrett's esophagus: The Prague C & M criteria. Gastroenterology. 2006;131:1392–9.
36. Spechler SJ, Zeroogian JM, Antonioli DA, et al. Prevalence of metaplasia at the gastro-oesophageal junction. Lancet. 1994;344:1533–6.

37. Wang KK, Sampliner RE. Practice parameters Committee of the American College of Gastroenterology. Updated guidelines 2008 for the diagnosis, surveillance and therapy of Barrett's esophagus. Am J Gastroenterol. 2008;103:788–97.

38. Shaheen NJ, Falk GW, Iyer PG, Gerson LB. ACG clinical guideline: diagnosis and management of Barrett's Esophagus. Am J Gastroenterol. 2015 Nov 3. doi:10.1038/ajg.2015.322. (Epub ahead of print).

39. Gupta N, Gaddam S, Wani SB, et al. Longer inspection time is associated with increased detection of high-grade dysplasia and esophageal adenocarcinoma in Barrett's esophagus. Gastrointest Endosc. 2012;76:531–8.

40. Graham DY, Schwartz JT, Cain GD, et al. Prospective evaluation of biopsy number in the diagnosis of esophageal and gastric carcinoma. Gastroenterology. 1982;82:228–31.

41. Marmo R, Rotondano G, Piscopo R, et al. Dual therapy versus monotherapy in the endoscopic treatment of high-risk bleeding ulcers: a meta-analysis of controlled trials. Am J Gastroenterol. 2007;102:279–89; quiz 469.

42. Laine L, Jensen DM. Management of patients with ulcer bleeding. Am J Gastroenterol. 2012;107:345–60; quiz 361.

43. Villanueva C, Piqueras M, Aracil C, et al. A randomized controlled trial comparing ligation and sclerotherapy as emergency endoscopic treatment added to somatostatin in acute variceal bleeding. J Hepatol. 2006;45:560–7.

44. Rubio-Tapia A, Hill ID, Kelly CP, Calderwood AH, Murray JA. ACG clinical guidelines: diagnosis and management of celiac disease. Am J Gastroenterol. 2013;108(5):656–77.

45. Barkun AN, Bardou M, Kuipers EJ, et al. International consensus recommendations on the management of patients with nonvariceal upper gastrointestinal bleeding. Ann Intern Med. 2010;152:101–13.

Index

© Springer International Publishing AG 2017
D.G. Adler (ed.), *Upper Endoscopy for GI Fellows*,
DOI 10.1007/978-3-319-49041-0

gastric varices, 26
   primary prophylaxis, 26–27
   salvage therapy, 27
   secondary prophylaxis, 27
Video capsule endoscopy (VCE), 152
   and DBE, 154
Video endoscopes, 125
Vitamin K, 12

W
Warfarin, 93
Whipple resection, 86, 90
   fluoroscopic appearance of forward-viewing endoscope after, 86*f*

Z
X-rays (plain radiography), 32
   abdominal, showing coin, 34*f*

Z
Z line, 4
   irregular Z-line, 169
Zargar's mucosal injury classification, 134, 134*t*